HUMAN PSYCHOPHARMACOLOGY

Volume 4

HUMAN PSYCHOPHARMACOLOGY
Measures and Methods

Volume 1

Edited by I. Hindmarch and P. D. Stonier

CONTENTS

ISBN 0 471 91238 7

HUMAN PSYCHOPHARMACOLOGY
Measures and Methods
Volume 2

Edited by I. Hindmarch and P. D. Stonier

CONTENTS

ISBN 0 471 91255 7

HUMAN PSYCHOPHARMACOLOGY
Measures and Methods

Volume 3

Edited by I. Hindmarch and P. D. Stonier

CONTENTS

ISBN 0 471 92743 0

HUMAN PSYCHOPHARMACOLOGY
Measures and Methods

Volume 4

Edited by

I. Hindmarch

*Human Psychopharmacology Research Unit, Milford Hospital,
University of Surrey, UK*

and

P. D. Stonier

*Medical Department, Hoechst UK Ltd,
Middlesex, UK*

JOHN WILEY & SONS
Chichester · New York · Brisbane · Toronto · Singapore

Other Wiley Editorial Offices

John Wiley & Sons, Inc., 605 Third Avenue,
New York, NY 10158–0012, USA

Jacaranda Wiley Ltd, G.P.O. Box 859, Brisbane,
Queensland 4001, Australia

John Wiley & Sons (Canada) Ltd, 22 Worcester Road,
Rexdale, Ontario M9W 1L1, Canada

John Wiley & Sons (SEA) Pte Ltd, 27 Jalan Pemimpin #05–04,
Block B, Union Industrial Building, Singapore 2057

Library of Congress Cataloging-in-Publication Data
(Revised for vol. 4)
Human psychopharmacology.
  Includes bibliographical references and indexes.
  1. Psychopharmacology. 2. Psychotropic
  drugs—Physiological effect. I. Hindmarch,
  I. (Ian), 1944–   II. Stonier, P. D.
  III. Series. [DNLM: 1. Behavior—drug effects.
  2. Psychopharmacology. QV 77 H918]
  RM315.H85   1987   615'.78   86–19125
  ISBN 0 471 91238 7 (v. 1)

British Library Cataloguing in Publication Data
Human psychopharmacology.
  Vol. 4
1. Psychopharmacology
I. Hindmarch, I. (Ian)   II. Stonier, P. D.
615.78

ISBN 0 471 93411 9

Typeset by Inforum, Rowlands Castle, Hants
Printed and bound in Great Britain by Biddles Ltd, Guildford and King's Lynn

Contents

List of Contributors

H. ALLAIN
Laboratoire de Pharmacologie Clinique, Faculté de Médecine, Avenue du Professeur Léon Bernard, 35043 Rennes Cédex, France

T. A. BAN
Department of Psychiatry, School of Medicine, Vanderbilt University, Nashville, Tennessee, TN 37215, USA

K. L. DAVIS
Department of Psychiatry, Mount Sinai Medical Center, New York, NY 10029-6574, USA

K. DENICOFF
NIMH, Building 10, Room 3N212, 9000 Rockville Pike, Bethesda, MD 20892, USA

H. ERZIGKEIT
Psychiatry Department, University of Erlangen–Nuremberg, Schwabach-anlage 6, D-8520 Erlangen, Germany

D. B. FAIRWEATHER
Human Psychopharmacology Research Unit, University of Surrey, Milford Hospital, Godalming, Surrey GU7 1UF, UK

O. K. FJETLAND
Department of Psychiatry, School of Medicine, Vanderbilt University, Nashville, Tennessee, TN 37215, USA

J.-M. GANDON
BIOTRIAL S.A. Drug Evaluation and Pharmacology Research, Technopole Atalante–Villejean, Rue du Professeur Jean Pecker, 35000 Rennes, France

M. S. GEORGE
NIMH, Building 10, Room 3N212, 9000 Rockville Pike, Bethesda, MD 20892, USA

C. R. GREEN
Department of Psychiatry, Mount Sinai Medical Center, New York, NY 10029-6574, USA

J. S. KERR
Human Psychopharmacology Research Unit, University of Surrey, Milford Hospital, Godalming, Surrey GU7 1UF, UK

T. A. KETTER
NIMH, Building 10, Room 3N212, 9000 Rockville Pike, Bethesda, MD 20892, USA

D. J. KING
Department of Therapeutics and Pharmacology, The Queen's University of Belfast, Whitla Medical Building, 97 Lisburn Road, Belfast BT9 7BL, UK

CH. KUSCHEL
Institut für Fahrzeugtechnik, Technische Universität Berlin, Gustav-Meyer-Allee 25, 1000 Berlin 65, Germany

M. KUTCHER
Department of Psychiatry, School of Medicine, Vanderbilt University, Nashville, Tennessee, TN 37215, USA

H. LEHFELD
Psychiatry Department, University of Erlangen–Nuremberg, Schwabach-anlage 6, D-8520 Erlangen, Germany

G. S. LEVERICH
NIMH, Building 10, Room 3N212, 9000 Rockville Pike, Bethesda, MD 20892, USA

A. LIEURY
Laboratoire de Psychologie Expérimentale, Université de Rennes II, 6 Avenue Gaston Berger, 35043 Rennes Cédex, France

M. E. MATTILA
Department of Pharmacology and Toxicology, University of Helsinki, Siltavuorenpenger 10, SF-0014 Helsinki, Finland

M. J. MATTILA
Department of Pharmacology and Toxicology, University of Helsinki, Siltavuorenpenger 10, SF-0014 Helsinki, Finland

K. MIKALAUSKAS
NIMH, Building 10, Room 3N212, 9000 Rockville Pike, Bethesda, MD 20892, USA

L. C. MOREY
Department of Psychology, Vanderbilt University, Nashville, Tennessee, TN 37215, USA

E. NUOTTO
National Medicines Control Laboratory, University of Helsinki, Siltavuorenpenger 10, SF-00170, Helsinki, Finland

H. OTT
Laboratorium Pharmakopsychologie, Schering AG, Berlin, Germany

R. M. POST
NIMH, Building 10, Room 3N212, 9000 Rockville Pike, Bethesda, MD 20892, USA

P. J. ROGERS
Consumer Sciences Department, AFRC Institute of Food Research, Reading Laboratory, Earley Gate, Whiteknights Road, Reading, RG6 2EF, UK

N. ROMBAUT
Quintiles UK Ltd, 56 Minster Street, Reading, Berkshire, UK

O. SCHULTHEIß
Psychiatry Department, University of Erlangen–Nuremberg, Schwabach-anlage 6, D-8520 Erlangen, Germany

N. SHERWOOD
Human Psychopharmacology Research Unit, University of Surrey, Milford Hospital, Godalming GU7 1UF, Surrey, UK

H.-P. WILLUMEIT
Institut für Fahrzeugtechnik, Technische Universität Berlin, Gustav-Meyer-Allee 25, 1000 Berlin 65, Germany

Preface

As in our earlier prefaces we begin by pointing out that these volumes are collations representing the activities and interests of practising psychopharmacologists and, except within this broad context of measures and methods, there is no theme to link the chapters or the volumes.

However, the contributors to this and previous volumes reflect the contemporary interests of clinicians, psychologists, pharmacologists, psychometricians and engineers, as well as the diversity of this ubiquitous speciality in the measurement of effects of drugs on human behaviour in health and disease. This volume in particular falls into the component parts of the subtitle of this series.

Drs Sherwood and Kerr begin with an investigation of reliability, validity and pharmacosensitivity of some psychometric tests based on information processing. Theirs is a timely reminder of the need to use only valid and reliable tests which are known to be sensitive to the types of drugs under investigation. Failure to appreciate this essential prerequisite of psychopharmacological investigations in man increases the risk of false positive results.

Professor Willumeit and his collaborators extend the objective measures of performance into the applied world of car driving. They show that laboratory measures of reaction time are useful to demonstrate the effects of psychoactive drugs, but they also warn that the perceived face validity of on-the-road tests is not reflected in their reliability or relevance to traffic safety.

Validation of psychometric measures is an acute problem when dealing with the measurement and definition of multidimensional disorders, and this is the concern of *Professor Erzigkeit and colleagues* in presenting their suggestions for measuring dementia and for assessing the effects of therapeutic intervention.

Of course, the psychometry of drug-induced change relies on providing firm baselines. This is particularly important in Alzheimer-type dementia and

Dr Green and Professor Davis demonstrate the basic clinical aspects of the diagnosis of this condition, and provide a patient protocol which emphasizes the necessary rigour to make a robust clinical assessment of dementia.

The differential diagnosis of psychological illness has never been easy due to overlapping aetiological factors and the co-morbidity of the presenting syndromes. *Professor Ban and his co-workers* describe the development of their polydiagnostic method for depressive disorders. They conclude that such diagnostic schemes are an essential component of multi-centre clinical investigations where patient populations are heterogeneous.

Appropriate methods allow the measurement of the efficacy and side-effects of medicines prescribed in the community, and this provides an extrapolation into the real world from laboratory measures and clinical trials. At the same time such methods facilitate the assessment of benefit and risk attendant on the use of a medicine. *Drs Fairweather and Rombaut* describe a novel method for a retrospective assessment of the effects of changes in prescribing on this benefit–risk assessment: in this case brought about by regulatory intervention.

Dr George, at almost the other end of the spectrum, describes the application of the new technologies for imaging brain structure and function in understanding psychopharmacological aspects of the neuroanatomy of obsessive-compulsive disorder.

As with dementia and depression, *Dr Rogers* shows that before we can truly evaluate the impact of therapeutic intervention on eating disorder, it is necessary to have a parsimonious and objective set of techniques and a method for measuring human eating behaviour *per se*.

Professor Allain and his colleagues illustrate how it is possible to quantify and evaluate the complex changes brought about in human memory following the administration of psychotropics. The same rigour that helps unravel some aspects of human mnestic function can be used to investigate the interactions between psychotropic agents on human skilled performance, as is well illustrated by *Professor Mattila and colleagues'* contribution.

In order to understand the intrinsic psychopharmacological effect of a psychotropic agent, one needs necessarily to use healthy volunteers, if for nothing more than the fact that the clinical state of the patient can greatly confound the interpretation of drug effects, this being particularly the case in schizophrenia. *Dr King* recognizes the importance of discovering the pharmacodynamic effects of neuroleptics intrinsic to the molecules themselves.

In the final analysis there is always a need to have appropriate methods and measures for assessing the effects of psychoactive drugs in patient populations. Often the variables are complex and seemingly too numerous to control. However, as is well illustrated by *Professor Post and his team*, even the most impenetrable combinations of drugs and changing neuropsychiatric status can be amenable to assessment, so long as appropriate strategies are employed.

Since the appearance of the first volume six years ago, human psychopharmacology has developed apace. The growth in the number of conferences, books and journals devoted to the specialty is almost exponential. Nevertheless, the underlying principles remain unchanged in that psychopharmacologists accept that the effects of psychotropic drugs can be measured by the changes they produce in behaviour. It remains the task of psychopharmacologists to develop valid and reliable psychometrics by which such drug-induced changes can be measured.

I. HINDMARCH
P. D. STONIER
Surrey 1993

1

The Reliability, Validity and Pharmacosensitivity of Four Psychomotor Tests

Neil Sherwood and John S. Kerr

Human Psychopharmacology Research Unit, University of Surrey, Milford Hospital, Godalming, UK

Introduction

The psychopharmacological approach to the assessment of psychoactive compounds has been to assume that psychological effects can be judged in behavioural terms. However, it is not sufficient simply to create *ad hoc* behavioural tests, administer psychotropics and record responses. Thorough psychometric assessment requires that a test system be created and used with due regard to established theoretical and methodological standards and provide information pertinent to questions of psychological health, behavioural toxicity and the quality of life.

A review by Hindmarch (1980) found that many of the tests used in psychopharmacology lacked a history of reliability and validity and were unlikely to provide useful data. These sentiments have recently been echoed in a series of articles by Parrott (1991a, 1991b, 1991c), who showed that little has changed in the past decade. Evidence to establish that important aspects of psychological function are measured in a stable and replicable manner is central to the utility of a psychometric test. In addition, it is essential that a test be sufficiently sensitive to the very subtle psychological changes brought about after the administration of a psychotropic.

Even if an appropriate selection of tests can be made, a complete understanding of the psychopharmacological profile of a drug further requires a careful consideration of investigative methods, since the choice of

Human Psychopharmacology, Vol. 4. Edited by I. Hindmarch and P. D. Stonier
© 1993 John Wiley & Sons Ltd

experimental variables determines the occurrence and extent of any effects which may be found. Controlled studies are essential to ensure that the influence of nuisance variables is kept to a minimum.

Research at the Human Psychopharmacology Research Unit (HPRU) has centred around the use of a preferred test battery in double-blind, placebo-controlled, repeated-measures experimental designs. To date, this approach has been used to profile over 200 different psychoactive compounds in both healthy volunteers and clinical populations.

The present chapter discusses the reliability, validity and pharmacosensitivity of the four most utilized tests from the HPRU battery (critical flicker fusion, choice reaction time, compensatory tracking and short-term memory scanning) and their capacity to differentiate both between and within various psychoactive groups. After a brief discussion of theoretical context, each of these tests is reviewed and information presented on their reliability, validity and pharmacosensitivity. Finally, the use of standardized measures and methods makes it possible to compare and contrast the psychopharmacological profiles of many different compounds on common theoretical constructs such as short-term memory and central nervous system (CNS) arousal. This is achieved through a comparison of the results of individual studies using an effect size analysis.

A Model of Cognition

To be relevant to our understanding of the actions of a drug on the CNS, psychopharmacological effects need to be considered in the context of a well-defined theoretical model of psychological processes and their relationship to overt behaviour. Cognitive psychology has developed descriptions of mental activity based upon empirical study. Common among these has been the suggestion that humans act as information processors, transforming data in a manner beneficial to their immediate or future needs by way of information-processing operations and strategies (Broadbent, 1971). The range of theoretical models onto which these processes have been mapped varies in their complexity and remit, but most make allowance for mechanisms of attention (the selection of information), cognition (the manipulation and processing of information), memory and behavioural response. To be sufficient, a model should include at least these processes.

Figure 1 presents a simple model of information processing adapted from Hindmarch (1980). The model isolates the major processes as separate mechanisms within a linear system. Information from the environment is attended to and passed to higher cognitive mechanisms, where it is analysed and, if required, integrated with information from memory. A decision concerning appropriate response is then reached and an order passes to the response output mechanisms.

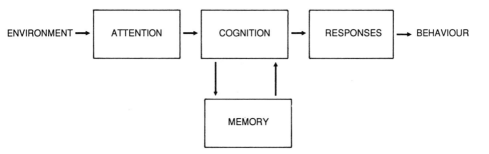

Figure 1. An information-processing model of cognition

The model serves three functions. First, it assists in the understanding of behaviour, which may be seen as the end result of a flow of information through the model, utilizing en route processes needed for appropriate responses. As such, overt behaviour becomes associated with a component set of information-processing operations. Second, these processing operations can then be targeted for investigation by a careful selection of appropriate tests which utilize particular aspects of behaviour. Third, the model provides a base upon which to map possible experimental effects.

Consequently the choice of psychomotor test is central to the understanding of any effects which are found. Thorough psychopharmacological assessment requires a range of tests to ensure that subtle or specific drug effects are not overlooked. The clear need is for chosen tasks to be representative of key, well-defined and accepted areas of cognition and psychomotor performance. Additionally such tests should be valid, reliable and have shown themselves to be sensitive to psychoactive compounds.

Critical Flicker Fusion Threshold (CFF)

CFF is one of the most widely used assessments in human psychopharmacological research, and is regarded as an index of overall CNS activity. Within the chosen model of information processing, an increase in CFF is associated with more efficient processing of discrete 'bits' of information (Hindmarch, 1982). A convenient analogy for CFF is the processing speed at which a computer operates.

The perception of flicker is believed to relate to a cortical process involved in the detection of movement (Simonson and Brozek, 1952). The use of this aspect of information processing as a preferred measure of CNS arousal has arisen almost by accident from the basic psychophysical measurements of flicker fusion made in the nineteenth century by Talbot (1834) and others.

CFF techniques in psychopharmacology have been reviewed extensively by Smith and Misiak (1976) and Hindmarch (1982). The advantages of the measure include the simple, non-invasive nature of the test, the short duration of the assessment and an absence of major practice effects. However, caution must always be exercised in interpreting the results of CFF measurements, in that thresholds are not specifically related to any one phenomenon. Rather, CFF is a function of the input parameters which, apart from the drug under investigation, may include (among others) age, sex, personality, circadian activity, and stage in menstrual cycle (Curran, 1990). Criticism of CFF techniques (Ott and Kranda, 1982) has often been aimed at the lack of control over these confounding factors.

CFF Apparatus

All CFF measurements are made using the Leeds Psychomotor Tester (LPT)—a stand-alone purpose-built instrument in CFF mode.*

CFF Procedure

Subjects are required to discriminate flicker from fusion, and vice versa, in a set of four red light-emitting diodes set at the corners of a 1 cm square in the centre of a 30 cm (height) × 40 cm (width) black background. Subjects sit at a 75 cm high table and the diodes are viewed binocularly in foveal fixation at 1 m in direct line of sight. The diodes flicker on and off at a 50/50 light–dark ratio according to a square waveform, and at a constantly increasing or decreasing rate of 1 Hz/s over a range of 12–50 Hz. Subject responses are obtained via a button held in the preferred hand. Individual thresholds are determined by the psychophysical method of limits as an average of responses on three ascending (flicker to fusion) and three descending (fusion to flicker) interspersed presentations (Woodworth and Schlosberg, 1958).

CFF Reliability

The assessment of CFF thresholds by the method of limits results in a high test–retest reliability, estimated at between $r = +0.85$ and $r = +0.90$ (Levander, 1982). CFF has similarly been shown to be internally consistent. Parrot (1982) gave split half reliability estimates of between $r = +0.92$ and $r = +0.97$ from a meta-analysis of 101 subjects in five HPRU studies.

CFF Validity

CFF has been shown to correlate highly with other non-performance measures of CNS arousal, including line analogue rating scales (Parrott, 1982) and the electroencephalogram (EEG) (Gortlemeyer and Weiman, 1982). Like

---

*Details from HPRU, University of Surrey, Milford Hospital, Godalming, Surrey GU7 1UF, UK.

many other measures which require the subject to attend and respond to a stimulus, CFF can confidently be said to reflect mental alertness. There is evidence of a strong relationship between raised CFF and improved performance on a range of tasks (Bobon *et al.*, 1982), although this may not hold at the extremes: amphetamine significantly raises CFF, but can also lead to inappropriate and uncoordinated behaviour (Parrott and Hindmarch, 1975).

CFF Pharmacosensitivity

CFF has been shown to differentiate clearly known sedating compounds, which lower thresholds, from stimulants which elevate thresholds. Additionally CFF is able to differentiate between drugs in the same therapeutic class such as the anxiolytic benzodiazepines (Hindmarch *et al.*, 1991a) and even different doses of the same drug such as alcohol (Hindmarch *et al.*, 1991b). These results confirm that CFF is pharmacosensitive, and provide further evidence to support suggestions that the measure closely reflects CNS activation.

Choice Reaction Time (CRT)

CRT is used as an indicator of sensorimotor performance, assessing the efficiency of the attentional and response mechanisms in the information-processing chain without the need for extended cognitive processing. The latency of a motor response to a critical stimulus is recorded, but since this stimulus is one of a number of possible alternatives, attentional monitoring abilities are also measured. After the method of Donders (1969), the total reaction time (TRT) is regarded as the sum of two separable components: the stimulus recognition reaction time (RRT) used as a measure of attentional monitoring, and the motor reaction time (MRT) used as a measure of the efficiency of the response output system.

The use of reaction time tasks in psychopharmacology has been extensively discussed in Hindmarch *et al.* (1988). Their widespread use can be attributed to the substantial body of theoretical literature discussing the measurement of reaction time and the simple task requirements which are quickly understood by subjects.

CRF Apparatus

The task is presented using the Leeds Psychomotor Tester (LPT) in CRT mode.*

---

*Details from HPRU, University of Surrey, Milford Hospital, Godalming, Surrey GU7 1UF, UK.

CRT Procedure

Subjects sit at a 75 cm high table with the LPT laid flat on the table top immediately to their front, 50 cm away from the subject's eyes so that their preferred hand can move freely over the surface of the equipment.

From a central starting position nearest to them, subjects are required on each trial to extinguish one of six equidistant red light-emitting diodes, illuminated at random, by touching the appropriate contingent response button. These light/button combinations are arranged in a 120° arc (24° between each light/button pair) of a 15 cm radius circle centred on and forward of the start button. The hand is clenched, with only the index finger extended. All buttons are touch sensitive, so there are no switches to engage.

Mean reaction times are obtained from the average of 20 consecutive trials. Both recognition (time taken to spot the light and to remove the finger from its starting position) and motor (time taken to reach the appropriate response button) components of the total reaction time are recorded automatically.

CRT Reliability

The reliability of a variety of choice reaction time tasks has been assessed by Krause and Bittner (1982). Once a performance plateau was reached, test–retest reliability coefficients in excess of $r = +0.58$ were found, and the task was recommended for repeated measure experiments.

CRT Validity

The laws which govern choice reaction are discussed in Teichner and Krebs (1974). Measurements of CRT provide information on the constant, very rapid adjustments individuals must make to their environment, which often require them to attend to several potential stimuli at once. This suggests that there is a high degree of construct validity inherent in reaction time measures.

CRT Pharmacosensitivity

CRT has been used successfully to assess performance changes following the administration of a wide range of substances, from the barbiturates which increase reaction times, through to stimulants like methylphenidate which reduce reaction times (Hindmarch *et al.*, 1990). The measure is also sensitive enough to discriminate between compounds of the same pharmacological class such as (again) the anxiolytic benzodiazepines (Hindmarch *et al.*, 1991).

Compensatory Tracking Task (CTT)

One criticism of the use of simple tests is that they allow the subject to reallocate cognitive resources and focus on the task in hand, masking effects which would be salient if the subject was required to undertake additional tasks. This trade-off of resources can be controlled by using laboratory analogues of skilled performance. Such tasks warrant particular attention because a drug-induced breakdown of a skill can have serious consequences.

Additionally, many psychomotor tests require only discrete responses and may not be sensitive to changes in performance where cognitive mechanisms are in constant use. A compensatory tracking task is used to investigate activities inherent in tasks such as car driving which require skilled motor activity in response to complex visual information.

CTT offers a means to assess the response output mechanisms required for fine motor control, in contrast to the gross motor activity required for CRT. Since attentional mechanisms are heavily utilized during tracking, peripheral responses (which are generally longer than those found under simple reaction time measures) reflect the need for the subject to divide their attention between the tracking and the reaction time task. The need to divide attention between competing stimuli is a requirement in many real-world situations.

CTT Apparatus

The compensatory tracking task is presented on a BBC model B microcomputer and 35 cm CUB monitor using software from the HPRU test battery. Subject tracking responses are made with an isometric (free-moving) joystick operated by the preferred hand. Reaction time measurements are recorded via the computer keyboard space bar. The program is currently being updated for use with PC-compatible systems.

CTT Procedure

Subjects are required to attend to two tasks: keeping a joystick-controlled cursor (an equilateral triangle with 2 cm sides) in line with a target (a similar triangle, inverted) moving along a horizontal axis in a pseudo-random fashion, while simultaneously responding to visual stimuli (filled white circles, 1 cm in diameter) presented at random in corners of the screen. The movement of the target is calculated by the computer as the sum of a number of sine waves. The root mean square (RMS) of the tracking error to four trials, each of 60 seconds duration and the mean reaction time (PRT) to 40 peripheral stimuli (10 per trial) are recorded at each presentation.

CTT Reliability

Kennedy *et al.* (1981) found a test–retest correlation among stabilized trials of $r = +0.78$ for compensatory tracking. The task was recommended for use in repeated-measures experiments.

CTT Validity

Compensatory tracking has a high degree of face validity in that it resembles real-world tasks such as vehicle handling (Hindmarch, 1988) and target pursuit (Kennedy *et al.*, 1981). Hindmarch (1986) reviewed the effects of various psychotropics on CTT against the results of 'on-the-road' tests of vehicle manoeuvring and braking. CTT was found to be as efficient as the on-the-road measures in identifying those drugs which impeded car-driving performance, suggesting a high degree of criterion validity.

CTT Pharmacosensitivity

Hindmarch *et al.* (1983) established the sensitivity of CTT to drug effects, and its ability to distinguish between the antidepressants amytriptyline (which impaired tracking) and zimeldine. The task has since been used to assess several compounds, including hypnotics (Harrison *et al.*, 1985), antidepressants (Alford and Hindmarch, 1990) and alcohol (Hindmarch *et al.*, 1991).

Short-term Memory Scanning (STM)

High-speed scanning and retrieval from short-term memory was assessed using a technique based upon a reaction time method pioneered by Sternberg (1966). The test involves making simple comparisons of a displayed probe digit against a set of stimuli digits held in short-term memory and indicating whether there is or is not a match to the probe in the stimulus set. Typically, subject reaction times increase as the size of the stimulus set grows, suggesting that some internal data comparison takes place before a response is initiated.

When a small stimulus set is used, the memory search task is relatively simple and consequently the final reaction time is dominated by the peripheral processes of perceiving and reacting to the probe. These processes are particularly affected by the level of drug-induced sedation. However, where a larger stimulus set is presented the reaction time contains greater central memory search and retrieval components, and it is possible to estimate specific effects on memory function.

STM Apparatus

The STM task is presented on a BBC model B microcomputer and 35 cm CUB monitor using software from the HPRU test battery. Subject responses are monitored via a hand-held response box which incorporates two response buttons operated by the thumbs. During training, subjects are given the choice of which button to press to signal the 'YES' response, and this is maintained for the remainder of the study. Subjects sat at a 75 cm desk with the computer screen 50 cm in front of them at eye level.

STM Procedure

Subjects are required to memorize a series of one to four digits (the stimulus set) presented sequentially at 1.2 seconds per digit. One second after the final digit an auditory warning signal (750 ms duration) sounds, followed by a series of up to 24 single probe digits. Subjects respond to the probes by pressing the 'YES' button (positive response) if the probe digit is contained in the memorized set, or the 'NO' button (negative response) if it is not. There are an equal number of positive and negative probe digits in each probe set. A new stimulus and probe set are presented at each assessment point.

STM Reliability

Carter *et al.* (1980) evaluated the reliability and stability of memory scanning as a performance measure. When used in a repeated-measures design, mean reaction times to set sizes of between one and four digits were found to be highly reliable performance measures, with test–retest correlation coefficients in excess of $r = +0.70$.

STM Validity

Memory scanning tasks have been used to investigate a range of phenomena, including chemical exposure (Smith and Langolf, 1981), brain damage (Harris and Fleer, 1974), age (Anders *et al.*, 1972) and environmental vibration (Sherwood and Griffin, 1990). The task has a high degree of construct validity in that it relates well to the commonly accepted two-process (short-term and long-term) model of memory proposed by Atkinson and Shriffin (1971).

STM Pharmacosensitivity

The sensitivity of the STM task to the effects of psychoactive compounds was established by Subhan and Hindmarch (1984). They investigated the amnestic effects of several hypnotics using the STM task, and found it able to clearly indicate impairments both 1 and 10 hours after drug administration. A similar finding with the anxiolytic benzodiazepines has recently been identified by Sherwood *et al.* (1992).

A Comparison of Drug Effects

An informative comparison of the results of several independent HPRU studies can be made using an effect size analysis which quantifies the 'strength' of each drug effect as compared to a placebo control as a standardized '*d*' value (Cohen, 1976). These values represent the peak acute responses of healthy volunteers and are derived from representative HPRU studies. The figures offered in Tables 1–4 are based upon individual studies, and it should be noted that the values are effectively samples from a population of possible scores. Unless indicated, all doses are in milligrams (mg).

Table 1. Ranked magnitude of drug effects on critical flicker fusion (CFF) and total choice reaction time (TRT)

Drug (dose)	d CFF	Drug (dose)	d TRT
Sertraline (100)	1.719	Sertraline (100)	0.648
Paroxetine (30)	1.153	Astemizole (10)	0.297
Astemizole (10)	1.052	Paroxetine (30)	0.276
Clobazam (30)	0.694	Nicotine (2)	0.157
Nicotine (2)	0.592	Nomifensine (100)	0.108
Caffeine (400)	0.128	Caffeine (400)	0.012
		Clobazam (30)	0.007
Placebo	0.000		
		Placebo	0.000
Zopiclone (7.5)	0.006		
Nomifensine (100)	0.152	Zopiclone (7.5)	0.017
Mequitazine (5)	0.178	Mequitazine (5)	0.061
Triprolidine (10)	0.367	Triprolidine (10)	0.149
Alcohol (0.5 g/kg)	0.370	Codeine (120)	0.494
Nitrazepam (2.5)	0.408	Morphine (20)	0.862
Codeine (120)	0.940	Nitrazepam (2.5)	1.030
Morphine (20)	1.272	Chlorpheniramine (12)	1.199
Dothiepin (50)	1.279	Alcohol (0.5 g/kg)	1.563
Lorazepam (1)	1.314	Dothiepin (50)	1.601
Chlorpheniramine (12)	1.473	Haloperidol (1)	1.834
Amitriptyline (25)	2.194	Amitriptyline (25)	2.300
Haloperidol (1)	2.326	Lorazepam (1)	2.442
Mianserin (10)	3.205	Mianserin (10)	3.286
Chlorpromazine (50)	6.172	Chlorpromazine (50)	6.172

Table 2. Ranked magnitude of drug effects on recognition reaction time (RRT) and motor reaction time (MRT)

Drug (dose)	d RRT	Drug (dose)	d MRT
Nicotine (2)	0.561	Nicotine (2)	0.853
Astemizole (10)	0.447	Nomifensine (10)	0.103
Mequitazine (15)	0.367	Zopiclone (7.5)	0.101
Nomifensine (100)	0.067	Clobazam (30)	0.040
Mianserin (10)	0.046	Placebo	0.000
Caffeine	0.043		
Sertraline (100)	0.043	Caffeine (400)	0.024
		Triprolidine (10)	0.030
Placebo	0.000	Sertraline (100)	0.032
		Astemizole (10)	0.037
Clobazam (30)	0.025	Mequitazine (5)	0.308
Zopiclone (7.5)	0.070	Nitrazepam (2.5)	0.719
Codeine (120)	0.180	Alcohol (0.5 g/kg)	0.744
Triprolidine (10)	0.310	Mianserin (10)	0.834
Morphine (20)	0.751	Morphine (20)	0.897
Nitrazepam (2.5)	0.791	Codeine (120)	0.949
Alcohol (0.5 g/kg)	0.804	Chlorphen (12)	1.285
Chlorphen (12)	0.827	Lorazepam (1)	1.468
Amitriptyline (25)	1.631	Amitriptyline (25)	1.863
Lorazepam (1)	1.821		

Table 3. Ranked magnitude of drug effects on tracker error (RMS) and tracker peripheral reaction time (PRT)

Drug (dose)	d RMS	Drug (dose)	d PRT
Nicotine (2)	0.884	Caffeine (400)	1.865
Caffeine (400)	0.624	Mequitazine (5)	1.217
Astemizole (10)	0.345	Nicotine (2)	0.467
Nomifensine (100)	0.061	Zopiclone (7.5)	0.134
Clobazam (30)	0.035	Nomifensine (100)	0.109
Placebo	0.000	Placebo	0.000
Sertraline (100)	0.012	Sertraline (100)	0.044
Paroxetine (50)	0.014	Astemizole (10)	0.081
Mequitazine (5)	0.043	Clobazam (30)	0.086
Zopiclone (7.5)	0.199	Alcohol (0.5 g/kg)	0.158
Alcohol (0.5 g/kg)	0.457	Paroxetine (30)	0.431
Chlorphen (12)	0.636	Chlorphen (12)	0.829
Dotheipin (50)	0.831	Mianserin (10)	1.103
Amitriptyline (25)	1.863	Dothiepin (50)	1.358
Lorazepam (1)	1.879	Amitriptyline (25)	1.631
Mianserin (10)	1.929	Lorazepam (1)	2.266

Table 4. Ranked magnitude of drug effects on short-term memory scanning (STM)

Drug (dose)	d STM
Nicotine (2)	0.158
Caffeine (400)	0.158
Nomifensine (100)	0.001
Placebo	0.000
Zopiclone (7.5)	0.020
Clobazam (30)	0.066
Sertraline (100)	0.098
Mianserin (10)	0.359
Amitriptyline (25)	0.655
Lorazepam (1)	1.256
Alcohol (0.5 g/kg)	1.766
Nitrazepam (2.5)	6.145

From this analysis it is clear that a large number of psychoactive compounds are behaviourally toxic in that they impair the performance of information-processing operations necessary for everyday psychomotor performance. This in part reflects the non-specific sedating effects of many compounds, but the differences in the magnitude of the effects for the same compound on different measures suggest that specific actions are also at work, i.e. the minor effect of nitrazepam on CFF compared to a much larger effect on STM. At the same time, compounds such as nicotine and caffeine demonstrate a favourable profile in that they show small positive effects on most dependent measures. Of particular interest is the large differences in the profile of those drugs of the same therapeutic class, i.e. the antidepressants paroxetine and dothiepin, or the anxiolytics lorazepam and clobazam.

These results confirm that the tests possess a wide response range, able to gauge either improvement or impairment with no evidence of an absolute 'ceiling' or 'floor' effect.

Summary

The use of a battery of psychomotor tests drawn from an acceptable model of cognition ensures that the effects of psychoactive compounds on overt behaviour can be understood in terms of their influence on aspects of psychological function. By combining these tests with a double-blind, repeated-measures, placebo-controlled methodology the effects of a range of psychoactive compounds on human psychomotor performance can be reliably identified and validly measured.

References

Alford, C., and Hindmarch, I. (1990). Measuring the effects of psychoactive drugs with particular reference to antidepressants. In: West, R., Christie, M., and Weinman, J. (eds), *Microcomputers, Psychology and Medicine,* Chichester: Wiley, pp. 85–95.

Anders, T.R., Fozard, J.L., and Lillyquist, T.D. (1972). Effects of age upon retrieval from short-term memory. *Dev. Psychol., 6,* 214–17.

Atkinson, R.C., and Shriffin, R.M. (1971). Recognition and retrieval processes in free recall. *Psychol. Rev., 79,* 97–123.

Bobon, D.P., Lecoq, A., Von Frenckell, R., Mormont, I., Laverque, G., and Lottin, T. (1982). La frequence critique de fusion visuelle en psychopathologie et en psychopharmacologie. *Acta Med. Belge, 82,* 1–112.

Broadbent, D.E. (1971). *Decision and Stress.* London: Academic Press.

Carter, R.C., Kennedy, R.S., Bittner, A.C., and Krause, M. (1980). Item recognition as a performance evaluation test for environmental research. In: *Proceedings of the Human Factors Society 24th Annual Meeting,* Santa Monica: Human Factors Society.

Cohen, J. (1976). *Statistical power analysis for the behavioral sciences.* New York: Academic.

Curran, S. (1990). Critical flicker fusion techniques in psychopharmacology. In: Hindmarch, I., and Stonier, P.D. (eds), *Human Psychopharmacology: Measures and Methods,* Vol. 3, Chichester: Wiley, pp. 21–38.

Donders, F.C. (1969). On the speed of mental processes (translated by W.G. Koster). *Acta Psychol., 30,* 412–31.

Gortlemeyer, R., and Wieman, H. (1982). Retest reliability and construct validity of critical flicker fusion frequency. *Pharmacopsychiatria, 15* (Suppl. 1), 24–8.

Harris, B., and Fleer, R. (1974). High speed memory scanning in mental retardates: Evidence for a central processing deficit. *J. Exp. Child Psychol., 17,* 452–9.

Harrison, C., Subhan, Z., and Hindmarch, I. (1985). Residual effects of zopiclone and benzodiazepine hypnotics on psychomotor performance related to car driving. *R. Soc. Med. ICCS, 74,* 89–95.

Hindmarch, I. (1980). Psychomotor function and psychoactive drugs. *Br. J. Clin. Pharmacol., 10,* 189–209.

Hindmarch, I. (1982). Critical flicker fusion frequency (CFF): The effects of psychotropic compounds. *Pharmacopsychiatria, 15* (Suppl. 1), 44–8.

Hindmarch, I. (1986). The effects of psychoactive drugs on car handling and related psychomotor ability: A review. In: O'Hanlon, J.F., and de Gier, J.J. (eds), *Drugs and Driving,* London: Taylor & Francis, pp. 71–9.

Hindmarch, I. (1988). The psychopharmacological approach: Effects of psychotropic drugs on car handling. *Int. Clin. Psychopharmacol., 3,* 73–9.

Hindmarch, I., Subhan, Z., and Stoker, M.J. (1983). The effects of zimeldine and amitriptyline on car driving and psychomotor performance. *Acta Psychiatr. Scand., 68,* 141.

Hindmarch, I., Aufdembrinke, B., and Ott, H. (eds) (1988). *Psychopharmacology and Reaction Time.* Chichester: Wiley.

Hindmarch, I., Kerr, J.S., and Sherwood, N. (1990). Psychopharmacological aspects of psychoactive substances. In: Warburton, D. (ed.), *Addiction Controversies.* Chur (Switz.): Harwood Academic, pp. 36–44.

Hindmarch, I., Haller, J., Sherwood, N., and Kerr, J.S. (1991a). Comparison of five anxiolytic benzodiazepines on measures of psychomotor performance and sleep. *Neuropsychobiology, 24,* 84–9.

14   *N. Sherwood and J. S. Kerr*

Hindmarch, I., Kerr, J.S., and Sherwood, N. (1991b). The effects of alcohol and other drugs on psychomotor performance and cognitive function. *Alcohol Alcoholism,* **26,** 71–9.

Kennedy, R.S., Bittner, A.C., and Jones, M.B. (1981). Video game and conventional tracking. *Percep. Mot. Skills,* **53,** 310.

Krause, M., and Bittner, A.C. (1982). *Repeated Measures on a Choice Reaction Time Task,* Research report NBDL-82R006, New Orleans: Naval Biodynamics Laboratory.

Levander, S.E. (1982). Computerised CFF: Reliability and validity of two psychophysical techniques. *Pharmacopsychiatria,* **15** (Suppl. 1), 54–6.

Ott, H., and Kranda, K. (eds) (1982). *Flicker Techniques in Psychopharmacology,* Weinhein and Basel: Beltz Verlag.

Parrott, A.C. (1982). Critical flicker fusion thresholds and their relationship to other measures of alertness. *Pharmacopsychiatria,* **15** (Suppl. 1), 39–44.

Parrott, A.C. (1991a). Performance tests in human psychopharmacology (1): test reliability and standardisation. *Human Psychopharmacology,* **6,** 1–9.

Parrott, A.C. (1991b). Performance tests in human psychopharmacology (2): content validity, criterion validity and face validity. *Human Psychopharmacology,* **6,** 91-98.

Parrott, A.C. (1991c). Performance tests in human psychopharmacology (3): construct validity and test interpretation. *Human Psychopharmacology,* **6,** 197–207.

Parrott, A.C., and Hindmarch, I. (1975). Arousal and performance—The ubiquitous inverted U relationship. Comparison of changes in response latency and arousal levels in normal subjects induced by CNS stimulants, sedatives and tranquilizers. *IRCS Med. Sci.,* **3,** 176.

Sherwood, N., and Griffin, M.J. (1990). Effects of whole-body vibration on short-term memory. *Aviation Space Environ. Med.,* **61,** 1092–7.

Sherwood, N., Haller, J., Kerr, J.S., and Hindmarch, I. (1992). Comparative effects of five anxiolytic benzodiazepines on two levels of difficulty in a short-term memory task. *J. Drug Dev.,* **5,** 35–41.

Simonson, E., and Brozek, J. (1952). Flicker fusion frequency background and applications. *Physiol. Rev.,* **32,** 349–79.

Smith, J.M., and Misiak, H. (1976). Critical flicker frequency and psychotropic drugs in normal human subjects: A review. *Psychopharmacology,* **47,** 175–82.

Smith, P.J., and Langolf, G.D. (1981). The use of Sternberg's memory scanning paradigm in assessing effects of chemical exposure. *Hum. Factors,* **23,** 701–8.

Sternberg, S. (1966). High speed scanning in human memory. *Science,* **153,** 652–4.

Subhan, Z., and Hindmarch, I. (1984). Effects of zopiclone and benzodiazepine hypnotics on search in short-term memory. *Neuropsychobiology,* **12,** 244–8.

Talbot, N.F. (1834). Experiments on light. *Phil. Magazine,* **5,** 321–34.

Teichner, W.H., and Krebs, M.J. (1974). Laws of visual choice reaction time. *Psychol. Rev.,* **81,** 75–98.

Woodworth, R.S., and Schlosberg, H. (1958). *Experimental Psychology.* London: Methuen.

2
Driving Performance Models: Comparison of a Tracking Simulator and an Over-the-road Test in Relation to Drug Intake

H.-P. Willumeit, *H. Ott and Ch. Kuschel

*Institut für Fahrzeugtechnik, Technische Universität Berlin, and
*Laboratorium Pharmakopsychologie, Schering AG, Berlin,
Germany*

Introduction

Analysis of traffic accidents reveals a dominating causative role of so-called 'human failure' (Statistisches Bundesamt, 1989). The concept of 'human failure', however, only means that the individual elements in the total system of driver, vehicle and traffic environment, as well as their interdependencies, are not in an optimal state of harmony. The significance of a total system not being optimally organized is underlined by the fact that a large number of system flaws leads only to 'near-accidents' which thus escape inclusion in accident statistics only by a narrow margin (Burger *et al.*, 1977).

Whereas *technical deficiencies* cause only a relatively small proportion of accidents, the environmental influences on traffic accidents is, astonishingly, not incorporated as a category in the German official statistics. A properly constructed *traffic environment*, consisting of appropriate road design, markings, signalling system, etc., would be an unlikely cause of accidents for the 'normal' driver, i.e. an operator whose driving abilities do not differ significantly from those of the average driving population. Within the category single-vehicle accidents the official statistics probably contain an unknown percentage of accidents caused neither by technical nor driver failures but by flaws in the quality of the traffic environment (Statistisches Bundesamt, 1989).

Human Psychopharmacology, Vol. 4. Edited by I. Hindmarch and P. D. Stonier
© 1993 John Wiley & Sons Ltd

In addition to environmental causes of accidents, there are a large number of causes which can clearly be traced to the *human components* of the total traffic system. In such cases, the driver shows substandard performance in responding appropriately to situations demanding rapid judgement and action. This may be due to the influence of fatigue, stress, illness, or drugs such as alcohol or medication (Treat *et al.*, 1977). In particular, the driving population under the influence of medication represents the largest group after that under the influence of alcohol (Hausmann *et al.*, 1988). This alone, however, does not prove the influence of the drug as a causative agent.

At present, there is no dependable analysis showing to what extent deficiencies in the above-mentioned three components of the traffic system, and/or incompatibilities between their points of interaction, contribute to the unreliability of the total system.

Considering the human component in inquiries into the causes of traffic accidents, it can be observed that hardly any validated correlations can be proven between features of human performance and the frequency of traffic accidents (Treat *et al.*, 1977). One exception was provided in a report by Enke (1979), who successfully demonstrated a correlation between one performance criterion—reaction time—and frequency of accidents. The detrimental effect of alcohol on human reaction time has also been reported in many publications (Hindmarch and Subhan, 1986). In addition, the relationship between driver intoxication and accident frequency has likewise been confirmed (Hausmann *et al.,* 1988). The fundamental lack of empirical investigations on this subject is altogether understandable, since no comprehensive correlations between the demands of driving and human performance have yet been demonstrated or verified.

Arising from this situation, two different test methods for investigating driving performance were developed independently in the late 1970s in Holland (O'Hanlon, 1983) and Germany (Willumeit and Neubert, 1979). The Dutch over-the-road test is based on a model which was developed largely to deal with the problems of stabilization in unstable aeroplanes, transferring this model to car driving. In this test, the subject attempts to drive a car at a given speed while staying within right lane boundaries. Speed and lateral position are then recorded and analysed to yield statistical results. In contrast, the second test method, the Tracking Simulator TS2, was developed primarily for driving-related tasks, which include not only the basic task of steering a car more or less perfectly in an unobstructed traffic environment, but also the mastering of an environment obstructed by other drivers or road hazards.

While the results obtained with the over-the-road test do not show a reliable relationship between driving performance and accident frequency, the reaction time measured in the Tracking Simulator can be clearly correlated with accident statistics. As in the over-the-road test, however, the frequency of mistakes in the instrumental, operative tasks of the Tracking Simulator test can be related to accident frequency only to a slight degree.

Parallel to these two test methods, psychological models were developed for the classification of car-driving tasks (Janssen, 1979), as were models for the interpretation of human information acquisition and processing which provide more appropriate and clearly defined criteria for driving performance. However, alternative test methods will be necessary in order to validate these models.

A direct comparison of the over-the-road and the Tracking Simulator tests was made in a study on the influence of a hypnotic drug (lormetazepam 1 mg) versus placebo and a different soporific (oxazepam 50 mg). The objective was to determine the hangover effect on the day following medication in a double-blind cross-over design with 18 healthy male volunteers. On the day following evening administration of a single dose, i.e. approximately 10 hours after application, the performance-impairing effect was tested with both methods. In this design, the same volunteers under the randomized medication conditions were tested on the driving simulator immediately after completion of the over-the-road tests.

Materials and Methods

In the over-the-road driving test (O'Hanlon, 1983), the subject has to drive 2 × 50 km in normal highway traffic in a medium-sized car equipped with special measuring instruments. The driver is to maintain a steady speed of approximately 90 km/h and to keep the vehicle on a straight course while staying on the right-hand lane of the road. During this test, the lateral deviations of the vehicle in relation to the continuous middle stripe on the road are recorded. The standard deviation of the mean lateral position (SDLP) was used as a criterion for driving performance. This includes only those driving segments in which the subject did not undertake any passing or braking manoeuvres; only the driving segments in which the subject maintains his course at a constant speed are included for evaluation. Additionally, the mean driving speed and its standard deviation are evaluated. Thus a high degree of real-life driving conditions is presumably achieved for the intended objective of the study.

Immediately after completion of the over-the-road test, the subject was tested on the Tracking Simulator TS2 (Willumeit and Neubert, 1979). The main requirements for this test with respect to real driving conditions are:

(1) To maintain the vehicle on roads with stochastic curvature (primary task).
(2) To react to rarely occurring external signals, e.g. sudden obstacles (secondary task).

For the evaluation of driving performance, the number of correctly executed primary tasks (tracking control, TC), as individually obtained within a period of 30 minutes, are calculated after subtracting the number of incorrectly executed tasks. The reaction time (RT) in the secondary task is determined as the mean of all individual reaction times.

Comparison and Evaluation of the Test Methods Using Theoretical Models

Psychological Models

In assessing these two tests according to the model of hierarchical structure of the driving task proposed by Janssen (1979) (Figure 1), the over-the-road test can be assigned exclusively to the lowest hierarchical level, i.e. the control level, since only the course-keeping tasks are evaluated. Furthermore, the maintaining of a steady course is to be accomplished in the rather undemanding environment of the highway, where there are wider lateral boundaries and the effort required to avoid lateral deviation is considerably less than in urban traffic. Furthermore, temporal or spatial variations of the nominal value (longitudinal curvature of the road) are practically impossible. In addition, because of the actual driving environment, a number of uncontrollable external parameters (light conditions, road surface conditions, side wind) are present which can influence the test results.

In evaluating the over-the-road test according to the human processing resources theory proposed by Wickens (1984) (Figure 2), the required information-processing functions can be assigned mainly to the 'visual' in terms of modality and to the 'spatial' in terms of processing codes. The response after completion of central processing is of 'manual' type.

According to Janssen (1979) (Figure 1), the experimental approach taken in the primary task of the Tracking Simulator TS2 test can also be assigned to

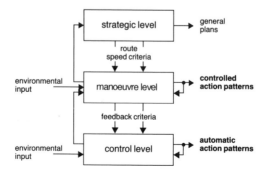

Figure 1. Scheme of hierarchical control levels in driving (modified from Janssen, 1979, and Sanders, 1986)

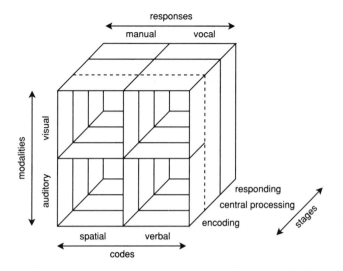

Figure 2. Four-dimensional model of human information processing in multiple time-sharing tasks (modified from Wickens, 1984). The different stages of human information processing during driving on a curved road, for example, are involved in the following manner:

1. Encoding the spatial input information in the visual channel
2. Central processing of input information and pattern recognition
3. Final transformation of the central decisions into manual response such as steering

During real driving, additional information from unexpected obstacles, traffic signs, dynamic states of the vehicle, etc., must be processed in parallel. Thus driving is a multiple time-sharing task and could be best conceptualized by a multiple resource model

the control level, while the occasionally occurring secondary task can be clearly placed at the manoeuvring level. In contrast to the over-the-road test, the Tracking Simulator TS2 allows highly variable spatial and temporal changes in the nominal values (longitudinal curvature of the road; Figure 3), and thus demands performance corresponding roughly to driving on a winding road at high speed. In order to increase the realism of this test, the subject is given a preview of the approaching changes in direction. This preview is generated by the simulator, as opposed to being generated by the driver in real road situations. The control mechanisms in this experimental approach corresponds to that shown in Figure 5. The transfer function of vehicle (H_2) is imitated by a realistic dynamic system of secondary order, and the side wind interference $r(t)$ is not realized in the present equipment.

According to the theory of human processing resources (Wickens, 1984; Figure 2) the encoding of input information in the TS2 can be assigned mainly to the 'visual' in terms of modality and, in terms of processing codes, mainly to the 'verbal'. The response after central processing of information is 'manual'. The highest level in the hierarchical driving task model proposed by Janssen (1979) (Figure 1), i.e. the strategic level, is encompassed neither by the over-the-road test nor with the TS2.

The differences between these two test types in terms of the 'cognitive–energetic model of stress and performance' (Sanders, 1983; Figure 4) at the processing level have been discussed above. On the level of energetic mechanisms, however, the TS2 approach has to be classified differently from the over-the-road test in terms of arousal effects and activation. The TS2 approach makes high demands on performance and motor adjustments, while in the over-the-road test there is a greater degree of monotony due to the low performance demands, and less activation due to the low motor adjustment (fewer steering wheel movements).

There are no great differences within the two approaches with respect to the evaluation and mechanisms which influence the degree of effort by comparisons of demands and accomplishment and classification of danger in addition to motivation by the promise of successful completion. In neither of the tests is there any real threat of danger by unsuccessful completion of the tasks.

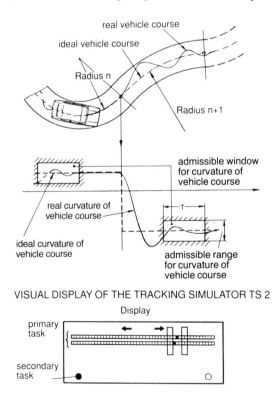

VISUAL DISPLAY OF THE TRACKING SIMULATOR TS 2

Table 1 shows a classification of the test methods and real car driving in terms of different theoretical models.

Theoretical Control Model

Both test methods can be depicted as a theoretical feedback model (Figure 5). For the Tracking Simulator TS2; however, this applies only to the primary task. The brake reaction time, i.e. the secondary task in the TS2, does not conform to this model.

The control task consists of manoeuvring the vehicle, represented by its characteristics H_2, along the given course $x(t)$ by the driver, whose constant controller characteristics are as seen under normal, i.e. placebo, conditions

Figure 3 (opposite). The tracking simulator, showing the ideal driving course and the visual display. The upper part shows a car on a curved road. The vehicle dynamics separate two different courses: the ideal vehicle course, given only by geometric road parameters; and the real vehicle course, influenced by road parameters as well as by the driving control activities at the steering wheel and by the dynamic behaviour of the car itself. The driver's control activities have to reflect the road condition as well as the vehicle's dynamic behaviour in order to minimize the accident risk in veering off the road. In the middle part of the figure the curvature of the vehicle course for the above driving situation is shown. The ideal curvature of the driving course during the change from a left to a right curve under ideal vehicle behaviour is shown as a dotted line, and the solid line marks the curvature of the vehicle course influenced by driver and vehicle for a given change in the road course. In order to avoid veering off the road and risking an accident the real curvature of the vehicle's course has to move within a certain time between the two border lines. This time space and the border lines define an admissible window for the curvature of the vehicle course. If the curvature exceeds this window the car driver risks an accident. In the lower part of the figure the visual display of the TS2 simulator can be seen. The upper row of 49 lamps presents the command signal as the ideal curvature of the vehicle course, and the lower row of 49 lamps displays the actual curvature of the vehicle course, which is almost proportional to the angle of the steering wheel but superimposed with the dynamics of the vehicle's behaviour at high speeds for lane-changing manoeuvre. At the left and right lower edges of the TS2 display, two lamps are seen which serve as visual signals for the secondary reaction task. Subjects in front of the visual display have to react to the command signal on the upper row of lamps by moving the steering wheel. A maximum time of 2.8 s is allowed for this task. If the subject succeeds in matching the light signals of both rows of lamps in a shorter period (admissible curvature of the vehicle course window) another task will be provided. Apart from this primary task the subjects have to stop the flashing of one or two extra lamps by pressing the respective pedal (left pedal if left light flashes, right pedal if right light flashes) or neither pedal if both lights flash simultaneously. That reaction time test serves as a secondary task. Referring to Figure 2 (multiple resource model) the input information of the road curvature within the primary task— which in a real driving situation is a visuo-spatial pattern—is reduced in the TS2 display, additionally supported by adequate instructions, to a one-dimentional visual–verbal code in the form of varying steps of command signal (modified from Willumeit *et al.*, 1984a)

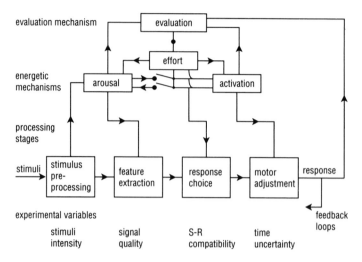

Figure 4. The cognitive–energetic model of stress and performance is described by Sanders (1986) as follows: 'Processing a signal demands an energy supply from at least two sources: a phasic arousal system, mediating perception and a tonic activation system, mediating motor preparation and execution. More energy is required as the demands increase as in the case of a bad signal quality or a high time uncertainty. Drugs and other adverse conditions such as sleep loss are supposed to suppress the energy supply which must be maintained by investing effort. Effort is a voluntary energetic mechanism, controlling the supply of the basal mechanisms. Investing effort to maintain performance has a major motivational aspect since it relies on a continuous evaluation of the equilibrium between demands and accomplishment' (modified from Sanders, 1983)

H_1. The medication-associated influence on the driver is added by a human drug-related noise q without changing H_1. The influence of side wind in the over-the-road test is likewise added as noise r to the lateral position y of the car. This results in the lateral displacement u relative to $x(t)$:

$$X - (Y + R) = U = \frac{W}{H_1} = \frac{Y}{H_1 H_2} - \frac{Q}{H_1} \tag{1}$$

where the capital letters represent the Fourier-transformed values

$$W = H_1 U \tag{2}$$

$$Y = H_2(W + Q) \tag{3}$$

Combining equations 1–3 results in the lateral displacement relative to the road:

$$U = \frac{1}{1 + H_1 H_2}(X - R - QH_2) \tag{4}$$

Table 1. Classification of test methods and real car driving according to theoretical models

Theoretical models	Over-the-road test	Tracking Simulator TS2	Real car driving
Control model	Constant operational parameter, uncontrollable external interference	Highly variable temporal operational parameter, at present without external interference (this could be included in a controllable form)	Variable temporal operational parameter which is discontinuously perceived and adjusted; intermittent steering functions
Hierarchical model of driving tasks (Janssen, 1979)	Control level only	Both control and manoeuvring level	Control, manoeuvring and strategic levels
Cognitive–energetic model (Sanders, 1983)	Low arousal (low vigilance level), neither constant nor controllable	High arousal (high vigilance level) constant and controllable over time	High or low vigilance level, depending on traffic environment and subject's conditions
Human processing resource model (Wickens, 1984)	Input: visual/spatial	Input: visual/verbal	Input: visual, kinaesthetic, auditory/spatial, verbal
	Response: manual	Response: manual	Response: manual

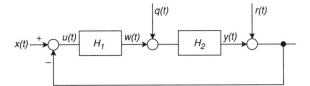

x(t) : course of the road
u(t) : vehicle's relative lateral position to the road
y(t) : vehicle's lateral deviation
w(t) : steer angle
q(t) : human drug-related steer noise
r(t) : sidewind related lateral deviation of the car
H_1 : transfer function of human controller
H_2 : transfer function of vehicle

Figure 5. Theoretical feedback model. For explanation see text

The auto power density of $u(t)$ is calculated by multiplying U by U^*, where U^* is the conjugated complex of U:

$$S_{uu} = UU^* = \frac{1}{(1 + H_1H_2)} \frac{1}{(1 + H_1H_2)^*} [X - R - QH_2][X^* - R^* - (QH_2)^*] \quad (5)$$

Because $x(t)$, $q(t)$ and $r(t)$ are statistically unrelated to each other, the result is:

$$S_{uu} = \frac{1}{(1 + H_1H_2)} \frac{1}{(1 + H_1H_2)^*} [S_{xx} + S_{rr} + S_{qq} |H_2|^2] \quad (6)$$

where S_{xx} = auto power density of the course, S_{rr} = auto power density of the side-wind noise, and S_{qq} = auto power density of the human drug-related steer noise.

With an identical driving course, S_{xx} is constant for all tests. The influence of medication on the SDLP results from S_{qq}. This overlaps with the non-controlled influence of the side wind S_{rr}, which should also be simultaneously measured during the road tests. The calculated standard deviation of lateral displacement is:

$$\sigma_u^2 = \int_0^\infty S_{uu}d\omega = (SDLP)^2 \quad (7)$$

The difference in power density of S_{uu}, for one subject in two following test drives under verum or placebo condition, is therefore:

$$\Delta = S_{uu_v} - S_{uu_p} = \frac{1}{(1 + |H_1H_2|^2)}[S_{rr_v} - S_{rr_p} + S_{qq}|H_2|^2] \quad (8)$$

where S_{rr_v} and S_{rr_p}, respectively, are the power spectral density of the wind during the verum and placebo test drives. This additionally shows that these results are also dependent on H_2, i.e. the vehicle characteristics. Thus, if the vehicle is substituted or, for that matter, even if the tyres are changed between tests, then the results of the different experiments will not be comparable.

Applying this model to the completed experiments, the power densities S_{xx}, S_{rr} and S_{qq} in equation 6 no longer appear as constant values, but as variables for each test. For the moment, the possibility that the controller characteristics H_1 might also behave as a variable is ruled out. The variable S_{uu} in equation 6 is thus the sum of the three variables S_{xx}, S_{rr} and S_{qq} (Table 2).

The variance of S_{uu} under placebo and verum conditions is therefore:

$$v(S_{uu})_p = K_1[v(S_{xx})_p + v(S_{rr})_p]; \, v(S_{qq})p = 0 \quad (9)$$

and

$$v(S_{uu})_v = K_1[v(S_{xx})_v + v(S_{rr})_v + v(S_{qq})_v K_2] \quad (10)$$

respectively, where K_1 and K_2 are constants from formula (8); subscripts v or p indicate verum or placebo condition.

Thus, resulting covariances between x, r and q disappear due to their lack of statistical relationship.

Table 2. Sources of variance v for each subject, and means $\bar{v}$ under placebo and verum conditions

Placebo:				
Subject 1	$v(S_{uu})_{p1}$	$v(S_{xx})_{p1}$	$v(S_{rr})_{p1}$	
Subject 2	$v(S_{uu})_{p2}$	$v(S_{xx})_{p2}$	$v(S_{rr})_{p2}$	
$\vdots$				
Subject n	$v(S_{uu})_{pn}$	$v(S_{xx})_{pn}$	$v(S_{rr})_{pn}$	
	$\bar{v}(S_{uu})_{p}$	$\bar{v}(S_{xx})_{p}$	$\bar{v}(S_{rr})_{p}$	
Verum:				
Subject 1	$v(S_{uu})_{v1}$	$v(S_{xx})_{v1}$	$v(S_{rr})_{v1}$	$v(S_{qq})_{v1}$
Subject 2	$v(S_{uu})_{v2}$	$v(S_{xx})_{v2}$	$v(S_{rr})_{v2}$	$v(S_{qq})_{v2}$
$\vdots$				
Subject n	$v(S_{uu})_{vn}$	$v(S_{xx})_{vn}$	$v(S_{rr})_{vn}$	$v(S_{qq})_{vn}$
	$\bar{v}(S_{uu})_{v}$	$\bar{v}(S_{xx})_{v}$	$\bar{v}(S_{rr})_{v}$	$\bar{v}(S_{qq})_{v}$

The difference of the variance for S_{uu} under placebo and verum is thus:

$$v(S_{uu})_v - v(S_{uu})_p = K_1[v(S_{rr})_v - v(S_{rr})_p + v(S_{qq})_v K_2] \tag{11}$$

under the assumption that $v(S_{xx})_p = v(S_{xx})_v$, since the course of the road does not change for the individual test drives.

The order of subjects is randomized by the randomization scheme of the experimental construct. In the execution of the test, however, a number of different practical aspects of the method cause the variance of the temporal distribution of the road tests under placebo $v(T)_p$ to diverge from the variance of temporal distribution of the road tests under verum. In a linear situation, their relationship to the variable S_{rr} can be expressed as:

$$H^2 v(T)_p = v(S_{rr})_p \tag{12}$$

for road tests under placebo, and

$$H^2 v(T)_v = v(S_{rr})_v \tag{13}$$

for tests under verum.

The following two cases should be distinguished:

(1) If the variances $v(T)_p$ and $v(T)_v$ are equal, then

$$v(S_{rr})_p = v(S_{rr})_v \tag{14}$$

as long as a linear relationship H exists between the variance of time of the road test and the variance of the power density of the wind. If this is the case, then the difference of the variances of the cross-deviation in equation 11 can indeed be clearly attributed to the variance of medication.

(2) If, however, the variances $v(T)_p$ and $v(T)_v$ are not equal in the randomiz-
      ation scheme, which is often the case, then the two side-wind variances
      in equation 11 will not cancel each other, and the test results for lateral
      position deviations are dependent upon the parameter of the difference
      of the side-wind variances in the placebo and verum road tests.

Under the conditions outlined in (2), the results obtained in different test
series, e.g. repetition of tests or test series using different medications, cannot
be reliably compared with each other, since these results contain the uncontrollable variable of the momentary side wind.

These arguments are only valid when the operator characteristics H_1 are
regarded as constant for the individual road tests, but not when they are
treated as variable. This should, and can, be investigated for each test.

In addition to the parameter of natural side wind, other factors that cause
wind-associated variances, such as oncoming traffic and road signs, should
also be considered, since an SDLP of up to 18 cm has been seen under placebo
conditions. Under medication conditions, SDLP has been given as only 1–8 cm
—less than one-third of the uncontrolled placebo effect. Replication tests also
showed differences of up to 2 cm SDLP. These discrepancies have not yet
been explained, and may be the result of the above-mentioned influences. It is
unlikely that the parameter SDLP alone is capable of yielding reliable information on the effects of medication on driving performance, because it is
uncontrollably admixed with the effects of external factors, as well as the
influences of the test substances.

Results and Discussion

The results of both test methods as obtained in a joint study are shown in
Figures 6–11.

Figure 6 shows the mean values and distribution of SDLP. Figures 8 and 10
show the mean values and distribution of TS2 results. In this joint study, the
parameter SDLP is the only significant parameter at the 5% level. In the
tracking control (TC) of the simulator, the same tendency can be seen, although it is evident from the broad standard deviations that differences between treatment and placebo tests were not significant.

The parameter reaction time (RT) shows a similar tendency, the main
difference being that performance was actually better under lormetazepam
than under placebo. The time course (Figure 11) shows a deterioration in RT
of about 0.06 seconds between the first and last 5-minute interval with varying
patterns under all three treatments during the trial. The average difference
between results obtained with placebo and oxazepam was 0.026 seconds,
which means really no differentiation in hangover effects.

In addition to Figure 6, Figure 7 gives an impression of the driving param-

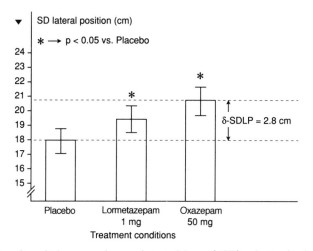

Figure 6. Results of the over-the-road test. Mean (±SE) of standard deviation of lateral position under the three treatment conditions, lormetazepam 1 mg, oxazepam 50 mg and placebo during the morning session (8.00–9.15 a.m.), $n = 18$ healthy male volunteers in a threefold cross-over design (modified from Volkerts *et al.*, 1990)

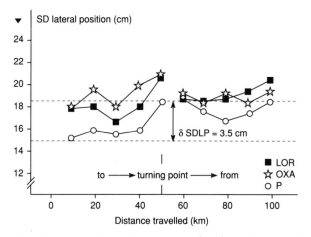

Figure 7. Results of the over-the-road test. Mean (±SE) standard deviation of lateral position under the three treatment conditions, lormetazepam (LOR) 1 mg, oxazepam (OXA) 50 mg and placebo (P) during the morning session (8.00–9.15 a.m.) as a function of travelled distance in kilometres; from start to turning point and back; $n = 18$ healthy male volunteers in a threefold cross-over design (modified from Volkerts *et al.*, 1990)

eter SDLP of the over-the-road test with values summarized at every 10 km of the 100 km distance travelled. At the 50 km position the vehicle turned back to the starting point.

According to Figure 7 two effects are obvious: on the one hand, the SDLP increased owing to the effects of medication; simultaneously, however, under all three treatments there is an increase of SDLP over the time required to drive the course. This may reflect a considerable influence on the driver's vigilance owing to monotony and lack of performance demands. At the end of the first 50 km course, the test procedure is interrupted by a turning

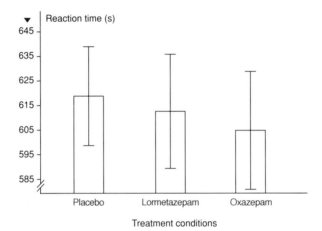

Figure 8. Results from the tracking simulator. Mean number of correct responses in the primary task under the treatment conditions, lormetazepam 1 mg, oxazepam 50 mg, and placebo during the morning session (9.30–10.00 a.m.); $n = 18$ healthy male volunteers in a threefold cross-over design (modified from Volkerts *et al.*, 1990)

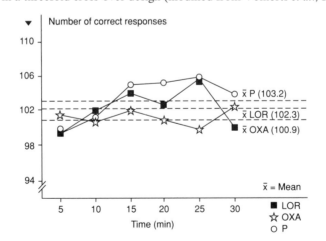

Figure 9. Results from the tracking simulator. Mean number of correct responses in the primary task over the time course of 30 minutes under the treatment conditions, lormetazepam (LOR) 1 mg, oxazepam (OXA) 50 mg, and placebo (P) during the morning session (9.30–10.00 a.m.); $n = 18$ healthy male volunteers in a threefold cross-over design (modified after Volkerts *et al.*, 1990)

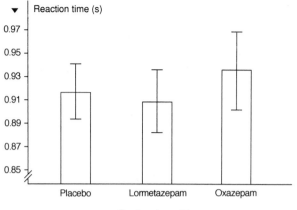

Figure 10. Results from the tracking simulator. Mean reaction times in the secondary task under the treatment conditions, lormetazepam 1 mg, oxazepam 50 mg, and placebo during the morning session (9.30–10.00 a.m.); n = 18 healthy male volunteers in a threefold cross-over design (modifed after Volkerts *et al.*, 1990)

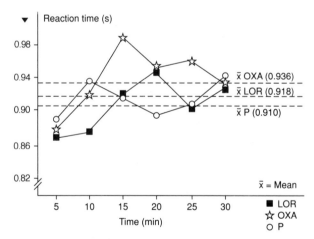

Figure 11. Results from the tracking simulator. Mean reaction times in the secondary task over the time course of 30 minutes under the treatment conditions, lormetazepam (LOR) 1 mg, oxazepam (OXA) 50 mg, and placebo (P) during the morning session (9.30–10.00 a.m.); n = 18 healthy male volunteers in a threefold cross-over design (modified after Volkerts *et al.*, 1990)

manoeuvre. Under placebo conditions, this has no influence on the SDLP. Following the turning manoeuvre, the first half of the 50 km return trip shows an increase in performance, whereas in the second half of the performance again decreases. These performance fluctuations may be an expression of underlying changes in the level of vigilance. Under medication, however, there is a clear improvement in performance, just after the manoeuvre, which then steadily decreases over the next 50 km.

In this test, the difference (δ-SDLP) between driving performance under placebo and medication averages 2.8 cm with oxazepam, i.e. 13.5% of the temporal mean value (see Figure 6), and the difference caused by vigilance-associated influence is 2.5 cm, i.e. 15.5% of mean value (see Figure 7), thus being higher than the effect of medication.

In the TS2 approach, one can also see a change in the results obtained over time (Figure 9). In this test, however, there is an increase in driving performance which may be caused by learning effects. The performance increase over 30 minutes under placebo conditions averages 36 tasks relative to 619 tasks (Figure 8), i.e. an increase of 5.8%. A decline in performance after 30 minutes testing, possibly the result of vigilance deterioration, is 11 tasks relative to 619 tasks, i.e. 1.8%. The influence of medication on driving performance in this test is 13 tasks over 30 minutes, i.e. a decrease of 2.1% in relation to placebo conditions.

It will not be attempted at present to quantify these results in terms of driving performance and its influence on traffic accident rates, since both experimental approaches have yet to be validated. But it seems that the over-the-road-test is more influenced by vigilance fluctuations than the TS2 driving simulator.

Results from Tests on Hypnotic Drug Influence

The study groups which proposed a correlation between results of the over-the-road test and driving ability made use, for lack of validation of this test method, of the performance results of over-the-road tests under acute alcohol intoxication. These alcohol tests, however, were performed under different test conditions (O'Hanlon, 1985) in terms of driving course, distance and environment. The proposed comparison of the effects of alcohol and drugs is shown in Figure 12 (after Brookhuis, 1989). Under consideration of the above-mentioned influence of vigilance deterioration on SDLP in this study, the variation δ-SDLP = 3.5 cm corresponds to 0.7‰ blood alcohol concentration (BAC).

In a further study by this group (Volkerts *et al.*, 1987), the change δ-SDLP under placebo conditions was 6 cm, i.e. 28.2% of BAC condition. In comparison to alcohol effects, this result would correspond to a BAC level of roughly 1.1‰. In other words, these studies suggest that performance after 100 km of highway driving should correspond to performance around the level of 0.7‰ BAC. This seems highly improbable.

The comparison of driving performance under drug, alcohol and vigilance-related effects in the TS2 test for the parameter TC yields results as shown in

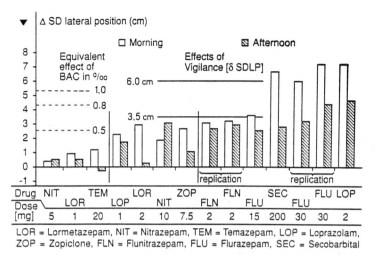

Figure 12. Results from the over-the-road test. Mean changes versus placebo of standard deviation of lateral position (SDLP) in the morning (10.00–11.00 a.m.) and the afternoon (4.00–5.00 p.m.) after application of the different compounds over two successive nights originating from diverse driving studies from different study groups. Additionally, on the left-hand side the effects on SDLP under acute alcoholic intoxication (BAC, mg/ml) and in the centre the effects of changes in vigilance on SDLP under placebo conditions are displayed as results from different driving studies (modified from Brookhuis, 1989)

Figure 13. The improvement in TC under placebo is +5.8% TC (Volkerts *et al.*, 1990). This can be interpreted as a learning effect, but may also be the result of enhanced vigilance or even a shift in task distribution between TC and RT, since RT lengthens during the course of the test. In contrast to the over-the-road test, decline in TC performance is minimal in the TS2 test at −1.8% (Volkerts *et al.*, 1990).

The effect of 0.6‰ BAC leads to a deterioration in performance of −12.2% TC (Willumeit *et al.*, 1984b), 0.7‰ BAC to −14.6% TC (Willumeit and Neubert, 1979), and 0.8‰ BAC to −25% TC (Ott *et al.*, 1990) or −15.7% TC (Willumeit *et al.*, 1984a). If the effect of vigilance on the alcohol scale is likewise included, this would result in a vigilance effect of about 0.1‰ BAC in the TS2 test, which seems much more plausible than calculations from the over-the-road test. Thus a reliable comparison between drug and alcohol effects on driving performance may be better achieved by the TS2 test.

In the Tracking Simulator TS2, the parameter RT, in contrast to the control parameters, operates on the manoeuvring level. The parameter RT shows a similar tendency as SDLP inasmuch as performance variability is less between the different medication trials than over the course of the study (Figure 11). The reason for this may lie in a change in the focus of attention between the two simultaneous tasks in the TS2 test. The RT task is given more attention at

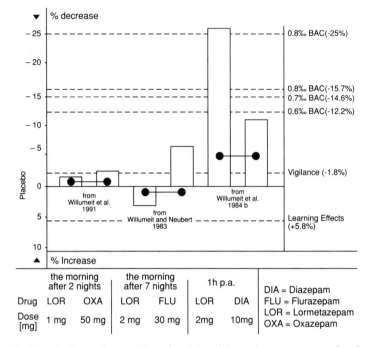

Figure 13. Results from the tracking simulator. Mean changes versus placebo of correct responses after application of different compounds originating from diverse driving simulator studies. Additionally, on the right-hand side the detrimental effects of acute alcohol intoxication (BAC, mg/ml) as well as of tiredness (vigilance decrements) and the improvements by learning under placebo conditions are displayed

the start of the trial because it is easier at first. After some practice, this task is mastered—there is also no feedback from the RT task—so that in the next phase attention is focused more on the TC task (Figure 9), in which successful completion is rewarded by perceptible feedback.

The futility of evaluating the test results absolutely, presenting them in a table, and comparing them with each other has been discussed above; this also applies to the parameter RT in the TS2 test.

The lesser pharmacosensitivity of the TS2 in this study might be explained by the fact that the TS2 tests began about 1.5 hours after the start of the over-the-road test, leading to a lower serum level and thus a higher state of alertness in the subject. The reason the TS2 results were not significant is the wide SD, which could be kept in bounds by a higher number of test subjects or a more homogeneous group.

A previous Tracking Simulator study (Willumeit *et al.*, 1984a) using short and long-acting control substances consistently showed significant results, at least at the 10% level.

Correlation of Results Obtained with the Two Test Methods

A comparison of the TS2 and over-the-road test methods in terms to seek tendentiously similar results in an identical test design can be made by correlative analysis. Based on the above classification of the test methods according to psychological models, however, no close similarities of test results can be expected, unless the effects of the applied substances are so strong that they can also be measured by other, completely different test methods. Table 3 shows the correlation of SDLP in the over-the-road test separately with the two independent results, TC and RT, in the TS2 test.

Table 3. Correlation coefficients between standard deviation of lateral position (SDLP) in the over-the-road test, reaction time (RT), and tracking control (TC) in the Tracking Simulator TS2 test

Drug	SDLP RT	SDLP TC	RT TC
Lormetazepam	−0.138	0.096	−0.368
Oxazepam	0.462	−0.589	−0.584
Placebo	−0.311	−0.160	−0.394

The correlation of SDLP with TC might be expected to show relatively higher values, since both parameters are based on the same operative level, i.e. the control level (Figure 1), albeit at extremely divergent vigilance levels. This is indeed confirmed by the correlative values given in Table 3, which show no relation under placebo and lormetazepam conditions, but do show the expected tendency toward higher values and with correct sign for the remarkably sedative effect of oxazepam. The correlation SDLP and RT show a similar correlative result, although the RT task extends into the manoeuvring level (Table 3).

The values TC and RT, exclusive to the TS2 in this context, show correlations under all three medications also with respect to their sign, which presents a cohesive preliminary picture whereby the results were most similar (as expected) for oxazepam.

These results show that the over-the-road test and the Tracking Simulator TS2 test apply to different psychological functions, despite their identical objectives.

Summary

In an investigation of the influence of benzodiazepine hypnotic compounds on driving performance, two different experimental approaches were used with the same subjects within a single design. The fundamental differences between these two approaches are demonstrated in relation to existing psychological models as well as a control model. While the over-the-road test is conducted with an instrumented vehicle in real traffic, the results of this method are bound to parameters that are of little relevance to traffic safety. In addition, the interference variables associated with the over-the-road test (wind vigilance) are not reliably measured. In contrast, the Tracking Simulator TS2 method is a pure laboratory experiment in which at least one of the parameters, i.e. reaction time, is related to traffic accident rates.

Under these experimental conditions, vigilance is kept stable at a high level and there are no interference factors. The idea of using the over-the-road test to calibrate drug effects based on a separate alcohol study is questionable. A comparison of drug and alcohol effects based on the TS2 test and its research strategy yields at least plausible results due to the fact that alcohol is included as a standard.

Correlations of the results of both experimental approaches show few similarities, though there are higher correlations, as expected, after the effect of a strong test substance. The two experimental methods compared in this chapter are not adequate to provide a comprehensive assessment of driving performance efficiency. In order to achieve this, the testing methods require further development on the basis of an analysis of driving tasks, which has yet to be adequately realized, and the performance criteria derived from such an analysis.

References

Brookhuis, K.A. (1989). Prüfung auf Verkehrstüchtigkeit unter Praxisbedingungen. *Fortschr. Med. Monographie Lormetazepam*, **8**, 9–12.

Burger, W.J., Smith, R.L., Queen, J.E., and Slack, G.B. (1977). *Accident and Near Accident Causation: The Contribution of Automobile Design Characteristics*. US Department of Commerce, PB-274 338, November 1977, 191 pp.

Enke, K. (1979). Möglichkeiten zur Verbesserung der aktiven Sicherheit innerhalb des Regelkreises Fahrer—Fahrzeug—Umgebung. *Proc. 7th Int. Conf. on ESV*, Paris.

Hausmann, E., Otte, D., and Möller, M.R. (1988). Alkohol/Arzneimittel und Drogen bei verkehrsunfallverletzten Fahrern. In: *Der Bundesminister für Verkehr Unfall- und Sicherheitsforschung Straßenverkehr*. vol. 65, Bremerhaven: Wirtschaftsverlag NW, pp. 56–59.

Hindmarch, I. and Subhan, Z. (1986). The effects of antidepressants taken with and without alcohol on information processing, psychomotor performance and car handling ability. In: O'Hanlon, J.F., and de Gier, J.J. (eds), *Drugs and Driving*, London: Taylor & Francis, pp. 231–40.

Janssen, W.H. (1979). Routeplanning en geleiding. In: *Literatuurstudie*, Rapport IZF 1979—C13, TNO Soesterberg: Institute of Perception.

O'Hanlon, J.F. (1983). Alcohol and hypnotic hangovers as an influence on driving performance. *Travel Traffic Med.*, **1**, 147–52.

O'Hanlon, J.F. (1985). The influence of different blood-alcohol levels on objectively measurable aspects of actual driving performance, *Annual Report*, University of Groningen, Traffic Research Center.

Ott, H., Rohloff, A., Kuschel, C., Willumeit, H.P., Voet, B. and Pennekamp, P. (1990). Potential reduction of driving skills at a driving simulator after acute combined intake of benzodiazepine-tranquillizer and alcohol. *10th European Winter Conference on Brain Research*, Les Arc, France, poster.

Sanders, A.F. (1983). Towards a model of stress and human performance. *Acta Psychol.*, **53**, 61.

Sanders, A.F. (1986). Drugs, driving and the measurement of human performance. In: O'Hanlon, J.F., and de Gier, J.J. (eds), *Drugs and Driving*, London: Taylor & Francis, pp. 3–16.

Statistisches Bundesamt (1989). *Verkehr*, Fachserie 8, Reihe 7, Verkehrsunfälle, Stuttgart: Metzeler-Poeschel.

Treat, J.R., Tumbas, N.S., McDonald, S.T., Shinar, D., Hume, R.D., Mayer, R.E., Stansifer, R.L., and Castellan, N.J. (1977). Tri-level study of the causes of traffic accidents. Report No. DOT-HS-034-3-535-77 (TAC), Indiana University, March 1977. Cited in: Shinar, D. (ed.) *Psychology on the Road: The Human Factor in Traffic Safety*, New York: Wiley, 1978, pp. 99–127.

Volkerts, E.R., and Abbink, F. (1990). Kater-effecten op de rijvaardigheid na slaapmiddelgebruik? Lormetazepam en oxazepam versus placebo. *J. Drug Therapy Res.*, **15**, 22–26.

Volkerts, E.R., Brookhuis, K.A., and O'Hanlon, J.F. (1987). Comparison of the effects of buspirone 5 mg and 10 mg, diazepam 5 mg and lorazepam 1 mg (t.i.d.) upon actual driving performance, *VK 87-02*, Traffic Research Centre, University of Groningen.

Volkerts, E.R., van Laar, M.W., and van Willigenburg, A.P.P. (1990). A methodical comparison of the acute residual effects of lormetazepam 1 mg, oxazepam 50 mg, and placebo on driving performance in an over-the-road driving test and in a driving-simulator, *Report, April 1990*, NIDDR, University of Utrecht.

Wickens, C.D. (1984). Processing resources in attention. In: Parasuraman, R., and Davies, R. (eds), *Varieties of Attention*, New York: Academic Press, pp. 63–102.

Willumeit, H.P., and Neubert, W. (1979). Überprüfung der Fahrtüchtigkeit unter dem Einfluß von Medikamenten und Alkohol. In: Bundesanstalt für Straßenwesen (ed.), *Unfall- und Sicherheitsforschung Straßenverkehr*, Heft 21, pp. 364–75.

Willumeit, H.P., and Neubert, W. (1983). Verkehrstüchtigkeitsprüfung am Fahrsimulator nach akuter und subchronischer Einnahme von Hypnotika und psychotropen Substanzen. In: Allgemeiner Deutscher Automobil club (ed.), *ADAC Schriftenreihe Straßenverkehr 27, Bericht über das 4. Symposium Verkehrsmedizin*, München, ADAC Verlag, pp. 102–111.

Willumeit, H.P., Ott, H. and Neubert, W. (1984a). Simulated car driving as a useful technique for the determination of residual effects and alcohol interaction after short- and long-acting benzodiazepines. In: Hindmarch, I., Ott, H., and Roth, T. (eds), *Sleep, Benzodiazepines and Performance/Psychopharmacology Supplementum 1*, Berlin: Springer, pp. 133–151.

Willumeit, H.P., Ott, H., Neubert, W., Hemmerling, K.G., Schratzer, M., and Fichte, K. (1984b). Alcohol interaction of lormetazepam, mepindolol sulphate and diazepam measuring by performance on the driving simulator. *Pharmacopsychiatry*, **17**, 36–43.

Willumeit, H.P., Ott, H., and Kuschel, C. (1991). Effects of lormetazepam and other benzodiazepine receptor ligands on car driving related skills. *Hum. Psychopharmacol.*, **6**, 209–18.

3

International Dementia Research: Comments on the Validation of Psychometric Measures and Proposals for the Definition of Clinical Relevance

H. Erzigkeit, H. Lehfeld, O. Schultheiß

Psychiatry Department, University of Erlangen–Nuremberg, Germany

Introduction

In the assessment of geriatric patients suffering from dementing disorders, psychometric tests and rating scales are administered mainly in order to determine the severity of the disease and—in the case of follow-up testing—to evaluate the effects of therapeutic interventions. As in general psychology, the accuracy with which the test instruments employed can yield information about the patient's competences and deficits, or their changes, depends largely on their validity. However, the development of valid tests and scales for clinical use requires the additional consideration of factors which do not play a major role in the examination of healthy persons, but may influence the validity of a test or a scale when administered to geriatric patients (Erzigkeit *et al.*, 1991). Moreover, since international comparisons of outcome measures in clinical studies aimed at proving the efficacy of therapeutic means have become increasingly important, test authors—besides adapting their instruments to clinical settings—also have to deal with the problems connected with validating a test for other cultural spheres.

In the following we would like to point out some of the difficulties to be faced in the construction of valid psychometric instruments suitable for use within international therapy evaluation studies. Nevertheless, tests and scales

Human Psychopharmacology, Vol. 4. Edited by I. Hindmarch and P. D. Stonier
© 1993 John Wiley & Sons Ltd

of even perfect validity cannot provide an answer to the question concerning the clinical relevance of improvements. Since, during recent years, discussions have increasingly focused upon the clinical relevance of therapeutic effects, we also make some suggestions for its possible demonstration by means of extended ADL and IADL measures.

Validation of Clinical Tests

Amongst the several classification possibilities of psychometric instruments, one is the subdivision into performance tests, observer-rating and self-rating scales. With respect to their application within the area of dementia, each of these categories bears, as far as validation is concerned, conceptual advantages and disadvantages of its own which impose different problems upon the test author.

Performance Tests

The group of measures probably most elaborated upon consists of performance tests which are widely used in clinical studies for the quantification of the patient's cognitive deficits, considered to be the core symptoms of dementia and related disorders. One of the invaluable advantages of cognitive performance tests can be considered to be their extensive independence of the investigator, which means they would fulfil the criterion of objectivity. Objectivity, defined as the extent to which the outcome of a test remains uninfluenced by the person applying it, forms a necessary—but not yet sufficient—prerequisite for the reliability and validity of a measure.

However, satisfactory validity coefficients of psychometric performance tests cannot be expected if authors do not adapt test materials and administration procedures to the specific demands of the test situation with patients in clinical everyday routine; it is a known fact that elderly people suffering from dementing disorders are more vulnerable to the stress a performance test imposes than healthy persons are. The ambition to perform well on the test hardly ever provides their motivational basis for undergoing a test procedure. Impairments regarded as being characteristic of the disease are very often accompanied by additional deficits, for example, reduced vision, motor abilities or motivation, with the effect that the administration of a test may be rendered far more difficult than in general psychology, if not impossible.

Since many of the psychometric tests frequently applied in clinical psychology were originally developed for testing healthy people, their employment in clinical settings raises the question of their 'ecological' or 'differential validity' which has to be answered whenever a test or scale is administered to persons belonging to a group for which normative data were not raised in the validation studies carried out. Due to the characteristics of dementing disorders and—what holds true for most psychometric instruments—the lack of norm values for samples of elderly patients, it would appear useful to catalogue some criteria which may bear positive effects on the validity of a performance test for patients suffering from dementing disorders.

An important condition for a test suitable for clinical routine is the economy of the procedure. Factors contributing to test economy are time required for application, evaluation and interpretation of the results. Easy handling of test materials, short time required to familiarize oneself with the theoretical basis of the test or the possibility to delegate the administration of the procedure to medical personnel may increase its acceptance on the part of the investigator. Results which are not distorted by a lack of motivation or increasing fatigue, thus yielding information about the patient's 'true' cognitive performance level, are most likely to be obtained when the test is well accepted by the patient. A brief testing time definitely contributes to its acceptance and the patient's willingness to cooperate in the testing session. Moreover, the attractiveness of the tasks to be carried out, the chance to do so successfully—which calls for tasks of low complexity—or an appealing design of the test material may help to maintain the patient's motivation during the test. We also gained the impression that the transparency of the specific requirements of the test may not be underestimated: this means that the purpose of the test should be obvious to the patient, and the atmosphere in which the testing takes place should prevent the patient from feeling under examination stress. As a consequence, the influence of potential sources of error such as lack of motivation to cooperate, weariness or exhaustion towards the end of the test will be reduced. The criteria discussed may be seen as prerequisites for valid results in clinical testing and should be taken into account in the construction phase of a performance test (Erzigkeit, 1989).

Deficits are most accurately measured during the early stages of dementia. In the case of dementing disorders, mild to moderate impairment as far as cognitive or intellectual functioning is concerned clearly forms the main area of interest. Therefore, in therapy control studies, cognitive performance measures often serve as the target variables. But, of course, they can never represent the clinical picture of a patient which may be dominated by changes in personality, emotionality or everyday behaviour. For the assessment of these aspects, rating scales are adequate methods.

Observer-rating Scales

Observer-ratings which require the assessment of the patient by a physician, a psychologist, a member of the nursing staff or a relative bear some principal advantages, and unlike performance tests they do not cause problems concerning economy or acceptance by the patient which may affect validity. Furthermore, they can be administered to severely disturbed patients unable to undergo a performance test. As a rule, the practicability of observer-rating scales has to be regarded as high; on the whole, they are easy to administer and can be repeated ad libitum since learning effects on the part of the patient are for the most part excluded.

The obvious advantages of observer-ratings are counterbalanced by the difficulties in proving the interrater reliability of these instruments, which, on the one hand, stem from the different clinical standards by which raters may judge patients. On the other hand, incompatible interpretations of the contents of an item due to different experiences or to the semantic vagueness of formulations may reduce concordance among raters. As the validity of a test cannot be higher than its reliability, these factors have to be regarded as crucial variables influencing the validity of observer-rating scales. In clinical studies, an attempt is made to eliminate these shortcomings by means of rater training sessions which serve the purpose of finding common standards of evaluation. However, this does not solve another problem, which is that the validity of any rating depends on the competence of the rater.

Self-rating Scales

Self-ratings are to be considered the most direct and economic approach to examining a patient. However, the disadvantages mentioned concerning observer-ratings generally hold true for self-ratings. It cannot be taken for granted that the patient will understand the questions in the same way the author of the scale meant them—a circumstance which will lower the validity of the instrument. A condition indispensable for self-ratings which will obstruct validity if not fulfilled is that the patient has to meet basic requirements with regard to linguistic competence. To avoid a loss of validity, the administration of self-rating scales is not recommended when a patient's IQ is below 85 (v. Zerssen, 1976). Other difficulties which refer mainly to self-ratings, but which cannot be excluded for observer-ratings, are so-called 'response sets'. This means that people filling out questionnaires may show a tendency towards, for example, mid-course or extreme answers or they fill out the form according to what they think is expected of them.

Bearing these conceptual properties of different kinds of psychometric instruments in mind, the next step will be the establishment of a validity coefficient which gives evidence of whether the test or the scale measures what is intended.

Concepts of Validity

The concepts of validity of psychometric tests have their roots in classical test theory, which also provides the theoretical basis for more recent formulations of validity like the ones to be found in the 'Standards for Educational and

Psychological Testing' (APA, 1985). In classical psychological test theory, two main aspects of validity are described: validity referring to theoretical constructs, and validity referring to a criterion. Both kinds of validity may be expressed as coefficients indicating the degree of statistical correlation between the test to be validated and other variables. These variables may be, for example, results obtained with other measures, i.e. criterion validity, or variables which are connected theoretically to what the test claims to measure, i.e. construct validity. As an exact differentiation between the varying aspects is not possible, these terms merely serve for indicating the dominant aspect. So-called therapy sensitivity, the ability of a test to document changes in the course of a disease caused by therapeutic effects, is the most important validation criterion for test instruments used in dementia research.

Outside the area of test theory, where the theoretical concepts of validity as well as empirical methods to establish validity coefficients have been elaborated, we often find that the understanding of the term 'validity' is rather imprecise. As the validity of a test—i.e. the accuracy with which the test measures what it is supposed to measure—should be regarded as the most important criterion in the selection of psychometric tools for any purpose, an uncritical interpretation of validity coefficients reported in test manuals may have severe consequences.

In clinical psychology as well as in psychiatry, it has become part of every-day routine to talk about the patient's personality, intelligence, affectivity or cognitive status in terms of test scores. However, this familiarity with test results makes one often forget that any test score obtained is valid only if the patient under assessment belongs to a diagnostic group for which the validity of the test has been proven in advance. As mentioned before, this well-known fact that a test instrument may be valid only for certain groups but not for others is called the 'differential validity' of a test. To give an example, it is quite unlikely that the WAIS (Wechsler, 1944), a psychometric instrument frequently used for testing intelligence, measures 'intelligence' understood to be a stable trait variable if administered to schizophrenic patients under neuroleptic medication or an intoxicated normal subject. In these cases, the WAIS may only serve for an approximate estimation of transient functional deficits, but does not allow an estimation or prediction of the level of intelligence as measured and defined by the test.

For many of the tests and scales in use, validation studies with elderly patients have either not been carried out at all or, if so, these studies included from a statistical point of view insufficient cases for establishing reliable correlation coefficients. Consequently, norm values for patients suffering from dementing disorders which could serve as guidelines in the interpretation of test results do not exist for most psychometric instruments. Therefore, test scores obtained with tests which have not yet been validated in the area of dementia have to be interpreted very carefully, because owing to moderator variables like the possible lack of motivation, fatigue and stress, it cannot be expected that the original validity coefficients computed on the data basis of other samples remain stable.

According to some statisticians, a more principal problem with regard to validating clinical tests has to be seen in the fact that it does not seem possible to define clinical populations such as patients suffering from dementing disorders or cognitive decline. In consequence, it is impossible to establish truly representative samples of patient groups (Lehrl, 1979) which would allow for an interpretation of test scores in a predictive or inferential sense, i.e. the interpretation of study results being valid not only for the analysed sample but for the whole population. However, one has learned to deal with these problems, and empirically satisfactory results have been published during recent years of test development. Even if it is not possible to fulfil these methodological basic requirements, a fair approximation of the validity of a test procedure may be obtained with an increasing number of congruent results on the basis of comparable patient samples.

Another problem for test authors concerning validity arises from the increasing demand for an international application of test instruments. It has become almost a standard procedure in dementia research to carry out international clinical studies for the proof of therapeutic effects.

International Validation

A large proportion of psychometric instruments employed today in clinical studies are translated versions of tests or scales developed in countries—and that also means in cultural spheres—different from those in which they originated. Of course, the validity of these tests and scales has been investigated in their countries of origin, but, as a rule, there is hardly any information available about the validity of their translations. Consequently, the quality of the results can be drawn into question; direct comparisons between data obtained with several versions of the same test procedure in different countries are—strictly speaking—not possible. In a way, the question of whether a test or a scale will maintain its validity if translated for application outside the culture in which it was developed resembles very much the problem of differential validity.

The demonstration of the international validity, besides final empirical proof, requires first of all the comparison of diagnostic concepts and criteria used in the different countries with the aim of defining comparable patient groups for inclusion in validation studies. In the area of dementia, the criteria established in DSM-III-R (APA, 1987) or by the NINCDS–ADRDA work group (McKhann *et al.*, 1984) or the ICD-10 (WHO, 1991) criteria represent examples for diagnostic orientation. The next step would be a thorough analysis of whether the contents of the scale items or tasks of the test to be translated are transferable to another culture without losing their original meaning or relevance. At first sight, this would seem easy to decide for performance tests measuring cognitive factors or speed of information processing; cross-cultural congruence of cognitive tasks has been approved in empirical studies. Nevertheless, one may also obtain unexpected results demonstrating the necessity to confirm this assumption. To give an example, we would like to refer to validation studies carried out for the SKT (Erzigkeit, 1989), a short cognitive performance test for the assessment of mnestic and attentional deficits of demented patients.

Compared to former editions, the new version of the SKT is distinguished by an improved design in order to enhance its acceptance and practicability and, in consequence, its validity. The new SKT is to be published in five parallel forms in an English and German test version (Erzigkeit, 1991). First results from reliability and validity studies obtained within clinical trials in Germany and the USA are encouraging and clearly show that both test versions can be regarded as parallel tests. The comparison of the US data with the German study results demonstrates the identity of the factorial structure of the SKT for both countries (Kim *et al.*, 1993; Overall and Schaltenbrand, 1992); as the samples participating in the validation studies comprised more than 600 patients the authors assume the international validity and, therefore, applicability of the SKT.

Nevertheless, there were some slight differences to be found concerning the mean scores of some subtests such as 'naming objects' or 'reversal naming'. In these subtests, the patient has to identify and name familiar objects (naming objects) as quickly as possible and to read single capital letters out loud (reversal naming) (cf. Erzigkeit, 1989). In the cross-cultural comparison, a dependence between language and the time needed to name the objects and letters could be established. Although in German studies no differences concerning the time required to fulfil the tasks were revealed between the five parallel forms of the SKT, the US data showed differing time scores, indicating a change of the difficulty of the tasks. These results, in the case of the naming objects procedure, can either be explained by the different length of the English and German names of some objects or by differences of their familiarity between the two countries and cultures. In the case of the reversal naming subtest, the combination of certain letters which are easy to pronounce in one language proved to be 'tongue-twisters' in another. It took more than 3 years after completion of the test materials to eliminate all the sources of error which would have been neither assumed nor detected on the basis of national validation data. In accordance with these experiences, we would like to point out the necessity of being sensitive towards expectations concerning the translation of even performance tests into other languages.

Perhaps even more problems will occur in the transfer of rating scales into other cultures. Before starting to translate an observer or self-rating scale, attention should first of all be paid to the analysis of the theoretical basis and the clinical concepts underlying the scale, which in some cases are not even published. It is of utmost relevance that the translator grasps the basic idea of an item which may be hidden behind its formulation. This, of course, may become a very difficult procedure requiring language capacities as well as clinical competence.

Due to the problems arising from cultural differences of the connotative and denotative meaning of terms, the success of a translation may often be difficult to evaluate. A prominent example for the divergent understanding of terms between cultures is the German word 'Einsamkeit', an accurate English translation of which would be 'lonesomeness'. Although this translation is absolutely correct, the connotative and denotative semantic profile investigated by Osgood *et al.* (1957) or Hofstätter (1966) showed a quite different understanding of the term. 'Lonesomeness' as it is used in the USA was found to be associated with negative emotions, weakness, social withdrawal or depression. The Germans when using the term 'Einsamkeit' associate being alone with more or less dominant aspects of inner peace and strength in a situation stimulating well-being. One may easily imagine to what extent these errors can influence psychopathologically oriented interviews or scores in clinical rating scales. Another difficulty has to be seen in the fact that some items would clearly lose relevance if transferred to another culture. For example, the ability to pay bills with credit cards or cheques can be considered an everyday competence in the USA, but this is definitely not true for Germany. On the other hand, being able to climb stairs is necessary for Europeans commonly dwelling in multi-storey houses without elevators, but this is less so the case for Americans. For rating scales, this must lead to finding 'analogous translations' or 'cultural equivalents'. They may perhaps contain operationalizations other than those in the original scale; the aim should not be a mere word-for-word translation of items.

The given examples may be well known to test constructors. Nevertheless, little effort has been made to avoid these types of error which occur when translating scales. Supposedly, this is mainly due to the additional inconveniences of international validation studies put to test authors after their efforts to validate their test instruments in the country of origin. However, we would like to stress the necessity of providing sufficient evidence for the international validity of tests and scales. But even if internationally validated dementia tests were at hand, a central problem concerning therapy evaluation would remain unsolved and that is the clinical relevance of therapeutic means.

Clinical Relevance

Generally speaking, in clinical studies aimed at proving the efficacy of therapeutic effects the assessment of patients is confined to demonstrating statistically significant differences between a treatment group and a control group. However, psychometric test results and levels of significance *per se* do not allow an evaluation of the clinical relevance of the treatment. For this purpose, additional information is required. So far, there has been no generally accepted definition of the term 'clinical relevance'. Paraphrases of clinically relevant changes such as 'increase in the patient's ability to cope with the demands of daily living' (Kanowski *et al.*, 1990) may convey an intuitive understanding of what is meant by clinical relevance; however, descriptions like this cannot be regarded as operationalizations: they do not contain precise instructions for the measurement of clinical relevance, thus preventing an evaluation of the psychometric outcome measures of clinical studies in terms of the direct benefits the patient received from the therapy.

During recent years, several proposals have been made as to how clinical relevance could be proved: the German Hirnliga, for example, recommended regarding the effects of therapeutic interventions as clinically relevant if statistically significant improvement can be documented on three levels of observation, including psychopathological, psychometric and behavioural aspects (Kanowski *et al.*, 1990). From a methodological point of view, this would seem to be a plausible approach, but considering our knowledge of the course of dementing disorders and clinical experience concerning therapeutic possibilities, the proposal may be too restrictive: at present, it would be too optimistic to expect a drug to improve the symptoms of a demented patient— especially in advanced stages—on all three levels of assessment. Since there is no medication of such a striking therapeutic effectiveness available, it would be sufficient to claim clinical relevance if it turns out to be superior to other medications or therapeutic strategies from a clinical point of view. In order to prevent this proposal from becoming an arbitrary criterion, a restrictive methodological design has to be set up, and the relevant evaluation criterion has to be defined in advance with regard to clinical expertise, i.e. the definition of clinical relevance used in a study must be given *a priori*. If the definition is compatible with international standards, statistically significant changes could be estimated as being clinically relevant even if observed on only one observation level. Of course, these changes should refer to variables or symptoms which are considered to be clinically meaningful.

Furthermore, there has been a proposal to accept the definition of clinical relevance as being either an improvement of more than half a standard deviation in test scores, or exceeding a threshold with regard to the number of symptoms improved or successfully treated patients. But these criteria appear on a methodological basis, as well as from clinical experience, to be too arbitrary to be of any use for a definition.

Quite a different approach to the definition of clinical relevance is described by Braun (1992), which is based on reliability concepts. The outcome measures of a given study are compared under the aspect of significance of group differences as well as with regard to the reliability coefficients of the assessment instruments. Test–retest differences in a repeated measurement design are to be considered 'relevant' if they extend the level of significance and reach beyond error margins caused by a lack of accuracy of the measures or, in other words, their reliability. With this proposal, Braun emphasizes the test instrument as a source for information on clinical relevance. Compared with the recommendations by the German Hirnliga, it has the advantage of a clear theoretical concept which may be approved for almost any test procedure. The Hirnliga proposal tends towards a more clinical approach with the advantage of a practice-orientated evaluation, but bears the disadvantage of, for example, requiring measures for the behavioural assessments which are as yet unavailable; this is at least true for instruments suitable for the early stages of dementia and related disorders.

As far as the documentation of clinical relevance of therapeutic effects in mild to moderate dementia is concerned, changes in activities of daily living seem to be a promising source of information. To demonstrate therapeutic influence on activities of daily living, so-called ADL scales could principally be administered. However, although we collected almost 100 ADL and IADL scales published in English, German or French in our literature study (ADL project group, 1990), we did not gain the impression that there is a scale available for the early stages of dementia appropriate for documenting therapy-induced improvements in everyday behaviour. As ADL scales for the assessment of everyday behaviour were originally developed for estimating the degree of care needed by chronically ill patients and the evaluation of rehabilitative means, most ADL scales at hand aim at the description of rather basic activities like bathing, toileting or eating. The competences assessed in ADL scales may not be considered sufficient to lead a self-supported life at home. Since patients suffering from mild to moderate dementia are, generally speaking, unimpaired with respects to 'classical' ADL, for these patients so-called IADL scales ('instrumental activities of daily living') referring to more complex activities, e.g. using a telephone or shopping, are regarded as being instruments of greater use for assessing therapy-induced improvements of behavioural aspects of everyday relevance.

Nevertheless, there are some critical points which do relate to ADL as well as to IADL scales. Since ADL and IADL scales were meant for application to geriatric patients irrespective of diagnosis, they are not specific enough to reveal deficits regarded as being typical for mildly to moderately demented patients. Furthermore, the sensitivity of the instruments available is too low to detect slight improvements in the course of therapy. A further disadvantage can be seen in the fact that—in order to demonstrate changes which bear direct relevance to the patient's life—ADL and IADL concepts have to be extended by further dimensions such as autonomy, social competence or 'quality of life'. If extended to areas like these, the behavioural assessment of patients in clinical studies would come closer to the WHO's definition of health, which takes into account not only physical health, but also aspects of mental and social well-being (WHO, 1958). Of course, several attempts have been made to develop psychometric tools for the broader assessment of everyday behaviour, but most of the resulting scales are considered impractical owing to the large number of items contained therein. Difficulties to be overcome by a scale suitable for the adequate description of behavioural aspects also arise from the numerous dependencies of everyday activities from intervening variables like gender, social status, multi-morbidity or biographic factors; in order to estimate the relevance of therapeutic effects for a given patient, these dependencies call for scales which ideally allow for individual descriptions. With this goal in mind, we established about 2 years ago a research project with the purpose of constructing a scale for the evaluation of therapeutic improvement on a behavioural level which should be appropriate for patients suffering from mild to moderate dementia (Sclan *et al.*, 1992).

A generally acceptable definition of clinical relevance would ease the evaluation of treatment effects documented in clinical trials. Even if we cannot make a satisfactory proposal and—as we have learned—a definition of clinical relevance cannot be expected on the basis of congruence between observation levels or statistical significance, we would nevertheless like to support these approaches. Prior to a more appropriate solution, they may serve as guidelines, although it may seem necessary in some cases to formulate exceptions. Until we are in a position to define clinically relevant changes in dementia, besides the approaches described we may also refer to global clinical judgements of patients like the CGI (Lehmann, 1984) as a source of information on the clinical relevance of therapeutic effects.

Final Remarks

By now, standardized or generally accepted procedures for the evaluation of the clinical relevance of therapeutic effects in dementia are not available. Recommendations of consensus conferences, clinical consultant groups or representatives of industry, universities or health authorities serve for some orientation (Amaducci *et al.*, 1990; Arbeitskreis 'Klinische Forschung Demenz', 1991; Bekanntmachungen des BGA, 1991). Although they cannot provide final solutions, they do support the discussion concerning clinical relevance and evaluation criteria for therapeutic effects in dementia within the scientific community.

The recent discussions based on FDA papers (Leber, 1990) may serve as an almost paradigmatic example for a vivid and constructive approach to a reasonable *modus vivendi*. We are watching this discussion with great interest. As there is basically very little difference, if any, between the German, European or American point of view concerning the evaluation of the therapeutic efficacy of anti-dementia drugs, we hope it will find resonance and provide an example which can be followed in future discussion in Germany and perhaps also throughout Europe.

One of the topics within the discussion concerned the validity of the CGI assessment procedure. Results published by Lehmann (1985), for example, demonstrate the sensitivity of the clinical global impression. The proposals concerning associated problems such as the independence or redundancy of the CGI within a clinical study remind us of the efforts to obtain higher transparency or objectivity of judgements within the area of 'Gestalt-psychologie' and the psychology of expressive behaviour. In this context, one has learned the risk of a loss of validity if an expert or rater is forced to explain decision steps or the strategies underlying the global impression. If it is true that the validity of global impressions depends on a 'natural' setting or a 'naive' rating procedure similar to a complex pattern perception process underlying, for example, Kraepelin's feeling of praecox, the FDA proposals for the operationalization of the CGI in order to avoid the obvious redundancy would probably not be very successful. However, there is reasonable doubt as to whether results of clinical trials—even if they were designed double-blind—can really prove the validity or sensitivity of the CGI towards changes in the course of the disease, since variables other than those intended may determine the global impression. One example often quoted is that of side-effects which allow the identification of patients treated with an active compound. This knowledge may have an impact on the expert's ratings and could cause a 'validation automatic', i.e. the rater's bias will probably lead to a more or less mutual influence on all measures and judgements.

In order to contribute to this discussion on the basis of empirical data we have established two work groups: the above-mentioned ADL project, and the 'Methoden-Forum' (Erzigkeit *et al.*, 1992). The ADL project is supervised by periodical meetings of interdisciplinary experts who are also participants in the Methoden-Forum. One of the goals within the work group of the Methoden-Forum is the establishment of empirically approved selection criteria for appropriate, internationally validated methods to enable the documentation of therapeutic effects in dementia. To this end, we have launched an international validation study with some selected dementia scales and tests which are already widely used. Of course, the CGI problem mentioned above played a relevant part within the discussion. One of the ADL project's issues is the evaluation of theoretical concepts, methodological basis and clinical experience underlying ADL or IADL scales and related instruments for the assessment of behavioural deficits, as well as activities which may contribute to a patient's autonomy or 'quality of life'.

The dimension and as we also believe the relevance of both projects reaches far beyond the capacities of our research group. Many of the work group consultants and colleagues from industry as well as hospitals or other universities in Germany and Austria support the projects not only by giving advice but also by establishing associated research centres; meanwhile 151 hospitals and universities have entered into the multi-centre study for the validation of international tests and scales in dementia. The Erlangen work group merely coordinates the study and expert meetings.

The ADL work group, aiming at an instrument for a sensitive assessment of changes in behaviour due to therapeutic interventions in the area of mild and moderate dementia, requires great effort and expertise, which in turn requires international cooperation. At least from the methodological point of view there should be a synergism between the projects, as both are concerned with problems of methods and measures in early dementia. After 2 years of extensive work we are still in a position to criticize almost every scale available, yet without an alternative. There is not even a preliminary ADL scale available which we could recommend for a clinical trial, and we can only contribute to discussions with some outlines containing ideas on how we intend to construct the scale. It is of utmost importance to discuss the results of literature research as well as conclusions derived from conferences such as the Methoden-Forum in order to increase the chances of success. As we believe and hope that these issues are of a broad interest, we would be glad if this chapter led to cooperation or further discussion on either the ADL project or our validation studies.

Summary

Basic research and drug evaluation require instruments which have been sufficiently elaborated upon in clinical practice and with approved international validity. The international validation of a test instrument is the *conditio sine qua non* for comparisons of studies carried out in different countries, or international multi-centre studies. Since international validation data are not available for most of the tests and scales, users refer to translations of scales and tests, leading sometimes to decisions between several available versions which for the most part have not yet been sufficiently validated. Informally imparted information on experience with a scale usually determines which one of—sometimes several available—translations will be favoured until there are sufficient validation data published.

It is often presumed that an 'authorized' translation, checked by translating back into the original language, ensures the maintenance of the ideas underlying the items as well as the reliability and validity coefficients originally obtained. This seems plausible for only some performance test procedures measuring cognitive functions such as memory and attention. Difficulties arise, however, when, for example, rating scales are translated for the description and assessment of psychopathological symptoms. Differing connotative and denotative associations may lead to inaccuracies or ambiguities which cannot really be compensated by translators attempting to improve the translation by means of 'translation–retranslation' procedures.

With this contribution, we would like to discuss some of the practical problems arising from our clinical experience. We have learned in clinical practice that we have to evaluate methods and measures more accurately with regard to their underlying validation concepts in order to allow a meaningful interpretation of data obtained in international studies. Consequently, for most of the scales and tests applied in international studies, reliability and validity scores have to be empirically approved for the translated versions. In order to attain the goal of equivalent international versions of a test, it is sometimes necessary to change test material and scale items in order to 'translate' not the written language but the underlying idea: internationally validated test forms will then perhaps change their character from a translation into an 'Analogon'.

Acknowledgement

We would like to thank Catherine Sheppard for her aid in translating this contribution.

References

ADL project group (1990). Alltagsaktivitäten im Alter. Unpublished literature review, Psychiatric Hospital of the University of Erlangen–Nuremberg, Department of Clinical Psychology.

Amaducci, L., Angst, J., Bech, P. *et al.* (1990). Consensus conference on the methodology of clinical trials of 'nootropics', Munich, June 1989. *Pharmacopsychiatry,* **23**, 171–5.

APA (1985). *Standards for Educational and Psychological Testing.* Washington, DC: American Psychological Association.

APA (1987). *Diagnostic and Statistical Manual of Mental Disorders* (3rd edn), revised. Washington, DC: American Psychiatric Association.

Arbeitskreis 'Klinische Forschung Demenz' der pharmazeutischen Industrie (1991). Empfehlungen zur klinischen Prüfung von Arzneimitteln in der Indikation dementieller Erkankungen. *Nervenarzt, 62,* pp. 256–9.

Bekanntmachungen des BGA (1991). Empfehlungen zum Wirksamkeitsnachweis von Nootropika im Indikationsbereich 'Demenz' (Phase III). Gemeinsames Papier der das Bundesgesundheitsamt beratenden Zulassungskommission für, neue Stoff (Kommission A) und der Aufbereitungskommission 'Neurologie, Psychiatrie' (Kommission B 3). *Bundesgesundheitsblatt* **7/91,** pp. 342–50.

Braun, W. (1992) Methodenkritische Analyse einer Langzeituntersuchung am Beispiel von Vinpocetin. In: Lungershausen, E. (ed.), *Demenz, Herausforderung für Forschung, Medizin und Gesellschaft,* Berlin: Springer, pp. 215–230.

Erzigkeit, H. (1989). *SKT, Ein Kurztest zur Erfassung von Gedächtnis- und Aufmerksamkeitsstörungen. Manual* (4th edn), Weinheim: Beltz.

Erzigkeit, H. (1991). The development of the SKT project. In: Hindmarch, I., Hippius, H., and Wilcock, G.K. (eds), *Dementia: Molecules, Methods and Measures.* Chichester: Wiley, pp. 101–103.

Erzigkeit, H., Lehfeld, H., and Branik, M. (1991). Überlegungen zur Anwendung von psychometrischen Verfahren bei der Diagnostik und Therapiekontrolle dementieller Erkrankungen. In: Möller, H.-J. (ed.), *Hirnleistungsstörungen im Alter. Pathobiochemie, Diagnose, therapeutische Ansatzpunkte,* Berlin: Springer, pp. 11–27.

Erzigkeit, H., Lehfeld, H., and Schaltenbrand, R. (1992). 1. Mitteilung des Erlanger Methodenforums: ADL-Konzepte zur Erfassung der klinischen Relevanz. *Geriatrie Forschung,* **2,** pp. 105–109.

Hofstätter, P.R. (1966). *Einführung in die Sozialpsychologie.* Stuttgart: Kröner.

Kanowski, S., Ladurner, G., Maurer, K. *et al.* (1990). Empfehlungen zur Evaluierung der Wirksamkeit von Nootropika. *Z. Gerontopsychol.-Psychiatrie,* **3,** pp. 67–79.

Kim, Y.S., Nibbelink, D.W. and Overall, J.E. (1993) Factor structure and scoring of the SKT test battery. *Journal of Clinical Psychology,* **49,** pp. 61–71.

Leber, P. (1990). *Guidelines for the Clinical Evaluation of Antidementia drugs.* First draft. Washington, DC: Food and Drug Administration.

Lehmann, E. (1984). Practicable and valid approach to evaluate the efficacy of nootropic drugs by means of rating scales. *Pharmacopsychiatry,* **17,** pp. 71–75.

Lehrl, S. (1979). Zur Abhängigkeit der psychopathometrischen Testkonstruktion und Analyse von neuropsychiatrischen Modellen. In: Fischer, B. (ed.), *Erste Klausenbacher Gesprächsrunde. Frühgeriatrie. Diagnostische und therapeutische Aspekte.* Reihe Aktuelle Medizin, Cassella Riedel Pharma GmbH, pp. 74–87.

McKhann, G., Drachman, D., Folstein, M., Katzman, R., Price, D., and Stadlan, E.M. (1984). Clinical diagnosis of Alzheimer's Disease: Report of the NINCDS–ADRDA work group under the auspices of Department of Health and Human Services Task Force on Alzheimer's Disease. *Neurology,* **34,** pp. 939–44.

Osgood, C.E, Suci, G.J., and Tannenbaum, P.J. (1957). *The Measurement of Meaning.* University of Illinois Press, Urbana.

Overall, J.E., and Schaltenbrand, R. (1992). The SKT neuropsychological test battery. *J. Geriatr. Psychiatry Neurol.,* **51,** pp. 220–227.

Sclan, S., Schmidt-Gollas, N., and Erzigkeit, H. (1992). *The Development of an International ADL Scale for Mildly to Moderately Demented Patients.* Dementia Congress, Rome 1991. Berlin: Springer, submitted.

Wechsler, D. (1944). *The Measurement of Adult Intelligence.* Baltimore: Williams & Wilkins.

WHO (1958). *The First Ten Years of the World Health Organization,* Geneva: WHO.

WHO (1991). *Tenth Revision of the International Classification of Diseases,* Chapter V (F): Mental and behavioural diseases (including disorders of psychological development). Clinical Descriptions and Diagnostic Guidelines. Geneva: WHO.

Zerssen, v., D. (1976). *Die Befindlichkeits-Skala. Parallelformen Bf-S und Bf-S'. Manual,* Weinheim: Beltz.

4

Clinical Assessment of Alzheimer's-type Dementia and Related Disorders

Cynthia R. Green and Kenneth L. Davis

Department of Psychiatry, Mt Sinai Medical Center, New York, USA

Introduction

The dementias may be grossly defined as organic diseases of the brain with onset in adulthood, where there is a resulting deterioration of functioning. Dementia is essentially characterized by impairment in memory. This disturbance in memory is associated with deficits in other areas of cognitive functioning, such as impaired judgement, abstraction ability, or language, or with changes in personality functioning. These disturbances may interfere significantly with the individual's usual level of functioning. Symptoms of dementia exist outside of a state of fluctuating consciousness or delirium. For a diagnosis of dementia to be made, there should be evidence of an underlying organic cause, or a lack of evidence for any other cause of the impairment, so that an organic cause of unknown aetiology can be presumed.

There are over 75 identified causes of dementia (see Table 1). In the United States, Europe, as well as in China, health statistics have suggested that approximately 15% of the population aged 65 years or older suffer from some form of dementia, with incidence increasing significantly with age (Hofman *et al.*, 1991; Kua, 1991; Schoenberg *et al.*, 1985; Yu *et al.*, 1989). Of these individuals, about 5% appear severely impaired, requiring either full-time supervision or institutionalization. The financial ramifications of such care is incredible. In the United States, the cost of institutional care for demented patients alone exceeds $25 billion dollars. When one considers that this is only a portion of the costs of caring for demented persons, the overwhelming financial implications of the illness become quite evident. In addition, both in

Human Psychopharmacology, Vol. 4. Edited by I. Hindmarch and P. D. Stonier
© 1993 John Wiley & Sons Ltd

Table 1. Causes of dementia

Degenerative
  Alzheimer's disease, senile and presenile forms
  Parkinson's disease[a]
  Pick's disease
  Huntington's chorea
Vascular
  Multi-infarct dementia[b]
    Carotid distribution
    Vertebrobasilar distribution
    Lacunar syndrome (basal ganglia, white matter, pons)
  Strategically placed large stroke
  Vascular inflammatory disease[a] (systemic lupus, periarteritis)
Toxic
Alcoholic cerebral atrophy[b]
  Chronic bromide or barbiturate intoxication[a]
  Metals: lead, mercury, manganese[a]
  Organic compounds: nitrobenzenes, organophosphates[b]
  Carbon monoxide[b]
Metabolic
  Hypothyroidism[a]
  Repeated hypoglycaemia[b]
  B_{12} deficiency[b] (possibly folic acid deficiency as well)
  Post-anoxic encephalopathy
  Chronic hepatic or portal systemic shunt encephalopathy[b]
  Wilson's disease[a]
  Uraemia[b]
  Non-metastatic effects of carcinoma
Mechanical
  Traumatic cerebral atrophy
  Hydrocephalus[a]: obstruction, subarachnoid infection, and haemorrhage
  Normal-pressure hydrocephalus[a]
  Chronic subdural hematoma[a]
Inflammatory
  General paresis of neurosyphilis[b]
  Chronic meningitis (fungal or tubercular)[b]
  Jakob–Creutzfeldt disease (and other slow virus diseases)
  AIDS encephalopathy
  Multifocal leucoencephalopathy
  Multiple sclerosis
Neoplastic
  Meningioma[a]
  Glioma
  Pituitary tumour[a]
  Metastatic tumour

[a]Potentially reversible cause.
[b]Condition that can be arrested.

From Horvath, T.B., Siever, L.J., Mohs, R.C. and Davis, K.L. (1989) Organic mental syndromes and disorders. In Kaplan, H.I. and Saddock, B.J. (eds), *Comprehensive Textbook of Psychiatry*, Vol. 1 (5th edn), Baltimore: Williams & Wilkins, 599–641.

Europe and in the United States, as well as in Japan, those individuals over 85 represent the fastest-growing portion of the population. Clearly, we can expect both the incidence of dementia and the costs of providing care for affected individuals to rise in coming decades.

Alzheimer's Disease

Of the many causes of dementia, Alzheimer's disease is the most common. It is estimated that Alzheimer's disease accounts for approximately half of all dementias. There are over 1 million persons afflicted with Alzheimer's disease in the United States alone. If one were to include cases with mixed presentations of Alzheimer's disease and another dementing illness, this number would be significantly higher. A recent community study in East Boston of the prevalence of Alzheimer's disease suggested an overall prevalence rate of the illness of about 10.3% in persons aged 65 years or older (Evans *et al.*, 1989). Prevalence studies both in the United States and Europe have shown that the incidence of Alzheimer's disease increases significantly with age, with figures nearly doubling with every 5 years of age increase (Jorm *et al.*, 1987; Rocca *et al.*, 1991; Schoenberg, *et al.*, 1987). Alzheimer's disease appears to be more prevalent in women than in men. At least half of all persons in nursing care facilities in the United States are thought to have dementia of Alzheimer's type (Kay and Bergmann, 1980; Brody *et al.*, 1984). Alzheimer's disease is listed as the fourth leading cause of death in persons over 75 years in the United States.

Alzheimer's disease is distinguished from other types of dementia in its insidious onset and progressive, deteriorating course. In its clinical presentation, the illness is marked by memory loss, and a variety of cognitive disabilities. Pathologically, Alzheimer's disease is characterized by the presence of senile plaques and neurofibrillary tangles. The quantity of senile plaques has been positively correlated with the degree of severity of dementia (Tomilson *et al.*, 1968). More recently studies have found that synapse loss is significantly correlated with the degree of cognitive impairment noted as well (Terry *et al.*, 1991). Other pathological evidence associated with Alzheimer's disease includes generalized cortical atrophy as well as neurochemical transmitter deficits. The disease appears to affect specific neurotransmitters and neuromodulators, with significant deficits in cholinergic functioning noted almost universally in patients with Alzheimer's disease. At this time, the exact cause of Alzheimer's disease is uncertain. Considerations of the aetiology of the illness have yielded several possible causes: a genetic vulnerability, a viral agent or agents, autoimmune causes, environmental toxins, or excesses or deficits in neurochemical systems. Research on the disease's aetiology continues to focus in these areas. A few risk factors associated with the illness have been identified. These include increased age, familial history of the disorder, as well as head trauma.

The onset of Alzheimer's disease may be seen as early as 40 years of age, but is most often seen after age 60. The average duration of Alzheimer's-type dementia from onset to death is approximately 12 years. However, this can vary greatly. The early stage of the illness is generally characterized by the appearance of cognitive impairment, most notably deficits in memory functioning. Memory loss appears to have a gradient effect, with the most recently learned information being lost first. In addition, there are impairments in new learning. Affected persons may also present with primary memory and attentional deficits. There may be a decreased ability to perform instrumental activities of daily living, such as household tasks, i.e. laundry, cooking or managing finances. Affected individuals may also complain of difficulties in complex tasks such as driving, or if they play a sport, such as golf or cards, in their performance. As the illness advances, there is further cognitive decline, which generalizes to other aspects of cortical functioning. Aphasic, apraxic, and other impairments associated with temporo-parietal and frontal lobe deficits are apparent. In addition, patients may present with symptoms of depression, apathy, agitation, or psychotic symptoms such as hallucinations or delusions. In the end stage of the disease, afflicted persons show extreme cognitive deterioration, with an inability to recognize family members, marked language impairment, and motor disturbance. Usually, they are completely dependent on others for even their most basic physical care.

Clinical Assessment of Alzheimer's Disease

Table 2 provides a list of those examinations and laboratory tests necessary for a complete assessment of Alzheimer's disease. Fundamentally, the diagnosis of Alzheimer's disease is a process which involves eliminating all other possible causes of dementia. First, it is necessary to obtain a complete history regarding the presentation of symptoms. In addition to the patient's report, it is essential to have family members (or close friends, if no family members are available) corroborate the history, as they may have observed changes in the person's functioning over time. In Alzheimer's disease, one expects to find a course of insidious onset, with decline that is progressive over time. In most cases, the earliest clinical symptom reported is that of recent memory loss, or an inability to learn new information. Patients and/or their informants may report that the patient forgets appointments, or has to write down information in order to remember it. However, in some cases, the earliest symptom may be a disturbance of language, such as word finding or naming difficulties, or visuo-spatial disturbance, such as getting lost in a family setting. In addition, patients and their families may report changes in the person's ability to manage activities of daily living (ADL). In the earlier stages of the illness, the individual will display marked losses in their ability to do complex independent activities of daily living, such as managing finances, travelling alone, or

Table 2. Clinical assessment for dementia

Complete history
Medical examination
Routine laboratory tests (CBC, SMA-18, UA)
Thyroid function tests
B_{12} and folate levels
VDRL
EEG
Neurological examination
Neuroimaging tests (CT, MRI)
Psychiatric examination
Neuropsychological examination

doing household chores such as the laundry or cooking. Later in the course of the disease, impairments in basic self-maintenance tasks, such as grooming, dressing, eating, and toileting are apparent. The approximate time since the first onset of symptoms is important in determining the course of illness and any decline that has occurred.

The assessment for Alzheimer's disease should include complete medical and neurological examinations. Medical examination should include an exhaustive medical history which covers contributing factors for other possible causes of dementia, such as a history of hypertension or other vascular disorders, alcohol use, head injury, malnutrition, as well as a history of exposure to toxins. Laboratory tests should be done in conjunction with the examination to exclude vitamin deficiencies, endocrine abnormalities, chronic infections, or carcinomas, all which could underlie a presentation of cognitive impairment. A neurological examination of persons in the early stages of Alzheimer's disease can be normal. However, this examination should be done to exclude other types of dementia, specifically the cerebrovascular and subcortical dementias. Special attention should be paid therefore to the presence of extrapyramidal signs or focal signs. This differential can be more difficult in the later stages of Alzheimer's disease, where affected individuals will show some of these signs. In addition, it is possible to have a mixed presentation of Alzheimer's disease and other types of dementia, such as Parkinson's disease and multi-infarct dementia. Therefore, it is crucial that the neurological examination be done with careful attention to the course of illness.

Electroencephalogram (EEG) studies can be helpful in differentiating between Alzheimer's disease and other causes of dementia. Whereas in the earlier stages of Alzheimer's disease one would expect EEG findings of normal activity or diffuse slowing, other dementing illnesses may present with focal presentations which would be noted on EEG.

Neuroimaging studies are an important part of the assessment for

Alzheimer's disease. Computed axial tomography (CT) and magnetic resonance imaging (MRI) studies of the brain may demonstrate generalized cortical atrophy. It is important to note that a normal CT or MRI examination
does not exclude the possibility of Alzheimer's disease. In addition, many
studies have shown that cerebral atrophy cannot reliably distinguish between
Alzheimer's disease and normal elderly persons (Elbe, 1990). However, these
techniques can be useful in distinguishing other possible causes of dementia.
In particular, CT or MRI studies can be very helpful in examining for focal
areas which could underlie other types of dementia.

Cerebral blood flow studies, using positron emission tomography (PET) or
single-photon emission computed tomography (SPECT) techniques, generally show decreased cerebral blood flow and metabolism in the posterior
temporoparietal cerebral cortex of Alzheimer's disease patients as compared
to age-matched normals. The usefulness of cerebral blood flow studies in the
diagnosis of Alzheimer's disease appears to be promising. Generally, the
accuracy rate of PET and SPECT is considered to be around 75%. While
there is concern that the accuracy of these techniques is limited by the significant variability seen in the distribution of metabolic reductions in afflicted
individuals (Elble, 1990), more recent findings indicate that Alzheimer's disease patients can be distinguished by the patterns of cerebral blood flow
changes seen (Holman *et al.*, 1992). Hopefully, further developments with
these techniques will make them clinically useful tools in the diagnosis and
early identification of Alzheimer's disease in the future, when they are ultimately validated against an autopsy-confirmed patient series.

Alzheimer's disease can present with a host of concomitant psychiatric and
behavioural symptoms, such as depression, agitation and restlessness, increased guardedness, and in some cases delusions or perceptual disturbances.
A psychiatric evaluation can be helpful in distinguishing between a primary
functional disturbance, such as depression or psychotic illness, and
Alzheimer's-type dementia. Careful attention should be paid to previous psychiatric history, to distinguish between a repeated episode of a psychiatric
illness presenting in late adulthood and a presentation of primary degenerative dementia.

Evaluation for Alzheimer's disease can be further aided by neuropsychological assessment for cognitive impairment. A battery of cognitive
tests can be useful in determining both the areas and patterns of cognitive
deficit. In many cases, cognitive testing can be the most sensitive tool in
detecting Alzheimer's disease during the early stages. Cognitive testing is
limited in its usefulness in diagnosing Alzheimer's disease at its earlier stages
by a dearth of data regarding normative cognitive functioning of the elderly,
especially in those over 75 years. However, on the whole, cognitive testing
remains of enormous value in the assessment of Alzheimer's disease. Screening tests which tap the cognitive areas where one would expect to see deficits,

such as orientation, memory, language, and praxis, are useful. The Blessed Test and the Mini Mental State Examination are two widely used screening instruments which provide this kind of information. However, screening instruments are limited in their ability to distinguish between Alzheimer's disease and other causes of dementia. For this purpose, a more extensive neuropsychological battery, administered by a trained neuropsychologist, is of tremendous value. A typical battery would include evaluation of major areas of cognitive function, such as attention, sensory perceptual and motor functions, verbal functions, visual functions, memory, executive functions and praxis. In Alzheimer's disease, one would expect to see deficits in memory, verbal and praxis functions, with a global worsening in other areas of cognitive performance over the course of the illness.

A rarely used method in assessment for Alzheimer's disease is brain biopsy. Biopsy of brain tissue to determine whether histopathology consistent with Alzheimer's disease is present is restricted to areas of brain from which tissue can be removed safely. In addition, the lack of clear-cut criteria for differential diagnosis between Alzheimer's disease-affected individuals and normals based solely on histological evidence even further limits the usefulness of this procedure. Studies suggest a failure to determine a definite diagnosis based on biopsy at rates of approximately 25%, while the procedure is associated with a mortality rate of approximately 1–3% (Sim *et al.*, 1966; Katzman *et al.*, 1988).

Diagnostic Criteria for Alzheimer's Disease

At this time, there is no valid and reliable means of definitively diagnosing Alzheimer's disease during life. A definite diagnosis of Alzheimer's disease can be made only post mortem, based on the pathological evidence at autopsy of senile plaques and neurofibrillary tangles, their distribution in the brain, in addition to a clinical history and examination consistent with the disease during life.

Because of the lack of any clear-cut markers for Alzheimer's disease during life, precise diagnosis of Alzheimer's disease has always been problematic. In the past, follow-up studies of patients diagnosed with Alzheimer's disease showed error rates from 20% to as high as 57% (Kendell, 1974; McKhann *et al.*, 1984; Nott and Fleminger, 1975; Ron *et al.*, 1979). A 1980 National Institute on Aging Task Force report found incorrect diagnosis of Alzheimer's disease ranging from 10% to 30% in the general medical population. Because of the obvious difficulties in diagnosing Alzheimer's disease during life, it is imperative that diagnostic criteria be utilized in the clinical assessment and diagnosis of Alzheimer's disease.

The most recent edition of the Diagnostic and Statistical Manual of the American Psychiatric Association (DSM-III-R) places Alzheimer's disease under the category of primary degenerative dementia of the Alzheimer's type.

Table 3. DSM-III-R diagnostic criteria for dementia

A. Demonstrable evidence of impairment in short- and long-term memory. Impairment in short-term memory (inability to learn new information) may be indicated by inability to remember three objects after 5 minutes. Long-term memory impairment (inability to remember information that was known in the past) may be indicated by inability to remember past personal information (e.g. what happened yesterday, birthplace, occupation) or facts of common knowledge (e.g. past Presidents, well-known dates)

B. At least one of the following:
   (1) Impairment in abstract thinking, as indicated by inability to find similarities and differences between related words, difficulty in defining words and concepts, and other similar tasks
   (2) Impaired judgement, as indicated by inability to make reasonable plans to deal with interpersonal, family and job-related problems and issues
   (3) Other disturbances of higher cortical function, such as aphasia (disorder of language), apraxia (inability to carry out motor activities despite intact comprehension and motor function), agnosia (failure to recognize or identify objects despite intact sensory function), and 'constructional difficulty' (e.g. inability to copy three-dimensional figures, assemble blocks, or arrange sticks in specific designs)
   (4) Personality change, i.e. alteration or accentuation of premorbid traits

C. The disturbance in A and B significantly interferes with work or usual social activities or relationships with others

D. Not occurring exclusively during the course of delirium

E. Either (1) or (2):
   (1) There is evidence from the history, physical examination or laboratory tests of a specific organic factor (or factors) judged to be aetiologically related to the disturbance
   (2) In the absence of such evidence, an aetiological organic factor can be presumed if the disturbance cannot be accounted for by any non-organic mental disorder, e.g. major depression accounting for cognitive impairment

Critieria for severity of dementia

Mild: Although work or social activities are significantly impaired, the capacity for independent living remains, with adequate personal hygiene and relatively intact judgement

Moderate: Independent living is hazardous, and some degree of supervision is necessary

Severe: Activities of daily living are so impaired that continual supervision is required, e.g. unable to maintain minimal personal hygiene; largely incoherent or mute

From *Diagnostic and Statistical Manual of Mental Disorders* (3rd edn), revised. Copyright American Psychiatric Association, 1987.

Table 4. DSM-III-R diagnostic criteria for Alzheimer's-type dementia

A. Dementia (meets DSM-III-R criteria for dementia)

B. Insidious onset with a generally progressive deteriorating course

C. Exclusion of all other specific causes of dementia by history, physical examination, and laboratory tests

Subtypes: with delirium; with delusions; with depression; uncomplicated

Note: Code 331.00 Alzheimer's disease on Axis III.
From *Diagnostic and Statistical Manual of Mental Disorders* (3rd edn), revised. Copyright American Psychiatric Association, 1987.

This is further characterized as having either presenile or senile onset, based conventionally on whether onset was before or after age 65. According to DSM-III-R criteria, a diagnosis of primary degenerative dementia of the Alzheimer's type requires that the DSM-III-R criteria for dementia be met (see Table 3), in addition to the presence of an insidious onset and progressive deteriorating course associated with Alzheimer's disease. The exclusion of all other specific causes of dementia, based on history, physical examination and laboratory tests, is also necessary. DSM-III-R criteria include as well subtypes of primary degenerative dementia: with delirium, with delusions, with depression, or uncomplicated. The criteria require that Alzheimer's disease be coded on Axis III as well (see Table 4).

In response to the difficulties in the accurate diagnosis of Alzheimer's disease, the National Institute of Neurological Communicative Disorders and Stroke (NINCDS) and the Alzheimer's Disease and Related Disorders Association (ADRDA) established a work group on the diagnosis of Alzheimer's disease. It was from this group that the NINCDS–ADRDA criteria for Alzheimer's disease were generated (McKhann *et al.*, 1984). These criteria are presented in Table 5. Reports concerning the validity and reliability of the NINCDS–ADRDA criteria have demonstrated a significant improvement in a diagnostic accuracy of early Alzheimer's disease with their use, with rates of accurate diagnoses with confirmation at autopsy ranging from approximately 80% to as high as 100% in some studies using more highly selected samples (Joachim *et al.*, 1986; Kawas, 1990; Morris *et al.*, 1988).

NINCDS–ADRDA criteria allow for a diagnosis of Alzheimer's disease on a definite, probable, or possible basis. A probable diagnosis of Alzheimer's disease may be made on the basis of dementia as documented by clinical examination and cognitive testing; deficits in at least two areas of cognitive functioning; progressive worsening of memory and other cognitive functions; absence of disturbed consciousness; and absence of other disorders or diseases which could account for the progressive deficits in memory or cognition. A diagnosis of probable Alzheimer's disease is further supported by progressive deterioration of specific cognitive functions such as language, motor

Table 5. NINCDS–ADRDA criteria for clinical diagnosis of Alzheimer's disease

I.   *The criteria for the clinical diagnosis of PROBABLE Alzheimer's disease include:*

      Dementia established by clinical examination and documented by the Mini Mental State Examination (MMSE), Blessed Dementia Scale, or some similar examination, and confirmed by neuropsychological tests

      Deficits in two or more areas of cognition

      Progressive worsening of memory and other cognitive functions

      No disturbance of consciousness

      Onset between ages 40 and 90, most often after age 65

      Absence of systemic disorders or other brain diseases that in and of themselves could account for the progressive deficits in memory and cognition

II.   *The diagnosis of PROBABLE Alzheimer's disease is supported by:*

      Progressive deterioration of specific cognitive functions such as language (aphasia), motor skills (apraxia), and perception (agnosia)

      Impaired activities of daily living and altered patterns of behaviour

      Family history of similar disorders, particularly if confirmed neuropathologically

      Laboratory results of:

           Normal lumbar puncture as evaluated by standard techniques

           Normal pattern or non-specific changes in EEG, such as increased slow-wave activity, and

           Evidence of cerebral atrophy on CT with progression documented by serial observations

III. *Other clinical features consistent with the diagnosis of PROBABLE Alzheimer's disease, after exclusion of causes of dementia other than Alzheimer's disease, include:*

      Plateaux in the course of progression of illness

      Associated symptoms of depression, insomnia, incontinence, delusions, illusions, hallucinations, catastrophic verbal, emotional, or physical outbursts, sexual disorders, and weight loss

      Other neurological abnormalities in some patients, especially with more advanced disease and including motor signs such as increased muscle tone, myoclonus, or gait disorder

      Seizures in advanced disease

      CT normal for age

IV.   *Features that make the diagnosis of PROBABLE Alzheimer's disease uncertain or unlikely include:*

      Sudden, apoplectic onset

      Focal neurological findings such as hemiparesis, sensory loss, visual field deficits, and incoordination early in the course of the illness

      Seizures or gait disturbances at the onset or very early in the course of the illness

V.   *Clinical diagnosis of POSSIBLE Alzheimer's disease:*

May be made on the basis of the dementia syndrome, in the absence of other neurological, psychiatric, or systemic disorders sufficient to cause dementia, and in the presence of variations in the onset, in the presentation, or in the clinical course

May be made in the presence of a second systemic or brain disorder sufficient to produce dementia, which is not considered to be the *cause of the dementia*

Should be used in research studies when a single, gradually progressive severe cognitive deficit is identified in the absence of other identifiable cause

VI.   *Criteria for diagnosis of DEFINITE Alzheimer's disease are:*

The clinical criteria for probable Alzheimer's disease and

Histopathological evidence obtained from a biopsy or autopsy

VII.   *Classification of Alzheimer's disease for research purposes should specify features that may differentiate subtypes of the disorder, such as:*

Familial occurrence

Onset before age of 65

Presence of trisomy-21

Coexistence of other relevant conditions such as Parkinson's disease

---

From McKhann, G., Drachman, D., Folstein, M., Katzman, R., Price, D. and Stadlan, E.M. (1984). Clinical diagnosis of Alzheimer's disease: Report of the NINCDS–ADRDA work group under the auspices of Department of Health and Human Services Task Force on Alzheimer's Disease, 1984.

skills, and perception; impairment in activities of daily living (ADL) functioning and behavioural changes; family history of memory disorder; and laboratory results consistent with Alzheimer's disease which do not suggest the presence of other disorders or diseases which could account for the memory and cognitive disturbance noted. A definite diagnosis of Alzheimer's disease requires histopathological evidence of Alzheimer's disease, based on autopsy or biopsy in addition to clinical evidence of probable Alzheimer's disease during life.

The NINCDS–ADRDA criteria also allow for a diagnosis of possible Alzheimer's disease. This diagnosis may be used where there appears to be an atypical presentation of Alzheimer's disease, in the absence of another known cause for the dementia. In addition, a diagnosis of possible Alzheimer's disease may be used when there is a second systemic disorder or brain disease that is known to cause dementia but is not thought to underlie the cognitive deterioration seen.

While the DSM-III-R and NINCDS–ADRDA criteria for Alzheimer's disease are similar in many respects, there are significant differences between them which should be considered. A drawback to the DSM-III-R criteria is the requirement, in the diagnostic criteria for dementia, that the cognitive disturbances present significantly interfere with the person's work performance or usual social activities or relationships. This can be difficult to assess, given that the impact of dementia on the affected person's usual functioning is mediated by their intellectual ability, previous level of functioning, and educational level, among other factors. Thus, one sees significant variation across individuals in the degree to which cognitive disturbance interferes with their everyday functioning, particularly in the early stages of the illness. Hence, the inclusion of this criterion as necessary for the diagnosis of dementia, and therefore Alzheimer's disease, is problematic. The NINCDS–ADRDA criteria do not require such changes in usual functioning for a probable diagnosis of Alzheimer's disease. Rather, such information is identified as supporting a probable diagnosis of the illness. In addition, while the DSM-III-R criteria for dementia implies that evidence of impairment in memory functioning be demonstrated, the NINCDS–ADRDA criteria require that that cognitive deficits be present in two or more areas of cognitive functioning rather than solely in memory functioning, and that these impairments be confirmed with neurocognitive tests.

Differential Diagnosis of Alzheimer's Disease

In considering the clinical assessment of Alzheimer's disease, it is perhaps most important to be concerned with the differential diagnosis of Alzheimer-type dementia from other types of dementing illness. Clinically, this distinction is essential, so that reversible causes of dementia can be identified and, where possible, treated. It is estimated that approximately 30% of those individuals presenting with symptoms of dementia may have a reversible illness (Cohen, 1984). In addition, mixed presentations of Alzheimer's disease with other types of dementia are possible, and not uncommon.

A careful assessment for Alzheimer's disease should include a differential evaluation for all possible causes of dementia. In most cases, a careful review of the patient's history, as corroborated by their family and/or close friends, in addition to a thorough physical examination and a thoughtful review of the laboratory results, will inform diagnostic decision making. In many cases, neuropsychological testing can be helpful in determining the patterns of cognitive deficits, which can aid in differential diagnosis. The evaluation should include consideration of risk factors, as well as the course of onset and clinical presentation, of other dementing illnesses. All causes of dementia should be considered, including relatively uncommon ones.

The cerebrovascular dementias, thought to be the second largest cause of dementia, with an estimated prevalence of about 10% of all dementias seen, are important to distinguish from Alzheimer's disease. Multi-infarct dementia is possibly the most common type of cerebrovascular dementia. As first identified by Hachinski *et al.* (1974), multi-infarct dementia is a dementia which is caused by discrete and multiple cerebral infarcts. Risk factors for multi-infarct dementia include increased age, a history of hypertension, previous cerebral or myocardial infarction, diabetes, or other vascular disorders. Multi-infarct dementia is characterized by an abrupt onset, fluctuating course, stepwise progression, and focal neurological signs, which distinguishes it from Alzheimer's disease. The Hachinski Ischaemic Score (Hachinski *et al.*, 1975) is a widely used instrument aimed at identifying those individuals with multi-infarct dementia, and is often used clinically by those attempting to differentiate between Alzheimer's disease and multi-infarct dementia (see Table 6). However, studies looking at the Hachinski scale have found that it has limited validity, and that its usefulness in the differential diagnosis of Alzheimer's disease and multi-infarct dementia may be restricted (Korczyn, 1991).

Table 6. Hachinski ischaemic score

Feature	Score
Abrupt onset	2
Stepwise orientation	1
Fluctuating course	2
Nocturnal confusion	1
Relative preservation of personality	1
Depression	1
Somatic complaints	1
Emotional incontinence	1
History of hypertension	2
History of strokes	1
Evidence of associated arteriosclerosis	1
Focal neurological symptoms	2
Focal neurological signs (including aphasia or apraxia)	2

In addition, an evaluation for memory disturbance should include consideration of alcohol-related causes, as well as iatrogenic causes of memory impairment. Alcohol-related dementia is the third most prevalent type of dementia seen in the United States. It is seen in about 10% of alcoholics, and typically presents in those individuals with at least a 10–15-year history of chronic alcohol abuse. A thoughtful history of alcohol use should be obtained in any patient complaining of memory disturbance to assist in the differential diagnosis of Alzheimer's disease from alcohol-related dementia. In other cases, possible iatrogenic causes of memory disturbance should be assessed. The elderly are particularly vulnerable to cognitive impairment secondary to iatrogenic causes, due to both the large number of medications they may receive for medical reasons as well as to their increased sensitivity to medications. Therefore, an assessment for memory disorder should include an evaluation of all medications the patient is currently prescribed, their dosage, and any possible interactions.

Other causes of dementia which may be confused with Alzheimer's disease include Pick's disease and the subcortical dementias. Pick's disease, characterized by marked frontotemporal atrophy, usually presents initially with marked behavioural changes. Later in the course of the illness, memory and language disturbances are seen. This is distinct from Alzheimer's disease, where the earlier stage of the dementia is usually distinguished by disturbance in memory functioning, followed later by changes in behaviour. Hence, a careful consideration of the history can be helpful in distinguishing between the two. In addition, neuroimaging techniques can be helpful in distinguishing between Pick's and Alzheimer's dementias. Alzheimer's disease can generally be discriminated from the subcortical dementias (Parkinson's disease; Huntington's chorea) based on a review of the course of illness and a careful neurological examination. While extrapyramidal signs may occur in Alzheimer's disease at the late stages of the illness, as noted above, one would expect to find a normal neurological examination in the early stages of dementia of the Alzheimer type.

Alzheimer's disease should also be distinguished from major depressive disorder, which may present in the elderly with symptoms of pseudodementia. This differential can be a difficult one, as it is not uncommon for persons afflicted with Alzheimer's disease to present with depressive disorder. Again, a careful history of the illness can be essential in making this distinction. Pseudodementia is more likely to be characterized by a prior history of depression in addition to a sudden, abrupt onset on symptoms. In some cases, however, it may be helpful to give a trial of antidepressant medication and to reassess following treatment, or to follow the person longitudinally to determine the course of illness.

Alzheimer's Disease Versus Age-related Changes in Memory

Alzheimer's disease must be distinguished as well from normative changes in memory functioning seen with ageing. The lack of normative data regarding memory changes associated with normal ageing can make this a difficult task, especially in the evaluation of persons over 75 years of age. In addition, methodological issues regarding the use of cross-sectional versus longitudinal techniques have raised questions regarding the normative data which are available (Craik, 1991; Zec, 1990).

Studies of memory functioning in normal ageing have suggested that older individuals experience age-related changes in secondary memory operations, while other areas of memory functioning appear to remain relatively stable (Albert, 1988; Craik, 1991; Zec, 1990). The term secondary memory is commonly thought to refer to long-term memory, or the memory store that can contain an unlimited amount of information for an unlimited amount of time (Albert, 1988). These changes are reflected in decreased ability in the encoding and retrieval of information. Normal elderly generally demonstrate improved performance on recognition versus recall of learned information, suggesting decline in retrieval functions rather than in learning (Craik, 1991; Zec, 1990). Craik (1991) suggests that the normal elderly are more dependent on external factors to cue secondary memory than their younger counterparts, and reports increased encoding and retrieval deficits for elderly subjects on tasks that are increasingly difficult and less supported by the environment. This is further supported by findings of less decrement with age on tasks which involve cueing, such as associational memory tasks.

Comparisons of the cognitive performance of normal elderly controls and Alzheimer's disease-affected individuals have shown that Alzheimer's disease subjects show impairments in all stages of memory, not just in secondary memory. Performance of Alzheimer's disease subjects is characterized by a rapid rate of forgetting when compared to normal controls (Zec, 1990). Zec (1990) suggests that cognitive measures which tap memory performance can be most useful in the differential diagnosis of Alzheimer's disease from age-related memory changes. In addition, Zec and his colleagues have found neurocognitive measures, such as the Alzheimer's Disease Assessment Scale (ADAS) (Rosen *et al.*, 1984) to effectively discriminate between mildly impaired Alzheimer's disease subjects and normal controls, as validated by their Mini Mental State Examination (MMSE) scale score (Zec, 1990).

The ability to differentiate between pathological changes in memory and age-related impairments has been made even more complex by the concept of 'age-associated memory impairment' (AAMI). The existence of AAMI as a separate clinical entity has been proposed (Crook *et al.*, 1986; Youngjohn *et al.*, 1992). The criteria suggested for this proposed classification are where persons at least 50 years of age experience a decline in memory functioning, as indicated by their subjective complaints and documented by performance on an objective memory test that falls at least one standard deviation below the mean performance on that test of young adults.

The establishment of a separate clinical diagnosis such as AAMI is a complex question. Several difficulties can be identified with the proposal for AAMI as it now exists. First, in order for any clinical diagnostic category to be valid, it should be distinguishable from normative findings. Given the dearth of information regarding normative changes in memory functioning during ageing, it seems perhaps hasty to classify as pathological changes which may be normal and universal. In addition, given that the available data suggest that changes in memory function occur normally with ageing, it is difficult to understand why the criteria for AAMI require that objective test performance be compared to that of young normals for diagnosis rather than to that of normal-age peers. It seems that this would lead to an over-diagnosis of AAMI in individuals with what are truly normative, age-related memory changes. Furthermore, the requirement that the individual's test performance fall at least one standard deviation below the mean of this younger sample is problematic. Given the variability one expects to see in performance on the proposed objective cognitive tests across a normative sample, a cut-off such as that proposed runs the risk of a high number of false positive findings, again leading to an over-diagnosis of AAMI. These concerns are substantiated by the findings of Smith *et al.* (1991), who found that in two large samples of cognitively normal elderly 77% and 98% of their samples, respectively, met the proposed criteria for AAMI. Clearly, these issues directly regard the validity of the proposed clinical criteria for AAMI and need to be addressed.

Other difficulties can be identified regarding the discriminant validity of AAMI as a clinical category. A diagnostic entity should have characteristics which set it apart from other diagnoses. One should be able to make such a distinction on the basis of information regarding the antecedent, concurrent, and predictive characteristics of the disorder. At this time, there does not appear to be this type of data to support the establishment of a unique diagnosis such as that proposed. For example, there is no available histo-pathological evidence post mortem to suggest that there is either a specific brain abnormality or a pattern of pathological cortical changes that distinguishes individuals with AAMI from normals. Lastly, it is most likely that individuals who have been identified with this proposed disturbance are actually a heterogeneous group who are suffering from some memory deficits for various reasons, many of which have not been identified, such as exposure to neurotoxins, undiscovered history of head trauma, or undiagnosed small strokes, and that others are early cases of common dementia. Longitudinal studies which have looked at the development of dementia in normative samples, such as that reported by Katzman and his colleagues (1989), have shown that those individuals with mild errors on objective cognitive tests, when followed over time, have a greater risk for the development of common dementias. Perhaps if some of the individuals identified as having AAMI were followed longitudinally, one would see that a significant number of them do ultimately meet diagnostic criteria for common dementing conditions.

Given the above concerns, it seems unjustified to establish a diagnosis of 'age-associated memory impairment' at this time. However, the questions raised by this proposed entity should be addressed further through longitudinal studies of both normative cognitive changes associated with ageing and of those individuals who present with mild memory loss.

Summary

Alzheimer's disease is the most common type of dementia, accounting for approximately half of all dementias seen. Alzheimer's disease is distinguished from other causes of dementia by its insidious onset and progressive, deteriorating course. Clinical assessment for Alzheimer's disease primarily involves the elimination of all other causes of dementia. An assessment for Alzheimer's disease should include a complete history, thorough medical examination, laboratory tests to assist in identifying other possible causes of cognitive disturbance, neurological examination, neuroimaging tests, psychiatric examination, and neuropsychological testing. Alzheimer's disease should be distinguished from other possible causes of dementia, such as multi-infarct dementia, Pick's disease, subcortical dementias such as Parkinson's disease and Huntington's disease, as well as from depression. Finally, attention should be paid to the differential diagnosis of Alzheimer's disease from normative changes in memory seen in ageing.

Bibliography

Albert, M.S. (1988). Cognitive function. In Albert, M.S. and Moss, M.B. (eds), *Geriatric Neuropsychology*, New York: Guilford Press, pp. 33–53.

Alzheimer, A. (1907). Uber eine eigenartige Erkrankung der Hirnrinde. *Allgemeines Zeitschrift für Psychiatire*, **64**, 146–8.

American Psychiatric Association (1987). *Diagnostic and Statistical Manual of Mental Disorders* (3rd edn, revised), Washington, DC: American Psychiatric Association.

Becker, R.E. (1990). Introduction. In Becker, R.E. and Giacobini, E. (eds), *Alzheimer Disease: Current Research in Early Diagnosis*, New York: Taylor & Francis, pp. 1–5.

Brody, E.M., Lawton, M.P., and Liebowitz, B. (1984). Senile dementia: Public policy and adequate institutional care. *Am. J. Pub. Health*, **74**, 1381–3.

Cattell, R.B. (1943). The measurement of adult intelligence. *Psychol. Bull.*, **3**, 153–93.

Cohen, G. (1984) Treatment of Alzheimer's disease and related disorders: Research, practice, and policy. In Kelly, W.E. (ed.), *Alzheimer's Disease and Related Disorders: Research and Management*, Springfield, IL: Charles C. Thomas, pp. 3–17.

Craik, F.I. (1991). Memory functions in normal aging. In Yanagihara, T., and Petersen, R.C. (eds), *Memory Disorders: Research and Clinical Practice*, New York: Marcel Dekker, pp. 347–67.

Crook, T.H., Bartus, R.T., Ferris, S.H., Whitehouse, P. *et al.* (1986). Age-associated memory impairment. Proposed diagnostic criteria and measurement of clinical change—Report of a National Institute of Mental Health work group. *Dev. Neuropsychol.*, **24**, 261–76.

Cummings, J.L. and Benson, D.F. (1986). Dementia of the Alzheimer's type: An inventory of diagnostic clinical features. *J. Amer. Geriatr. Soc.*, **34**, 12–19.

Elble, R.J. (1990). Early diagnosis of Alzheimer's disease. In Becker, R.E., and Giacobini, E. (eds), *Alzheimer's Disease: Current Research in Early Diagnosis*, New York: Taylor & Francis, pp. 19–30.

Evans, D.A., Funkenstein, H.H., Albert, M.S. *et al.* (1989). Prevalence of Alzheimer's disease in a community population of older persons: Higher than previously reported. *JAMA*, **262**, 2551–6.

Fischbach, R.L. (1990). Early identification of demented persons in the community. In Becker, R.E., and Giacobini, E. (eds), *Alzheimer's Disease: Current Research in Early Diagnosis*, New York: Taylor & Francis, pp. 49–74.

Hachinski, V.C., Lassen, N.A., and Marshall, J. (1974). Multi-infarct dementia: A cause of mental deterioration in the elderly. *Lancet*, **ii**, 207–9.

70   *C. R. Green and K. L. Davis*

Hachinski, V.C., Iliff, L.D., Phil, M. *et al.* (1975). Cerebral blood flow in dementia. *Arch. Neurol.,* **32**, 632–7.

Hofman, A., Rocca, W.A., Brayne, C. *et al.* (1991). The prevalence of dementia in Europe: A collaborative study of 1980–1990 findings. *Int. J. Epidemiol.,* **20**, 736–48.

Holman, B.L., Johnson, K.A., Gerada, B., Carvalho, P.H., and Satlin, A. (1992). The scintigraphic appearance of Alzheimer's disease: A prospective study using TC-99M HMPAO SPECT. *J. Nuclear Med.,* **33**, 181–5.

Horvath, T.B., Siever, L.J., Mohs, R.C., and Davis, K.L. (1989). Organic mental syndromes and disorders. In Kaplan, H.I., and Saddock, B.J. (eds), *Comprehensive Textbook of Psychiatry,* Vol. 1 (5th edn), Baltimore: Williams & Wilkins, pp. 599–641.

Hovaguimian, T., Henderson, A.S., Khachaturian, Z., and Orley, J. (eds) (1989) *Classification and Diagnosis of Alzheimer's Disease: An International Perspective.* Toronto: Hogrefe & Huber.

Jablensky, A. (1989). The tenth revision of the International Classification of diseases (ICD-10). In Hovaguimian, T., Henderson, A.S., Khachaturian, Z., and Orley, J. (eds), *Classification and Diagnosis of Alzheimer's Disease: An International Perspective,* Toronto: Hogrefe & Huber, pp. 53–7.

Joachim, C.L., Morris, J., and Selkoe, D.J. (1986). Autopsy neuropathology in 76 cases of clinically diagnosed Alzheimer's disease. *Neuropathology,* **36** (Suppl. 1), 226.

Jorm, A.F., Korten, A.E., and Henderson, A.S. (1987). The prevalence of dementia: A quantitative integration of the literature. *Acta Psychiatr. Scand.,* **76**, 465–79.

Katzman, R., Lasker, B., and Bernstein, N. (1988). Advances in the diagnosis of dementia: Accuracy of the diagnosis and consequences of misdiagnosis of disorders causing dementia. In Terry, R.D. (ed.), *Aging and the Brain,* New York: Raven Press, pp. 17–62.

Katzman, R., Aronson, M., Fuld, P., Kawas, C. *et al.* (1989). Development of dementing illnesses in an 80-year-old volunteer cohort. *Ann. Neurol.,* **25**, 317–24.

Kawas, C.H. (1990). Early clinical diagnosis: Status of the NINCDS–ADRDA criteria. In Becker, R.E., and Giacobini, E. (eds), *Alzheimer's Disease: Current Research in Early Diagnosis,* New York: Taylor & Francis, pp. 9–18.

Kay, D.W.K., and Bergmann, K. (1980). Epidemiology of mental disorders among the aged in the community. In Birren, J.E. and Sloane, B. (eds), *Handbook of Mental Health and Aging,* Englewood Cliffs, NJ: Prentice-Hall, pp. 34–56.

Kendell, R.E. (1974). The stability of psychiatric diagnoses. *Br. J. Psychiatry,* **24**, 352.

Khachaturian, Z.S. (1985). Diagnosis of Alzheimer's disease. *Arch. Neurol.,* **42**, 1097–1105.

Kua, E.H. (1991). The prevalence of dementia in elderly Chinese. *Acta Psychiatr. Scand.,* **83**, 350–2.

Lieberman, M.A., and Kramer, J.H. (1991). Factors affecting decisions to institutionalize demented elderly. *Gerontologist,* **31**, 371–4.

McKhann, G., Drachman, D., Folstein, M., Katzman, R., Price, D., and Stadlan, E.M. (1984). Clinical diagnosis of Alzheimer's disease: Report of the NINCDS–ADRDA work group under the auspices of Department of Health and Human Services Task Force on Alzheimer's Disease. *Neurology,* **34**, 939–44.

Merriam, A.E., Aronson, M.K., Gaston, P., Wey, S.L., and Katz, I. (1988). The psychiatric symptoms of Alzheimer's disease. *J. Am. Geriatr. Soc.,* **36**, 7–12.

Morris, J.C., McKeel, D.W., Fulling, K. *et al.* (1988). Validation of clinical diagnostic criteria for Alzheimer's disease. *Ann. Neurol.,* **24**, 17–22.

Moss, M., and Albert, M. (1988). Alzheimer's disease and other dementing disorders. In Albert, M.S., and Moss, M.B. (eds), *Geriatric Neuropsychology,* New York: Guilford Press, 145–78.

National Institute on Aging Task Force Report (1980). Senility reconsidered: Treatment possibilities for mental impairment in the elderly. *JAMA,* **244,** 259–63.

Nott, P.N., and Fleminger, J.J. (1975). Presenile dementia: The difficulties of early diagnosis. *Acta Psychiatr. Scand.,* **51,** 210.

Perry, E.K., Tomilson, B.E., Blessed, G., Bergman, K., Gibson, P.H., and Perry, R.H. (1978). Correlation of cholinergic abnormalities with senile plaques and mental test scores in senile dementia. *Br. Med. J.,* pp. 1457–9.

Price, D.L. (1984). Neuropathology of Alzheimer's disease. In Kelly, W.E. (ed.), *Alzheimer's Disease and Related Disorders: Research and Management,* Springfield, IL: Charles C. Thomas, pp. 81–104.

Rocca, W.A., Hofman, A., Brayne, C. *et al.* (1991). Frequency and distribution of Alzheimer's disease in Europe: A collaborative study of 1980–1990 prevalence findings. *Ann. Neurol.,* **30,** 381–90.

Ron, M.A., Toone, B.K., Garalda, M.E. *et al.* (1979). Diagnostic accuracy in presenile dementia. *Br. J. Psychiatry,* **134,** 161.

Rosen, W.G., Mohs, R.C., and Davis, K.L. (1984). A new rating scale for Alzheimer's disease. *Amer. J. Psychiatry,* **141,** 1356.

Schoenberg, B.S., Anderson, D.W., and Haerer, A.F. (1985). Severe dementia: Prevalence and clinical features in a biracial US population. *Arch. Neurol.,* **42,** 740–3.,

Schoenberg, B.S., Kokmen, E., and Okazaki, H. (1987). Alzheimer's disease and other dementing illnesses in a defined United States population: Incidence rates and clinical features. *Ann. Neurol.,* **22,** 724–9.

Sim, M., Turner, E., and Smith, W.T. (1966). Cerebral biopsy in the investigation of presenile dementia. *Br. J. Psychiatry,* **112,** 119–25.

Smith, G., Ivnik, R.J., Petersen, R.C. *et al.* (1991). Age-associated memory impairment diagnoses: Problems of reliability and concerns for terminology. *Psychol. Aging,* **6,** 551–8.

Terry, R.D., Masliah, E., Salmon, D.P., Butters, N. *et al.* (1991). Physical basis of cognitive alterations in Alzheimer's disease: Synapse loss is the major correlate of cognitive impairment. *Ann. Neurol.,* **30,** 572–80.

Tomilson, B.E., Blessed, G., and Roth, M. (1968). Observations on the brains of non-demented old people. *J. Neurol. Sci.,* **7,** 331–56.

Youngjohn, J.R., Larrabee, G.J., and Crook, T.H. (1992). Discriminating age-associated memory impairment from Alzheimer's disease. *Psychol. Assessment,* **1,** 54–9.

Yu, E.S., Liu, W.T., Levy, P. *et al.* (1989). Cognitive impairment among elderly adults in Shanghai, China. *J. Gerontol.,* **44,** S97–106.

Zec, R.F. (1990). Neuropsychology: Normal aging versus early AD. In Becker, R.E., and Giacobini, E. (eds), *Alzheimer Disease: Current Research in Early Diagnosis,* New York: Taylor & Francis, pp. 105–17.

5

CODE-DD: Development of a Diagnostic Scale for Depressive Disorders

*Thomas A. Ban, *Olaf K. Fjetland, *Mark Kutcher and †Leslie C. Morey

*Department of Psychiatry, School of Medicine, and †Department of Psychology, Vanderbilt University, Nashville, Tennessee, USA

Introduction

The Composite Diagnostic Evaluation (CODE) system is one of the polydiagnostic methods with an integrated criteria list and standardized data collection. It consists of a set of diagnostic instruments (referred to as CODEs)—each dealing with a different category of illness—which, by specially devised algorithms, can simultaneously assign a diagnosis from several diagnostic systems to a patient.

To achieve its objective, each CODE within the system is comprised of a set of symptoms (codes) which can provide diagnoses in all the component diagnostic systems; a semi-structured interview suitable for the elicitation of all the symptoms in terms of 'present' or 'absent'; and a set of diagnostic decision trees which organize the symptoms into distinct psychiatric illnesses in the component diagnostic systems.

The CODE system differs from other polydiagnostic evaluations in that each CODE includes all the diagnostic formulations which are relevant to the conceptual development of the diagnostic category, and each decision tree within the system is constructed with consideration to the theory that each classification in psychiatry represents a polythetic taxonomy in which different psychopathological symptoms may lead to the same diagnostic structure. A third differential characteristic of the CODE system is the capability to provide readily accessible information relevant to the diagnostic process, from the lowest to the highest level of decision making.

Human Psychopharmacology, Vol. 4. Edited by I. Hindmarch and P. D. Stonier
© 1993 John Wiley & Sons Ltd

Table 1. The 90-item Rating Scale for Depressive Diagnoses (RSDD) with its 40-item subscale, the Rating Scale for the Assessment of Severity in Depressive Disorders (RSADD). Variables comprising the ten 'functional areas' of the RSADD are indicated by the first superscript (1–10). Weights are assigned according to the hierarchical order, i.e. $1 = 1, 2 = 2, 3 = 3$ and $4 = 4$. The order of hierarchy is indicated by the second superscript (1–4). (In the second 'functional area', i.e. Depersonalization/Disorders of the experience of the self, the presence of any of the following variables is given a weight of 4: Thought broadcasting, Thought withdrawal, Thought insertion or Other feelings of alien influence)

1. Genetically on spectrum
2. Genetically pure
3. Impairment of social adaptation in past
4. Medical illness
5. Treatment with mood-depressant medication
6. Precipitating factor
7. Temporal connection
8. Early onset
9. Acute onset
10. Subacute onset
11. Disturbance of concentration[3-1]
12. Hallucinations[2-3]
13. Bodily misperceptions[2-2]
14. Rumination[3-2]
15. Retarded thinking[3-4]
16. Inhibited thinking
17. Constricted thinking[3-3]
18. Tangential thinking
19. Incoherence
20. Ideas of reference[4-3]
21. Delusions[4-4]
22. Thought broadcasting[2-4]
23. Thought withdrawal[2-4]
24. Thought insertion
25. Other feelings of alien influence[2-4]
26. Derealization
27. Depersonalization[2-1]
28. Hypochondriasis
29. Suspiciousness
30. Phobias[4-1]
31. Obsessive thoughts[4-2]
32. Anxious mood
33. Reactive mood changes
34. Depressive mood[5-3]
35. Unmotivated depressed mood
36. Depressive evaluations
37. Parathymia
38. Anxiety[5-1]
39. Dysphoria[8-4]
40. Unmotivated dysphoria
41. Constricted affect[6-1]
42. Anhedonia[6-2]
43. Apathetic indifference[6-4]
44. Feeling of loss of feeling[6-3]
45. Feelings of inadequacy[7-1]
46. Feelings of guilt[7-2]
47. Feelings of impoverishment
48. Lack of interest
49. Displeasure[8-1]
50. Hopelessness[7-4]
51. Self-incrimination[7-3]
52. Irritability[5-2]
53. Hostility[5-4]
54. Vegetative manifestations[9-1]
55. Asthenia[9-2]
56. Corporization[8-3]
57. Felt loss of vitality[9-3]
58. Disturbance of vital balance
59. Complaintiveness[8-2]
60. Driven complaintiveness
61. Lack of drive
62. Decreased sex drive[10-1]
63. Loss of desire to live[10-3]
64. Suicidal tendencies[10-4]
65. Histrionics
66. Motor restlessness[1-4]
67. Abulia[9-4]
68. Motor retardation[1-2]
69. Negativism
70. Parakinesis
71. Diurnal variations
72. Worse in the morning
73. Early insomnia[1-1]
74. Middle insomnia
75. Late insomnia[1-3]
76. Hypersomnia
77. Decreased appetite[10-2]
78. Excessive appetite
79. Indecisiveness
80. Time still
81. Mood congruent psychotic symptoms

82. First episode
83. Manic/hypomanic episode in past
84. Seasonal pattern
85. Prolonged duration
86. Continuous presence in past

87. Responsiveness to somatic treatment in past
88. Full recovery in past
89. Excessive alcohol consumption
90. Impairment of social adaptation

Description of CODE-DD

The prototype of the CODE system is CODE-DD, the CODE that deals with the classifications of depressive disorders. It consists of an integrated criteria list presented in a 90-item Rating Scale for Depressive Diagnoses (RSDD) and its subscale, the Rating Scale for the Assessment of Severity in Depressive Disorders (RSASDD) (Table 1); a Semi-Structured Interview for Depressive Disorders (SSIDD) suitable for the elicitation of the presence or absence of each of the 90 variables of the RSDD; and decision trees which provide diagnoses within 25 diagnostic classifications of depressive disorders (Ban, 1989a, 1989b, 1989c).

Administration of CODE-DD is completed during a 30–40-minute interview which can be carried out with or without computer prompting. (The computer program employed was written in the FORTRAN programming language for the MS–DOS operating system.)

Severity Scale

The RSASDD, the subscale of the RSDD, consists of 40 items. These are grouped under ten headings (functional areas), each representing a different affected area (or different dimension within an affected area) of mental functioning in depressive illness. The four items included in each of the ten functional areas are ranked in hierarchical order with each item assigned a score (weight) from 1 to 4. In the ultimate analysis, however, the RSASDD provides one interpretable score only. This total score is based on the sum of the ten component scores, i.e. one score—the highest score—from each of the functional areas. Accordingly, the severity score of RSASDD ranges from 0 to 40, with 0 representing the lowest and 40 the highest degree of severity of the depressive disorder.

Diagnostic Classifications

To attain a diagnosis in each of the 25 classifications of CODE-DD, symptoms in the component classifications were transformed in a manner to correspond to variables of the RSDD; and diagnostic decision trees were constructed in a manner to be based exclusively on symptoms included in the RSDD. Since administration of the SSIDD elicits the information necessary for the scoring—in terms of present or absent—of each variable on the diagnostic decision trees, by employing the SSIDD and scoring the variables of the diagnostic decision trees—by hand or computer—25 diagnoses are obtained. Of the diagnostic systems included in CODE-DD, three are based on the conceptual development of the classifications of depressive disorders (and syndromes) in Europe and three on the conceptual development of the classifications of depressive disorders (and syndromes) in North America; two are consensus-based classifications, one based primarily on the consensus of experts in Europe (ICD-10) and the other on the consensus of experts in North America (DSM-III-R); ten are empirical classifications, the result of factor or cluster analyses of psychiatric rating scales; six are miscellaneous classifications; and one is a composite diagnostic classification (CDC), based on the different classifications included in CODE-DD (Table 2).

Table 2. The 25 classifications (identified by the authors) included in the Composite Diagnostic Evaluation of Depressive Disorders (CODE-DD)

Conceptual development	Empirically deprived	Miscellaneous
Europe	Lewis (1934)	Berner *et al.* (1983)
Kraepelin (1896, 1921)	Hamilton and White	Kielholz (1972)
Schneider (1920, 1959)	(1959)	Klein (1973, 1974)
Leonhard (1957, 1979)	Kiloh and Garside (1963)	Pollitt (1965)
	Pilowsky *et al.* (1969)	Taylor (1986)
North America	Mendels and Cochrane	Winokur (1974, 1979)
Robins and Guze (1972)	(1968)	
Feighner *et al.* (1972)	Foulds (1973, 1976)	*Composite*
Spitzer *et al.* (1978)	Overall *et al.* (1966)	Ban (1989a, 1989b, 1989c)
	Paykel (1971)	
Consensus	Raskin and Crook (1976)	
Europe	Wing *et al.* (1974)	
WHO (1988)		
America		
APA (1987)		

The three classifications included under the conceptual development of European classifications are Kraepelin's (1896, 1921), Schneider's (1920, 1959) and Leonhard's (1957, 1979); and the three classifications included under the conceptual development of North American classifications are Robins and Guze's (1972), the St Louis Criteria of Feighner *et al.* (1972), and the Research Diagnostic Criteria of Spitzer *et al.* (1978).

In the European development, Kraepelin's (1896, 1921) unitary concept of depressive states, an integral part of manic-depressive insanity, was extended by Schneider (1920, 1959) into the trichotomy of vital depression, reactive depression and depressive psychopathy; and Schneider's (1920, 1959) unitary concept of vital depression was divided by Leonhard (1957, 1979) into bipolar and unipolar depression with the separation of pure (complete) melancholia from the five distinct subforms of pure (incomplete) depression in the unipolar group. There was also a shift in emphasis in terms of the cardinal symptoms from thought retardation and decreased drive in depressive states (Kraepelin, 1896, 1921), through corporization in vital depression (Schneider, 1920, 1959), to apathetic indifference in pure melancholia (Leonhard, 1957).

In the North American development, somewhat similar to the European development, Kraepelin's (1921) unitary concept of depression was extended by Robins and Guze (1972) into the dichotomy of primary and secondary depressive disorders. These, in turn, were divided in the St Louis Criteria by Feighner *et al.* (1972) into probable and definite primary and secondary depressions, respectively. In a further step, the primary and secondary dichotomy was replaced in the Research Diagnostic Criteria of Spitzer *et al.* (1978) by the dichotomy of major and minor depression.

Development of empirically derived classifications was triggered by the publication of Lewis's (1934) clinical survey of depressive states in which, on the basis of a detailed analysis of 61 cases, he put forward a unitary concept of melancholia. Nevertheless, in subsequent years by employing factor and cluster analyses on different rating scale data, Lewis's (1934) unitary concept of melancholia was divided into two to four distinct depressive syndromes (Table 3).

Among the miscellaneous classifications, Kielholz's (1972) is a pragmatic, aetiologically orientated classification in which somatogenic, psychogenic and endogenous depressions are separated; Winokur's (1974, 1982) is a genetically orientated classification in which pure depression, depressive spectrum disease and sporadic depression are separated; and Pollitt's (1965) is a target-orientated classification based on the separation of psychological type J depression from physiological type S depression.

Of the remaining miscellaneous classifications, Klein's (1973, 1974) trichotomy of endogenomorphic depression, acute dysphoria and chronic neurotic dysphoria shows some resemblance to Schneider's (1959), whereas, the Berner *et al.* (1983) dichotomy of endogenomorphic–depressive and endogenomorphic–dysphoric axial syndromes, i.e. the Vienna Research Criteria (Berner *et al.*, 1983), is distinct from all other classifications, by its strong emphasis on biorhythmic and sleep disturbances. Finally, Taylor's (1986) classification—based on publications by Taylor and Abrams (1978) and Taylor *et al.* (1981)—seems to provide a bridge between European and American classifications of depression.

Reliability of CODE-DD

An essential prerequisite of a diagnostic instrument to be used in clinical practice and psychiatric research is that it yields similar (i.e. reliable) diagnoses when employed by different assessors. The level of reliability is a good

Table 3. Depressive syndromes divided by factor and cluster analyses. (The one in parentheses is not included in CODE-DD)

Lewis (1934)	Melancholia			
Mendels and Cochrane (1968)	Endogenous depression			
Hamilton and White (1959)	Retarded depression	Agitated depression		
Kiloh and Garside (1963)	Endogenous depression	Neurotic depression		
Pilowsky *et al.* (1969)	Class A Endogenous depression	Class B Neurotic depression		
Foulds (1976)	Psychotic depression	Neurotic depression	Dysthymic depression	
Overall *et al.* (1966)	Type A Anxious depression	Type B Hostile depression	Type C Retarded depression	
Wing *et al.* (1974)	Class D Depressive psychosis	Class R Retarded depression	Class N Neurotic depression	
Paykel (1971)	Group 4A Psychotic depression	Group 4B Anxious depression	Group 4C Hostile depression	(Group 4D Young depressive with personality disorder)
Raskin and Crook (1976)	Type 1 Agitated depression	Type 2 Neurotic depression	Type 3 Endogenous depression	Type 4 Poor premorbid personality depression

indicator of to what extent assessor bias is outweighed by the rules set for deriving diagnostic decisions. Since testing for reliability may also focus attention on hidden shortcomings, in the development of CODE-DD reliability studies have played an important role.

First Study

Although the original CODE-DD manual (Ban, 1989a) was written in English, development of CODE-DD (from the time of its inception) took place in an international setting. Accordingly, in the first reliability study—in which seven psychiatrists viewed seven videotaped interviews (conducted in English) of depressed patients—the primary languages of the assessors were Hungarian, Italian and Spanish. In spite of this, there was an 87.8% median inter-rater agreement regarding the presence or absence of the 90 CODE-DD variables. Only for five variables, i.e. impairment of social adaptation in the past, delusions, thought broadcasting, driven complaintiveness and first episode, did the level of reliability fail to exceed that which one would have expected by chance.

Since reliability of the different diagnostic systems in CODE-DD is a function of the reliability of the component variables of the respective system, there was a considerable variation in reliability in the different diagnostic systems. Nevertheless, the median percentage agreement for the 25 diagnostic systems was 72%, with a median overall kappa coefficient of 0.439.

It was noted that the CODE-DD Severity Score had an intraclass correlation of 0.706 (Morey, 1991a).

Second Study

On the basis of findings in the first reliability study, CODE-DD was revised before conducting a second reliability study. In this second study, five videotaped interviews of depressed patients were viewed by four assessors, i.e. two qualified psychiatrists and two psychiatric residents. In variance with the first reliability study, however, the primary language of all the assessors in the second study was English.

There was a considerable difference in terms of reliability measures between the results of the first and second studies. This was to the extent that median percentage agreement on the 90 CODE-DD variables improved from 87.8% to 100%. Nevertheless, reliability of five variables, including first episode, family history of affective illness, temporal connection (as relevant to precipitating factor), dysphoria and apathetic indifference, remained below a desirable level.

Improvement in reliability of variables was reflected in the improvement of reliability in the different diagnostic systems. Accordingly, median percentage agreement for the 25 diagnostic systems was 74%, with a median overall kappa coefficient of 0.519. In variance with expectations, reliability was not found to be a function of the level of experience.

It was noted that the CODE-DD Severity Score in the second study had an intraclass correlation of 0.790.

Third Study

On the basis of findings in the second reliability study, CODE-DD was further revised and its computerized version finalized. Consequently, the third reliability study was conducted with the use of the computer to derive the final diagnoses.

In variance with the first and second reliability studies, in the third reliability study two psychiatrists participated in live interviews with seven depressed patients, one conducting and the other observing the interview, while each used the CODE-DD computer program independently to arrive at the final diagnoses. As a result, median percentage agreement on the 90 CODE-DD variables was 100%, with a median percentage agreement of 100% for the 25 diagnostic systems and a median overall kappa coefficient of 1.00. Only in 9 of the 25 diagnostic systems was there less than perfect diagnostic agreement; the lowest diagnostic agreement for any of the diagnostic systems was 71.4%.

It was noted that the CODE-DD Severity Score in the third study had an intraclass correlation of 0.992, i.e. a correlation substantially greater than that of the second study.

With consideration of findings in the third study, it was concluded that the objective of reliability studies had been achieved and that the revised CODE-DD (on the basis of the first and second reliability studies), can be used in a highly reliable manner.

Validity of CODE-DD

In the absence of generally recognized standards, validation studies with CODE-DD have been directed primarily at establishing relationships between CODE-DD measures and measures of different assessment instruments commonly employed in the study of depressive disorders.

The CODE-DD Severity Scale was constructed with the hope that it would reflect the severity of depressive disorder. To fulfil its purpose, one would expect that its severity score would be consistent with the total scores of widely accepted depression scales employed primarily in the assessment of change in these disorders.

First Study

To study the consistency between the CODE-DD Severity Score and the total scores of the Hamilton Rating Scale for Depression (HAM-D; Hamilton, 1960) and the Beck Depression Inventory (BDI; Beck and Steer, 1987), the CODE-DD, HAM-D and BDI were administered to 66 adult inpatients with a clinical diagnosis of depressive disorder. As a result, it was found that there were significant ($p < 0.001$) and strong associations between the CODE-DD Severity Score and the total score of the 17-item HAM-D (correlation = 0.785), the total score of the 21-item HAM-D (correlation = 0.815) and the total score of the BDI (correlation = 0.689).

A subsample of 28 patients of the 66 patients included in the first validity study were re-evaluated with the same assessment instruments after an average interval of 16 days from the initial assessment. As a result, it was found that correlations between the CODE-DD Severity Score and the total score of the 17-item HAM-D, the total score of the 21-item HAM-D and the total score of the BDI were even higher (i.e. 0.912, 0.894 and 0.775, respectively) at follow-up than at the time of the initial evaluation.

In Table 4 the mean CODE-DD Severity Score and the mean total scores of the HAM-D (17-item) and BDI are presented at the time of the initial and at the time of the follow-up assessment, with the percentage of change between the two assessments. As shown in the table, the extent of change was quite comparable. The correlation between the percentage change of the CODE-DD Severity Score and the percentage change of the total score of the HAM-D was 0.866, and the correlation between the percentage change of the CODE-DD Severity Score and the percentage change of the BDI total score was 0.692. Each of these correlations was highly significant ($p < 0.001$).

Table 4. Mean CODE-DD Severity Score and mean total scores of the HAM-D (17-item) and BDI at the time of the initial and at the time of the follow-up evaluation, with the percentage of change between the two assessments. Note that only 24 patients completed the BDI at both assessment periods

Assessment instruments	N	Mean scores		
		Initial evaluation	Follow-up evaluation	Percentage change
CODE-DD Severity Score	28	30.46	15.36	49.4
HAM-D (17-item) total score	28	23.14	11.04	52.6
BDI total score	24	33.13	13.00	60.9

Second Study

To study the consistency between the CODE-DD Severity Scale and the depression scale or subscale of assessment instruments which were not developed exclusively for the assessment of depression, the CODE-DD, the Brief Psychiatric Rating Scale (BPRS; Overall & Gorham, 1962) and the Personality Assessment Inventory (PAI; Morey, 1991b) were administered to 44 patients in a second study. As a result, it was found that there is a highly significant correlation between the CODE-DD Severity Score and the score of the depressed mood scale of the BPRS (0.7401, $p < 0.001$); the score of the depression scale of the PAI, and scores of the three subscales of the depression scale (i.e. affective, cognitive and physiological) of the PAI (Table 5).

Table 5. Mean CODE-DD Severity Score and mean scores of the BPRS depressed mood scale and the PAI depression scale and its three subscales

CODE-DD	BPRS	PAI			
	Depressed mood	Depression scale	Affective subscale	Cognitive subscale	Physiological subscale
Severity score	0.740**	0.789**	0.725**	0.721**	0.677**

**p < 0.001.

Table 6. Correlations between functional area scores of CODE-DD Severity Scale and scores of specific scales of the BPRS, and scores on the three subscales of the depression scale of PAI

CODE-DD	BPRS		PAI		
Functional areas	Guilt feelings	Motor retardation	Depression—affective	Depression—cognitive	Depression—physiological
Early insomnia/ Motor restlessness	0.308	0.258	0.349	0.312	0.649**
Depersonaliza-tion/Disorders of the experience of the self	0.205	0.315	0.341	0.359	0.290
Disturbance of concentration/ Retarded thinking	0.312	0.448*	0.578**	0.525*	0.677**
Phobias/ Delusions	−0.157	0.396*	0.514*	0.498*	0.251
Anxiety/ Hostility	0.340	0.519**	0.741**	0.803**	0.595**
Constricted affect/ Apathetic indifference	0.360	0.409*	0.566**	0.560**	0.422
Feelings of inadequacy/ Hopelessness	0.476*	0.429*	0.613**	0.629**	0.568**
Displeasure/ Dysphoria	0.557**	0.382	0.493*	0.533*	0.488*
Vegetative manifesta-tions/Abulia	0.331	0.473*	0.651**	0.600**	0.505*
Decreased sex drive/Suicidal tendencies	0.340	0.647**	0.612**	0.603**	0.545**

*p < 0.01; **p < 0.001.

In the same study, as shown in Table 6, there were also significant correlations between some of the functional area scores of the CODE-DD Severity Scale and scores on some of the specific scales of the BPRS, as well as on scores of one or another subscales of the depression scale of the PAI.

Concluding Remarks

In the foregoing development of CODE-DD, a polydiagnostic evaluation of depressive disorders was outlined, and findings of reliability and validity studies with CODE-DD were briefly reviewed. It was pointed out that CODE-DD can be used in a highly reliable manner, and that the severity score of CODE-DD shows consistency with the severity score of scales employed in the assessment of change of depressive disorders.

At present, CODE-DD is employed in nosological research and in multi-centre clinical investigations with potential antidepressants. To facilitate its use (in addition to the English original), CODE-DD is available in Italian and Polish, and several additional translations, including Estonian, French, Portuguese, Russian and Spanish, are in advanced stages of their development.

References

American Psychiatric Association. (1987). *Diagnostic and Statistical Manual of Mental Disorders* (3rd edn), Washington: American Psychiatric Association.
Ban, T.A. (1989a). *CODE-DD: Composite Diagnostic Evaluation of Depressive Disorders*, Brentwood: J.M. Productions.
Ban, T.A. (1989b). CODE-DD: *Composite Diagnostic Evaluation of Depressive Disorders*, translated by E. Aguglia,, Padova: Liviana Editrice SpA.
Ban, T.A. (1989c). CODE-DD: *Composite Diagnostic Evaluation of Depressive Disorders*, translated by S. Pużyński, M. Jarema and J. Wdowiak, Poland: Prasowe Zaklady Graficzne w Koszalinie.
Beck Depression Inventory Manual. San Antonio: Psychological Corporation.
Berner, P., Gabriel, E., Katschnig, H., Kieffer, W., Koehler, K., Lenz, G., and Simhandl, C. (1983). *Diagnostic Criteria for Schizophrenia and Affective Psychoses*, Washington: World Psychiatric Association and American Psychiatric Association.
Feighner, J.P., Robins, E., Guze, S.B., Woodruff, J.P., Winokur, G. and Munoz, R. (1972). Diagnostic criteria for use in psychiatric research. *Arch. Gen. Psychiatry*, **26**, 57–63.
Foulds, G.A. (1973). The relationship between the depressive illnesses. *Br. J. Psychiatry*, **122**, 531–3.
Foulds, G.A. (1976). *The Hierarchical Nature of Personal Illness*, Orlando, FL: Academic Press.
Hamilton, M. (1960). A rating scale for depression. *J. Neurol Neurosurg. Psychiatry*, **23**, 56–62.
Hamilton, M., and White, J.M. (1959). Clinical syndromes in depressive states. *J. Ment. Sci.*, **150**, 985–90.
Kielholz, P. (1972). Diagnostic aspects in the treatment of depression. In: Kielholz, P. (ed.), *Depressive Illness*, Bern: Hans Hubert.

Kiloh, L.G., and Garside, R.F. (1963). The independence of neurotic depression and endogenous depression. *Br. J. Psychiatry,* **109**, 451–63.

Klein, D.F. (1973). Drug therapy as a means of syndromal identification and nosologic revision. In: Cole, J.O., Friedman, A.M., and Friedhoff, A.J. (eds), *Psychopathology and Psychopharmacology,* Baltimore: Johns Hopkins University Press.

Klein, D.F. (1974). Endogenomorphic depression. *Arch. Gen. Psychiatry,* **31**, 447–54.

Kraepelin, E. (1896). *Psychiatrie* (5th edn), Leipzig: Barth.

Kraepelin, E. (1921). *Manic-depressive Insanity and Paranoia,* translated by R. Mary Barclay, Edinburgh: Livingstone.

Leonhard, K. (1957). *Aufteilung der endogenen Psychosen,* Berlin: Akamedie-Verlag.

Leonhard, K. (1979). *The Classification of Endogenous Psychoses,* translated by Russell Berman, New York: Irvington.

Lewis, A. (1934). Melancholia: A clinical survey of depressive states. *J. Ment. Sci.,* **80**, 277–378.

Mendels, J., and Cochrane, C. (1968). The nosology of depression: The endogenous-reactive concept. *Am. J. Psychiatry,* **124** (Suppl.), 1–11.

Morey, L.C. (1991a). Reliability considerations in the development of CODE-DD. In Aguglia, E., and Ban, T.A. (eds), *International Symposium on Functional Psychoses Today,* London: John Libby, pp. 297–304.

Morey, L.C. (1991b). *The Personality Assessment Inventory Professional Manual.* Odessa, FL: Psychological Assessment Resources.

Overall, J.E., and Gorham, D.R. (1962). The brief psychiatric rating scale. *Psychol. Rep.,* **10**, 799–812.

Overall, J.E., Hollister, L.E., Johnson, M., and Pennington, V. (1966). Nosology and depression and differential response to drugs. *JAMA,* **195**, 946–8.

Paykel, E.S. (1971). Classification of depressive patients: A cluster analysis derived grouping. *Br. J. Psychiatry,* **118**, 275–88.

Pilowsky, I., Levine, S., and Boulton, D.M. (1969). The classification of depression by numerical taxonomy. *Br. J. Psychiatry,* **115**, 937–945.

Pollitt, J.D. (1965). Suggestions for a physiological classification of depression. *Br. J. Psychiatry,* **111**, 489–95.

Raskin, A., and Crook, T. (1976). The endogenous–neurotic distribution and a predictor of response to antidepressant drugs. *Psychol. Med.,* **6**, 59–70.

Robins, E., and Guze, S.B. (1972). Classification of affective disorders: The primary-secondary, endogenous–reactive and the neurotic–psychotic concepts. In: Williams, T.A., Katz, M.M., and Shield, J.A. (eds), *Recent Advances in Psychobiology of the Depressive Illnesses,* Washington, DC: US Government Printing Office, pp. 283–293.

Schneider, K. (1920). Die Schichtung des emotionalen Lebens und der Aufban der Depressions Zustande. *Z. Ges. Neurol. Psychiat.,* **58**, 281–5.

Schneider, K. (1959). *Clinical Psychopathology,* translated by M.W. Hamilton, New York: Grune & Stratton.

Spitzer, R.L., Endicott, J., and Robins, E. (1978). *Research Diagnostic Criteria (RDC) for a Selected Group of Functional Disorders* (3rd edn), New York: New York State Psychiatric Institute (updated 1980).

Taylor, M.A. (1986). *The Neuropsychiatric Mental Status Examination,* New York: Pergamon Press.

Taylor, M.A., and Abrams, R. (1978). The prevalence of schizophrenia: A reassessment using modern diagnostic criteria. *Am. J. Psychiatry,* **135**, 945–8.

Taylor, M.A., Redfield, J., and Abrams, R. (1981). Neuropsychological dysfunction in schizophrenia and affective disease. *Biol. Psychiatry,* **16**, 467–8.

Wing, J.K., Cooper, J.E., and Sartorius, N. (1974). *Measurement and Classification of Psychiatric Symptoms*, Cambridge: Cambridge University Press.

Winokur, G. (1982). The development and validity of familial subtypes in primary unipolar depression. *Pharmacopsychiatria,* **15**, 142–6.

Winokur, G. (1974). The division of depressive illness into depressive spectrum disease and pure depressive disease. *Int. Pharmacopsychiat.,* **9**, 5–13.

Winokur, G. (1979). Unipolar depression: Is it divisible into autonomous subtypes? *Arch. Gen. Psychiatry,* **36**, 47–52.

World Health Organization (1988). ICD-10, 1987 Draft of Chapter V, Categories F00–F99, *Mental, Behavioral and Developmental Disorders: Clinical Descriptions and Diagnostic Guidelines.* Geneva: World Health Organization, Division of Mental Health (WHO/MNH/MEP/87.1 Rev. 2).

6

Assessing the Consequences of Regulatory Intervention on Psychotropic Drugs

*D. B. Fairweather and †N. Rombaut

*Human Psychopharmacology Research Unit, University of Surrey, and †Quintiles UK Ltd, Reading, UK

Post-marketing Surveillance

Success in development of new medicines to combat disease is the lifeblood of the ethical R&D-based pharmaceutical industry. An innovative product with preliminary evidence of an improved risk/benefit profile is a source of hope for clinicians and for patients. No responsible ethical pharmaceutical manufacturer believes that the duty of the company to clinicians and the patient community ends with the authorization to market the product. In the period after the grant of a product licence, medical and marketing aims must find common ground to ensure that the use of the medicine by physicians worldwide is appropriate and effective, based on continuous, rapid dissemination of up-to-date knowledge of the product profile. Information on usage, therapeutic profile, incidence of side-effects and drug–drug interactions has to be clearly and rapidly incorporated into the product data-sheet as the evolution of use progresses and more information becomes available.

Post-marketing surveillance (PMS) studies are a part of this process. The term PMS as used here describes observational, non-interventional cohort studies undertaken after the launch of a new medicine into the market. PMS, in the pharmacoepidemiological sense, describes methods based on anonymized data from a number of sources, including patients' clinical histories, government agencies such as the UK Prescription Pricing Authority (PPA) who contribute data for Prescription Event Monitoring (PEM), and record linkage systems of various kinds, e.g. Medicines Evaluation and Monitoring Organization (MEMO) and the UK-based VAMP Research group. Well

Human Psychopharmacology, Vol. 4. Edited by I. Hindmarch and P. D. Stonier
© 1993 John Wiley & Sons Ltd

planned and conducted PMS studies can contribute to knowledge of the safety and effectiveness of a drug treatment, but a report by UK Committee on Safety of Medicines (CSM) representatives in the *British Medical Journal* (Waller *et al.*, 1992) criticized the efforts of pharmaceutical companies in this area: 'Our data suggest that company-sponsored post marketing surveillance studies, as conducted under the quadripartite guidelines, have made little contribution to regulatory monitoring of drug safety over the past four years'. Recently, a senior member of the UK CSM commented to an international pharmaceutical industry audience, 'I would advocate that PMS be placed in the hands of an independent institute of medicines monitoring jointly funded by the industry and government. Such a body could set standards, approve and monitor all PMS studies. It would report its findings to the UK Licensing Authority. Until such a system is established, PMS is likely to gain little scientific credibility' (Asscher, 1992).

Product safety requires an efficient programme of information exchange, post-marketing surveillance, and updating and consulting between the company, the medical profession as well as national and international regulatory authorities. This dialogue is essential in the event of the occurrence of adverse events not identified in the pre-licensing clinical programme. A significant amount of this information comes from surveillance methods based on spontaneous ADR reporting to the national data collection centre. National drug surveillance schemes in the US, Japan and Europe and those of the WHO, the International Medical Benefit–Risk Foundation (IMBRF) and the newly formed German Drug Safety Foundation, source their information from reports from hospital-based clinicians and those 'in the field', and encourage direct adverse drug reaction (ADR) reporting by drug manufacturers. While complex, expert systems have been designed to record and process data collected through spontaneous ADR reporting, there are differences of opinion on how the data should best be interpreted and used. With the forthcoming harmonization of the EC regulatory system for pharmaceuticals, the need for efficient monitoring systems is a matter of urgency. Spriet-Pourra and Auriche (1988) commented in a review of drug withdrawals from 1961 to 1987: 'International consultation between regulatory authorities should be the rule. These authorities should act in liaison with manufacturers and experts. More objective methods of drug benefit/risk assessment should be developed to make the decision-making process codified and explicit'.

Case History—Summary Account of a Drug Withdrawal

The 'second-generation' tricyclic antidepressant nomifensine (Merital) was voluntarily withdrawn from the world-wide market, in all dosage forms, by the manufacturer (Hoechst AG) on 21 January 1986 (Stower, 1992). This compound was indicated for a wide range of depressive illnesses including that accompanied by anxiety. The product was launched in Germany (1976), in the UK (1977) and six other world markets by the end of 1977. By 1980, Merital was available in 52 countries for the treatment of depression and by 1985 over a million prescriptions had been issued in the UK alone. Evidence from clinical trials, post-marketing product monitoring and side-effects comparisons of the marketed agents indicated that nomifensine demonstrated an acceptable side-effect profile compared with other antidepressant agents in use, with the advantage of low cardiotoxicity in overdose (Dawling and Braithwaite, 1979). 'Second generation' tricyclics such as nomifensine were developed to reduce the incidence of sedative, cardio- and hepatotoxic effects so often seen with MAOIs and 'first generation' tricyclics and to ensure a greater margin of safety in overdose. Comparator products in clinical trials included imipramine, amitriptyline, clomipramine, nortriptyline, doxepin, desipramine, viloxaxine, mianserin and maprotiline.

Adverse Reactions

Two years after the launch of nomifensine in the UK, the manufacturer received two reports of haemolytic anaemia in patients who were being treated with nomifensine; the mechanism causing these immune-based reactions was unknown and the patients recovered without sequelae. The rare ADR triggered a six-month, post-marketing immunological investigation by the manufacturer, conducted as a prospective study in patients treated with nomifensine and designed with the assistance of the UK Department of Health, the parent company and a UK academic immunology department. A retrospective study was also carried out by the parent company. One aim of these studies was, if possible, to characterize the basis of any immune reaction. None was found as a result of the prospective study and the manufacturer continued to follow up any similar reports when they occurred, using the same laboratory assays. Equally important was the aim of identifying those patients treated for depression who would be more likely than others to develop the syndrome, and assist the clinician to make a risk/benefit assessment of nomifensine based on the fullest data on its immunogenic potential. In 1983, a new 5-HT uptake inhibitor (zimeldine) was withdrawn world-wide, mainly as a result of Guillain–Barré syndrome ADR reports. A high level of these reports (473) were received in one year. One of the characteristic descriptions was of an 'influenza-like syndrome' and hepatic reactions were also common, including reversible liver damage due to 'a sensitivity reaction'. This was to influence the perception of the safety profile of nomifensine, as a few ADR reports received in the period 1984 onwards described a similar pattern.

Increasing numbers of reports of cases of haemolytic anaemia in patients treated with nomifensine were reported to the UK CSM in 1984 and 1985, making a total of 43 UK reports, of which three were fatal. This prompted a

CSM 'Current Problems' briefing on antidepressants (including nomifensine). In January 1986 nomifensine was withdrawn world-wide, with concomitant media publicity. The decision to withdraw the product was accompanied by 'heavy consumer pressure in the (then) Federal Republic of Germany and the UK' (Spriet-Pourra and Auriche, 1988). Hoechst AG's decision was made prior to the hearing with Health Authorities of France and the UK, scheduled for 30 January 1986, and was due in a significant part to the alteration made to the perceived risk/benefit ratio of nomifensine, as a result of the intensive pressure by consumer organizations and the media. However, the French authorities decided to go ahead with their assessment of the production on the evidence they had gathered from the company and academic sources. Their decision was that nomifensine was able to demonstrate a positive risk/benefit ratio and their recommendation was that the licence for the product should be maintained. In large measure, this was due to the evidence from studies of the clinical experience with the drug in depressed patients, showing that where the risk of suicide was present, nomifensine contributed to patient safety by being non-toxic in overdose.

Risk/Benefit Profiles

In 1987, a year after the withdrawal of nomifensine, Cassidy and Henry reported that nomifensine carried a significantly lower level of fatal risk than all other antidepressants in cases of self-poisoning (Cassidy and Henry, 1987). It had proved difficult to identify a predisposing factor, either pathological or drug-related, that would help to explain why a few out of the many patients treated with nomifensine were susceptible and had developed haemolytic anaemia while on drug treatment. These events occurred prior to a similar scenario with the antidepressant mianserin (Bolvidon, Organon), again involving haematological ADRs, leading to suspension of the product licence by the licensing authority in the UK. An independent assessment of the risk/ benefit profile of mianserin was mounted through the PEM post-marketing surveillance of method developed by the independent trust, the Drug Safety Research Unit (DSRU). Following the publication of the results of the survey (Inman, 1988), the company concerned were successful in bringing into the risk/benefit equation the subject of safety in overdose by means of legal action taken in the UK courts against the decision of the Health Authority's Committee on Safety of Medicines. Mustill (1990) said, 'It must therefore be taken that the references to "administered" and "purposes" extend beyond circumstances which involved strict compliance with the intended use of the drug and that the risks attaching to misuse can properly be brought into account'. Inman commented, 'The UK CSM's hands may be tied by the Medicine Act 1968, which does not permit consideration of the comparative efficacy of drugs in normal use nor the comparative safety of drugs in abnormal situations, such as those presented by suicide attempts. It is to be hoped that new European legislation will allow both sides of a safety and efficacy equation to be taken into consideration' (Inman, 1991).

The Implications of Drug Withdrawal for the Psychiatric Patient

From the point of view of the anxious and/or depressed patient, the sudden news that their prescribed treatment is no longer available may cause bewilderment and worry, exacerbating symptoms already present. Patients as well as clinicians need to be told why a sudden withdrawal has happened, the risks involved, and how best a patient who may have been on long-term treatment may be transferred to another drug. Where this information is not made available, problems can arise. General practitioners (GPs) and hospital-based clinicians in psychiatric medicine are aware that such situations are best met by counselling patients on the need to transfer to another drug in the same class, and this requires advice from the manufacturer: 'To ban a drug overnight without any instructions as to what to do is surely not a good thing for GPs and their patients'. A television debate broadcast in the UK in October 1991 (*The Time, The Place*, 1991) examined the problems posed for patients by the sudden unavailability of their prescribed medicine, in this case a benzodiazepine. The participants in the programme included a consultant psychiatrist, a GP, representatives of patient support organizations and an audience of patients including those who had been long-term users of that particular benzodiazepine. All agreed that they could not think what they were to do now it was withdrawn. A consultant psychiatrist commented that abrupt withdrawal from drug treatment in these patients can cause severe problems and that 'there must be some way of maintaining people on their treatment'. A GP noted that in his experience, 'A month's supply (what the patient on average has left) is hardly enough to wean a patient off'. Transferring patients to another benzodiazepine could incur more problems if a patient does not do well on it. If patients were allowed to be maintained on their medicine for a period of time that would permit a gradual transfer to an alternative drug treatment by a controlled decrease in dosage. It was felt that this would be preferable to discontinuing treatment with the drug in question.

Some part of the problem in conveying to patients the necessity of making a risk/benefit assessment for their drug treatment is due to the public perception of the role of psychoactive agents. A MORI poll conducted in the UK on behalf of the Royal College of Psychiatrists in December 1991 revealed that the general public regard depression as a social rather than a biological problem. Given this attitude, it is not surprising to find that in the population surveyed, there was little distinction in their minds between tranquillizers and antidepressants. Both drug classes were regarded as 'short-term' treatments. Significantly, both were regarded as 'addictive' by 78% of those taking part in the MORI poll, a perception undoubtedly reinforced by the publicity given to the action of the benzodiazepine class. In the rapidly developing field of psychopharmacology, representatives of new and established classes of psychoactive medicines are waiting in the wings. Each will have a safety and efficacy database derived from clinical studies, hopefully carried out according to GCP (Good Clinical Practice). But this early clinical experience, although the basis for the submission to the licensing authority, is only the beginning of the history of a new psychopharmacological agent.

The means to monitor the progress of a new medicine in clinical use, based on good scientific methods, are becoming increasingly well defined. Against this background, a decision to remove a drug from the market, on the basis of spontaneous ADR reports collated from a number of national sources, has far-reaching, international implications. While it is essential to report ADR data centrally, collection and subsequent interpretation of such data should be carried out nationally, and pooling of international data avoided, as this can lead to flawed decision-making. In a case of drug withdrawal, there is no 'no-risk option'. What are the effects of taking a psychoactive agent off the market? What is patients' experience on a new drug and what is happening to those who now have no treatment at all? The consequences of drug withdrawal for patients and their clinicians should not be neglected (Lis et al., 1992). Studies that address this important aspect are urgently required.

The Consequences of Regulatory Intervention—An Example

The benzodiazepine hypnotic Halcion (triazolam) was suspended by the UK regulatory authorities on 2nd October 1991. This precipitous suspension provided the opportunity to investigate the effects of such a decision on clinical practice. The main objective was to formulate a parsimonious method which would assess how patients and GPs judged treatment with triazolam versus alternative therapies in a setting where substitution was forced by external rather than clinical factors.

Methodological Considerations

There are several problems encountered when performing this type of study, the major one being that there are various predetermined factors which cannot be controlled. As this study was retrospective in nature, the investigators had no influence over the number of patients to be switched to a particular alternative, or indeed, what the comparative medication would be. Drug doses, duration of treatment, concurrent medication and patient demography were also predetermined.

Direct access to the patients was impossible, therefore a method had to be developed which would take into account reports made by GPs, who had few data to assess the effects of drugs upon mood, feelings and states of awareness other than verbal reports of the patient receiving the treatment. Subjective awareness of drug activity is an important determinant of behavioural response (Hindmarch, 1980) and it is necessary to have a reliable method of evaluating the activity of psychotropic drugs on an individual's feelings.

One such method to be considered is that of rating scales. On the basis of earlier work (Freyd, 1923; Hayes and Patterson, 1921), Aitken (1969) argued in favour of 10 cm line visual analogue scales. The validity and reliability of such measures have since been demonstrated in drug evaluation studies (Bond and Lader, 1974), in mood assessment of psychiatric patients (Luria, 1975) and in measuring early morning performance following nocturnal administration of hypnotics (Hindmarch, 1975, 1976, 1977).

Considering the above points, the present study was designed as a retrospective multicentre postal survey where GPs were asked to complete questionnaires and visual analogue rating scales according to patient records and spontaneous reports by comparing global impressions and side effects associated with triazolam and substitute therapies.

General Methodology

Selection criteria In order to avoid geographic bias based on clinical practice style or location, the UK was divided into regions, covering metropolitan, urban and suburban practices. GPs from these areas were invited to participate in the survey, and were required to indicate the number of eligible patients in their practice. Participating GPs were paid a small fee for their time in accordance with the BMA (British Medical Association) guidelines.

Patient eligibility Patients were regarded as eligible if they had been successfully treated with triazolam and, because of the UK suspension of triazolam, had been prescribed an alternative treatment. Only those patients whose medication had been changed after 2 October 1991 were included. If the reason for the switch was other than the suspension of triazolam, or if medical records were incomplete, subjects were excluded from the study.

Patient numbers No more than 15 patients were accepted from any individual GP. If more than 15 cases were presented, a random selection was made using the first 5 eligible cases from an alphabetical listing of patients, together with the last 5 and a similar number from the middle of the list.

Ethical approval Ethical approval was not required as patient identity was not disclosed. However, the study protocol was submitted to the Ethics Committee to ensure that, if required, source document checks could be carried out.

Procedure The patients themselves did not take part in this survey. GPs with eligible patients were asked to complete questionnaires based upon reviews of patient records. Case record forms were completed using information from the patients' medical records, including any concurrent medication, and the GPs' knowledge of each individual case.

Data verification GPs were informed that on-site spot checks would take place. In addition, any conflicting or ambiguous results were verified by telephone.

Assessments Day-time functioning and feelings were assessed using a set of 10 cm line visual analogue scales (VASs) which were completed by the GP. These VASs were designed to compare triazolam with the substitute hypnotic regarding tiredness, memory problems, anxiety, depression, agitation and other adverse events.

Adverse events The term 'adverse event' included any symptom or abnormality which developed or increased in severity during the course of treatment. Events experienced during the last (up to 90) days of triazolam treatment and during the first 90 days of alternative hypnotic treatment were recorded. These events were rated as mild (causing no limitation of usual activities), moderate (causing some limitation of usual activities) or severe (causing inability to carry out normal activities).

Global assessments The Clinical Global Impression (CGI) and the Physician's Preference (PP) for either triazolam or substitute therapy were assessed using 10 cm visual analogue scales. GPs were also asked if they agreed with the suspension and whether or not they felt that the suspension had benefited general practice prescribing for the insomniac patient.

Statistical methods Summary statistics were based on all patients from the different investigators combined and no adjustment for investigator was made in the analysis. All statistical tests for treatment comparisons are presented using two-sided *P*-values (with 95% confidence limits).

Thirteen VAS scores were presented for each patient, eleven measuring daytime effects, one measuring GP global clinical impression and one the GP's preference. Global distress was derived as the sum of the eleven individual day-time scores. The VAS responses were described by splitting the 10 cm line into 10 mm categories and the percentage and frequency of patients in each category was calculated. Between-treatment comparisons were made for the complete set of patients by performing a paired *t*-test on the data in their continuous form.

Results

One thousand, one hundred and ninety-three (333 male and 860 female) patient records were obtained for analysis. The patients' ages ranged from 21 to 94 years with a mean of 66.4 years (age was calculated relative to the withdrawal date of triazolam). The duration of treatment with triazolam and substitute therapy was also recorded, and if the substitute therapy was on-going, the duration of treatment was calculated up until the time that the GP signed the case report form.

The most popular alternative treatment on the cessation of triazolam was temazepam, which was given to 67.6% of patients. Other substitute therapies included loprazolam, nitrazepam, lormetazepam, chloral betaine, zopiclone, antidepressants, antipsychotics and anxiolytics (Figure 1).

Adverse events Adverse events (AEs) were reported in 24% of subjects while receiving triazolam and in 32% of subjects whilst on substitute medication. The relative differences were greater when the central nervous system (CNS) AEs were examined: 18% of subjects receiving substitute therapy compared to 9% receiving triazolam reported CNS AEs.

When the CNS AEs were broken down by comparator (Figure 2), triazolam continued to have the lowest overall reported rate followed by loprazolam, chloral betaine, temazepam and zopiclone. The highest rates

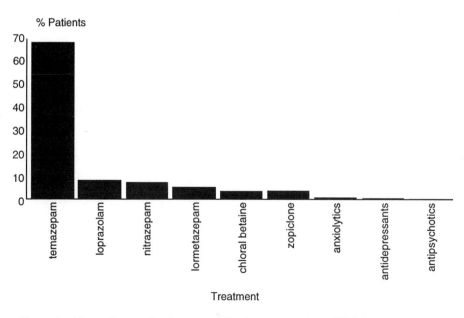

Figure 1. Alternative medications prescribed on suspension of Halcion

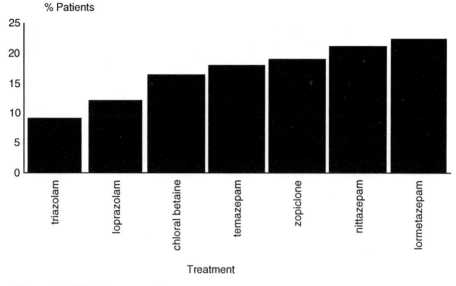

Figure 2. CNS adverse events

were reported with nitrazepam and lormetazepam. 1.2% of patients had mild, moderate and severe CNS AEs which were thought to be related to triazolam, whereas the number of patients experiencing CNS AEs related to substitute therapy was 10.5%. Of the patients on triazolam 0.2% reported non-CNS AEs which were related to triazolam, whilst on substitute therapy 1.6% patients experienced non-CNS AEs which were related to treatment.

Global assessments   In the CGI assessment triazolam was reported as being significantly better than substitute therapy. When individual comparators were examined the mean ratings again showed preference for triazolam. This pattern was repeated in the PP and Global Distress scales.

    The results from this survey show that GPs strongly disagreed with the decision to suspend triazolam and did not believe that the suspension was beneficial to patients. In addition, the consensus of opinion was that the suspension had compromised GP prescribing flexibility.

Discussion

This was a retrospective study designed to examine the effects of the regulatory suspension of triazolam on clinical practice. The main objective was to devise a method which would compare the side-effects and physician-assessed global impressions associated with triazolam and other comparator hypnotics.

The data presented here are contrary to the assertion that triazolam has a narrower risk/benefit ratio than other hypnotics. Instead, the results from this study suggest that while the patients were on triazolam fewer CNS and non-CNS adverse events were experienced than when they were taking the substitute prescription. In addition to appearing favourable in its side-effect profile, GPs preferred triazolam to the alternative treatments as measured by visual analogue scales. The opinion of the GPs was that the action of the regulatory bodies compromised their prescribing flexibility and had narrowed their treatment options.

However, it is not the purpose of this chapter to examine the results in detail (this will be published elsewhere), but to discuss the possibility of adopting such a method in assessing the impact of regulatory decisions on clinical practice.

Criticisms and suggestions   The major disadvantage in performing this study was that it was retrospective rather than prospective and therefore could not be carried out in a double blind fashion. This meant that it was impossible to control for all variables. A relatively small population of patients' records were analysed due to time constraints, therefore it would be advantageous for future studies to enrol bigger numbers. However, using a multicentre trial design allowed for a representation of a large population it was not feasible to include a control group in the study and so within-patient comparisons were made. This was advantageous in that assessments were made on the effect that the suspension had on each *individual* patient.

If the main purpose of this investigation was simply to compare medications, then a significant criticism would be that, by definition, patients and GPs were satisfied with the existing treatment, i.e. triazolam, and if not an alternative medication would have been prescribed prior to the regulatory decision. However, the aim of this survey was not to evaluate the efficacy of triazolam, but to assess the consequences of regulatory suspension on patients who were being successfully treated with triazolam.

Concluding Remarks

The decision by the UK regulatory bodies to suspend Halcion provided the opportunity to devise a simple method to obtain information on how such an action affects GPs and their patients. Despite the criticisms of such studies, the results obtained provide an indication of how GPs regard such intervention on their prescribing flexibility and, most importantly, if they feel that their patients have benefited.

Finally, when assessing the risk/benefit ratio of the suspension of a psychotropic drug, results of investigations along these lines should be taken into consideration.

References

Aitken, R.C.B. (1969). Measurement of feelings using visual analogue rating scales. *Proceedings of the Royal Society of Medicine*, **62**, 989–97.

Asscher, W. (Chairman, Committee on Safety of Medicines, Department of Health, UK), 1992. Promoting Therapeutic Innovation: Management Forum, 5th Annual Pharmaceutical Conference 1992, London, UK, 20–21 October.

Bond, A., and Lader, M. (1974). The use of analogue scales in rating subjective feelings. *British Journal of Medical Psychology*, **47**, 211–18.

Cassidy, S., and Henry, J. (1987). Fatal toxicity of antidepressant drugs in overdose. *British Medical Journal*, **295**, (6605), 1021–24.

Dawling, S., and Braithwaite, R. (1979). Nomifensine overdose and plasma drug concentration. *Lancet* (letter), Jan 6 1979.

Freyd, M. (1923). The graphic rating scale. *Journal of Educational Psychology*, **14**, 83.

Hayes, M.H., and Patterson, D.G. (1921). Experimental development of the graphic rating method. *Psychology Bulletin*, **18**, 98.

Hindmarch, I. (1975). A 1,4-benzodiazepine, temazepam (K3917): its effect on some psychological parameters of sleep and behaviour. *Arzneim. Forsch. (Drug Research)*, **25**, 1836–9.

Hindmarch, I. (1976). A sub-chronic study of the subjective quality of sleep and psychological measures of performance on the morning following night-time medication with temazepam. *Arzneim. Forsch. (Drug Research)*, **26**, 2113–16.

Hindmarch, I. (1977). A repeated dose comparison of three benzodiazepine derivatives (nitrazepam, flurazepam and flunitrazepam) on subjective appraisals of sleep and measures of psychomotor performance the morning following night-time medication. *Acta Psychiatrica Scandinavica*, **56**, 373–81.

Hindmarch, I. (1980). Psychomotor function and psychoactive drugs. *British Journal of Clinical Pharmacology*, **10**, 189–209.

Inman, W.H.W. (1988). Blood disorders and suicide in patients taking mianserin or amitriptyline. *Lancet*, **2**, 90–2.

Inman, W.H.W. (1991). *PEM News*, **7**, 36, August 1991.

Lis, Y., Chukwujindu, J., and Cockburn, I. (1992). Addressing drug discontinuation using the VAMP Research data bank. Second European Pharmacovigilance Symposium, Nov 1992.

Luria, R.E. (1975). The validity of the visual analogue mood scale. *Journal of Psychiatry Research*, **12**, 51–7.

Mustill, Lord Justice (1990). *Re Organon Laboratories Ltd v. Department of Health and Social Security* (referring to UK Medicines Act 1968, Section 28(3)(g)).

Spriet-Pourra, C., and Aurich, K. (1988). *Drug Withdrawal from Sale*. PJB Publications, London.

Stonier, P.D. (1992). Nomifensine and haemolytic anaemia—experience of a post-marketing alert. *Pharmacoepidemiol. Drug Safety*, **1**, 177–185.

The Time, The Place, ITV Birmingham, October 1991.

Waller, P.C., Wood, S.M. *et al.* (1992). Review of company post-marketing studies. *British Medical Journal*, **304**, 1470–72.

7

The Contributions of Positron Emission Tomography and Single-photon Emission Computed Tomography Toward a Psychopharmacological Neuroanatomy of Obsessive-compulsive Disorder

Mark S. George

National Institute of Mental Health, Bethesda, Maryland, USA

Introduction and Aims of the Chapter

Within the past decade, the field of psychiatry has undergone a radical change. Once confined to ignoring the brain and concentrating solely on behaviour or the mind, psychiatry has rediscovered the brain and its mechanisms. The new methodologies of imaging brain structure (computed tomography (CT) or magnetic resonance imaging (MRI)) initially kindled this change. Psychiatrists no longer had to wait until autopsy in order to analyse brain changes in psychiatric disease. CT and MRI scanning effectively allowed one to bypass the skull.

Imaging an organ's structure, while quite important, nevertheless leaves unanswered questions concerning how well the organ functions. An often-quoted but somewhat misleading statement is that, on CT or MRI, a dead brain looks the same as a living one. Consequently, the next step, following the advances of MRI and CT, has taken place in the field of functional neuroimaging. As never before, scientists can observe the function of the living working brain. Positron emission tomography (PET) and single-photon

Human Psychopharmacology, Vol. 4. Edited by I. Hindmarch and P. D. Stonier
© 1993 John Wiley & Sons Ltd

emission (computed) tomography (SPECT or SPET) allow important insights into the functioning human brain in both health and disease.

These revolutionary new technologies have led to important breakthroughs in understanding several previously enigmatic psychiatric disorders. It is the aim of this chapter to discuss and explain how new findings using PET and SPECT are providing clues into the abnormal function of the brain in patients with obsessive-compulsive disorder (OCD). In the short span of 20 years the field has gone from little understanding of OCD or its mechanism and no effective treatment, to having effective ameliorative therapies and a clearer understanding of the genetics and underlying brain pathology of the disorder.

In what follows, OCD will serve as the background for a discussion of how the new methodologies of functional neuroimaging can yield important information about neuropsychiatry. As part of this discussion, PET and SPECT methodologies and limitations will be reviewed. Finally, these new functional neuroimaging findings will be incorporated into a composite, if incomplete, theory of the psychopharmacological neuroanatomy of OCD. Throughout, emphasis will be placed on the methods and measures of PET (Phelps *et al.*, 1986) and SPECT (George *et al.*, 1991a) imaging, and how these emerging techniques have opened up new areas of understanding about OCD.

An Overview of OCD and Related Disorders

Within the past 10 years, the fields of neurology, biological psychiatry and nuclear medicine have rediscovered OCD. Despite the fact that it was well described over 150 years ago, and that early clinicians thought it was a brain-based illness (Gilles de la Tourette, 1885; Jellife, 1927, 1932), for most of the twentieth century it was relegated to the class of 'incurable' illnesses of presumed psychoanalytic origin. Partly because of the lack of a cure and proper understanding of the illness, the incidence of OCD was grossly underestimated. We now know that OCD occurs in approximately 2% of all US adults and is thought to exist at similarly high rates in other cultures (Rasmussen and Eisen, 1990).

OCD consists of recurrent intrusive thoughts (obsessions) or senseless repetitive actions (compulsions). OCD is distinguished from mere habits or psychotic thinking by the necessary qualification that in OCD the obsessions or compulsions must be ego-dystonic (unpleasant), recognized as coming from the person's own mind, and result in significant dysfunction. Usually beginning in the second or third decade of life, OCD is found equally in men and women. Some have combined different types of obsessions and compulsions into various phenomenological symptom clusters: (1) washers, (2) checkers, (3) patients with pure obsessions, and (4) people without marked obsessions or compulsions but who are obsessionally slow and unable to make decisions (Hymas *et al.*, 1991).

In the majority of cases, there is a large genetic component to OCD, with an increased prevalence in first-degree relatives of OCD, tics, or the neuropsychiatric movement disorder, Gilles de la Tourette syndrome (GTS) (Pauls and Leckman, 1986a; Pauls *et al.*, 1986a, 1986b). Additionally, OCD is frequently accompanied by other psychiatric problems. For example, Rasmussen and Eisen (1990) found that 30% of OCD patients suffered from a major depressive episode, 27% at one point had simple phobias, 5% had GTS, 14% had panic disorder and 9% had agoraphobia.

Many neuropsychiatrists divide OCD cases into two types. Some cases of OCD appear to have strong genetic component, and arise in the absence of gross antecedent structural brain pathology. This is sometimes referred to as *primary or essential OCD*. There are, on the other hand, numerous cases where OCD arises in conjunction with a change in brain structure—*secondary OCD* (George *et al.*, 1992; Grimshaw, 1964; Cummings and Frankel, 1985). The other diseases which result in secondary OCD will be reviewed below as they may hold important clues into the aetiology and pathophysiology of primary OCD.

In addition to classical OCD consisting of obsessions and compulsions, there is an interesting collection of OCD-like disorders which share the feature of repeated behaviour which is recognized by the individual as senseless and to some degree unpleasant, but over which they have reduced control. Many of these disorders respond pharmacologically in a manner similar to OCD and display related functional brain changes on PET and SPECT (see Table 1) (for a review see George, 1992a). In attempting to understand the phenomenology of OCD, and thus its neurobiological underpinnings, it is important to bear these related conditions in mind. OCD may represent an aberration or dysfunction of normal behaviours such as grooming that have an ethological importance (Insel, 1988; Rapoport, 1990; Maclean, 1990; Marks, 1987). By examining the neuropharmacological systems involved with grooming or checking, one can begin to piece together the underlying neuropharmacology of OCD (Grindlinger and Ramsay, 1991; Insel, 1988; Pitman, 1989).

OCD and Related Disorders

The interesting thing about the collections of diseases in Table 1 is that they are irrational recurrent impulses which respond, at least in part, to manipulation of the 5-hydroxytryptamine (serotonin, 5-HT) system with 5-HT reuptake blockers. The exact relationship between these disorders and primary OCD remains to be solved using genetic and functional neuroimaging studies. Functional neuroimaging studies to date, which will be reviewed below, have shown both similarities (George *et al.*, 1991c) and differences (Swedo *et al.*, 1991) between some of these disorders and primary OCD.

Table 1. OCD and obsessional-compulsive spectrum disorders

Disorder	Description	Response to 5-HT?	Reference
OCD	Recurrent obsessions and compulsions	Yes	George (1992)
Trichotillomania	Recurrent hair pulling	Yes	Alexander (1991)
Bulimia nervosa	Recurrent bingeing and purging	Yes	Jenike (1989)
Gilles de la Tourette syndrome (GTS)	Recurrent motor and vocal tics	Yes	George et al. (1991d)
Dysmorpho-phobia	Recurrent thoughts of an abnormal body part	Yes	Hollander et al. (1989) Brady et al. (1990)
Excessive moral and religious scrupulosity	Recurrent thoughts that one has sinned	Yes	Fallon et al. (1990)
Voyeurism	Recurrent urges to look at others	Yes	Kafka and Coleman (1991)
Monosymptom-atic hypo-chondriasis	Recurrent abnormal thought that one is ill	Yes	Jenike (1989)

Known Structural Neuroanatomical Changes Associated with OCD

Before examining how PET and SPECT have given increased understanding about the neuroanatomy of OCD, it is useful to review the known brain structural changes associated with primary or secondary OCD.

Pathological and CT/MRI Studies

There are limited autopsy data available concerning OCD. This is due to numerous factors, including the fact that only until recently have most clinicians adequately recognized the disease. Several studies have employed either MRI or CT to examine brain structures in subjects with primary OCD, with a lack of clear-cut findings (see Table 2). However, two studies have found differences that are neuroanatomically intriguing. Luxenberg et al. (1988)

Table 2. Brain structural changes in primary OCD

Region	Abnormality	Methodology	Reference
Caudate nuclei	Decreased volume	CT scans	Luxenberg *et al.* (1988)
Frontal white matter	Increased prolongation of T1	MRI scans	Garber *et al.* (1989)

used CT scans to measure brain regions in male subjects with OCD onset prior to age 18. Compared with controls, they found a significant decrease in volume of the caudate nucleus bilaterally in OCD subjects. Other studies (Kellner *et al.*, 1991; Garber *et al.*, 1989) have failed to confirm the decreased caudate volume using OCD subjects with mixed age of onset. Interestingly, Garber and colleagues found increased T1 relaxation times in the right frontal white matter in OCD subjects, the significance of which is unclear. Spin-lattice relaxation time (T1) reflects interactions between excited protons and an excited molecular environment. This finding could possibly be related to increased blood flow in the right frontal region—a fairly consistent finding in the PET and SPECT work.

In summary, there are no consistent structural abnormalities yet identified with primary OCD, either at autopsy or using CT of MRI. There are interesting hints that the caudate nuclei may be decreased in size and that the frontal white matter may also be involved. Unfortunately, these findings are tantalizing and have not been easily replicated.

Secondary OCD Produced by Specific Brain Diseases and Localized Pathology

OCD may result from any number of lesions or conditions that involve either the *basal ganglia* or *frontal white matter* (George *et al.*, 1992). There are few reports of diseases which result in OCD that do not involve one or the other of these two key regions. Although a lengthy review of these conditions is beyond the scope of this chapter, a quick overview can set the stage for the discussion of functional neuroimaging that follows (see Table 3).

Mass lesions of the right frontal (Seibyl *et al.*, 1989), frontal (Cambier *et al.*, 1988) and caudate regions (Tonkonogy and Barriera, 1989) can ablate tissue and result in secondary OCD. Similarly, infarctions of the striatum have been reported to result in OCD (Weilburg, 1989). However, the most interesting category of secondary OCD consists of infectious diseases which produce basal ganglia damage, presumably through an immune-mediated process. Schilder (1938), Jellife (1932) and most recently Sacks (1982) have described

Table 3. Secondary OCD

Disease class	Disease	Brain region	Reference
Lesions	Tumours	Temporal lobe	Brickner (1940)
		Right frontal	Seibyl et al. (1989)
		Frontal	Cambier et al. (1988)
		Caudate	Tonkonogy and Barriera (1989)
	Infarction	Striatum	Weilburg et al. (1989)
Closed head injury		Diffuse	McKeon et al. (1984)
Post-infectious	Post-encephalitic Parkinsonism	Striatum	Schilder (1938)
	Wasp sting	Basal ganglia	Laplane et al. (1981)
	Von Economos	Basal ganglia	Wohlfart et al. (1961)
	Sydenham's chorea	Basal ganglia	Swedo et al. (1989a)
Others	Multiple sclerosis		George et al. (1989)
	Gilles de la Tourette syndrome	Basal ganglia	Gilles de la Tourette (1885); Lees et al. (1984)
	Epilepsy	Temporal lobe	Bear and Fedio (1977)
		Frontal lobe	Ward (1988)
	Amphetamine psychosis		Ellinwood (1967)

the interesting OCD-like characteristics of patients who contracted von Economo's post-infectious encephalitis during the epidemic of the 1920s and 1930s. Autopsy studies of these subjects showed extensive basal ganglia involvement (Von Economo, 1931). This same disease continues to occur sporadically (Wohlfart et al., 1961) and can produce secondary OCD. Other post-infectious processes can cause basal ganglia damage and produce OCD. Laplane et al. (1981) described a patient who developed OCD following an allergic reaction to a wasp sting and bilateral necrosis of the basal ganglia. Another interesting disease with resultant secondary OCD is Sydenham's chorea, an immune-mediated basal ganglia disease developing after streptococcal infections. OCD-like characteristics of these patients have been sporadically described. Swedo et al. (1989a) sampled patients suffering from rheumatic fever with rheumatic carditis or Sydenham's chorea. Those with chorea had a markedly elevated rate of OCD compared with controls who merely had carditis and no central nervous system (CNS) involvement. Some postulate that Sydenham's chorea develops along with antibody production to the caudate nuclei (Husby *et al.*, 1976). This theory holds that the body attempts to fight off the streptococcal infection immunologically with antibody production. In some individuals cross-reacting antibodies produce valvular heart disease or caudate damage (Husby *et al.*, 1976; George *et al.*, 1987). Preliminary results from an ongoing study at the National Institute of Mental Health (NIMH) indicate that patients with acute Sydenham's chorea may have enlarged caudates on MRI and increased levels of anti-caudate antibodies (Swedo, personal communication).

A pot-pourri of other diseases have been reported with associated OCD. In reviewing these case reports it is always a challenge to decide whether the link between OCD symptoms and the other disease is causal or merely coincidental. Because OCD is so common (2% of the general population), many OCD patients will naturally have associated diseases that may have no association with OCD symptoms. In general, the more convincing case reports of OCD stemming from another disease commonly involve damage to the basal ganglia or frontal white matter (George *et al.*, 1992).

The most important category of secondary OCD may be those cases associated with GTS. As mentioned above, OCD occurs in 30–60% of patients with GTS (Cummings and Frankel, 1985; Frankel *et al.*, 1986; Comings, 1990; Trimble, 1989; Sacks, 1982). It is an important question whether OCD as it occurs in GTS is a form of secondary OCD, or whether GTS is merely the end of the spectrum of primary OCD. In essence, the question is whether OCD and GTS represent different phenotypes of the same or similar underlying neurobiological dysfunction, or whether they are truly separate diseases with different CNS pathology. GTS is an idiopathic disorder involving migratory motor and vocal tics over time. More common in males, it is thought to involve a disorder of dopamine and the basal ganglia (George *et al.* 1991b abstract). GTS tics respond to treatment with dopamine-blocking agents such as haloperidol and pimozide. Recently, George *et al.* (1991d) demonstrated that in subjects with concurrent OCD/GTS, fluvoxamine, a 5-HT reuptake blocker, may be nearly as effective as sulpiride (a D_2-blocker) in reducing tics as well as OCD symptoms. Thus it appears that OCD and GTS are pharmacologically as well as genetically linked. Functional neuroimaging studies are beginning to shed new light on this question.

In summary, many diseases which involve damage to the frontal white matter or basal ganglia may produce secondary OCD.

Surgical Treatments of OCD

For most of this twentieth century, it has been known that surgical excision of key brain regions can reduce OCD symptoms (Mitchell-Heggs *et al.*, 1977;

Tippin and Henn, 1982; Kurlan *et al.*, 1990; Jenike *et al.*, 1991). Several different neurosurgical procedures have been used with moderate success: anterior capsulotomy, bilateral anterior cingulotomy and bimedial orbital leucotomy. In the modern era this procedure is reserved for severe OCD patients refractory to conventional pharmacological and behavioural treatments.

Ballantine's group at Harvard favours lesioning the fibres projecting from the anterior cingulum to the frontal cortex. Jenike *et al.* (1991) recently reviewed the 25-year history of psychosurgery for OCD at the Massachusetts General Hospital, Boston, USA. Thirty-five patients had undergone bilateral anterior stereotactic cingulotomy for OCD, with 25–30% receiving substantial benefit.

In the UK, Bridges *et al.* (1973) have tended to favour bilateral stereotactic tractotomy (also known as a subcaudate tractotomy), with some relief of obsessions and compulsions. Historically, some patients who received a prefrontal leucotomy probably suffered from severe OCD, when examined retrospectively. A prefrontal leucotomy severs fibres projecting from the thalamus to the frontal lobe. In a review of the experience at the Maudsley Hospital in London from 1951 to 1965, Tan *et al.* (1971) demonstrated that frontal leucotomy was generally safe and effective, with few side-effects in these OCD patients.

In summary, three neurosurgical procedures demonstrate that interruption of fibres in the loop from the caudate to thalamus to cingulate to orbital frontal cortex can reduce OCD symptoms. This is in many ways an unbiased and independent confirmation of the importance of this loop in producing OCD. These neurosurgical data supplement the brain lesion and structural

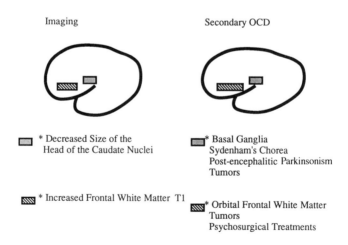

Figure 1. Brain areas implicated in OCD pathogenesis by structural imaging with CT or MRI (left) and secondary diseases associated with OCD symptoms (right). Both categories demonstrate the important role of the orbital frontal cortex and basal ganglia in regulating obsessional-compulsive behaviours

imaging studies previously described, and the rapidly emerging functional neuroimaging data to follow.

Summary Sketch and Diagram of Structural Neuroanatomy of OCD

Thus neuroimaging studies in primary OCD implicate pathology in the heads of the caudate and right orbital frontal white matter. Secondary causes of OCD all involve either the basal ganglia, thalamus, cingulum, or frontal white matter. Finally, neurosurgical cases from the past 30 years demonstrate that one can decrease OCD symptoms by lesioning interconnecting tracts in this circuit. Figure 1 summarizes many of these findings.

These three divergent fields—structural neuroimaging, secondary causes of OCD, and psychosurgery—have sketched the neuroanatomy of OCD. With this as background, it is now important to shift the focus and examine which neurotransmitters have been implicated in OCD. Then, with a firm understanding of the neuroanatomy and neuropharmacology of OCD, one can integrate the new information emerging from PET and SPECT.

The Current Psychopharmacology of OCD

Studies into abnormalities of brain structure are a necessary beginning on the road to understanding OCD. Yet understanding brain structural problems is somehow incomplete and lifeless. Structural abnormalities are the black and white sketch upon which one must eventually place the 'colour' of pathology. What neurotransmitters have been implicated in OCD treatment and pathogenesis? The answers stem mainly from CSF studies, neurotransmitter challenge studies, and clinical treatment trials.

CSF Studies

Well-conducted prospective studies looking at cerebrospinal fluid (CSF) metabolites in OCD are lacking. In one study, Thoren *et al.* (1980) identified a group of OCD subjects with high CSF 5-hydroxyindoleacetic acid (5-HIAA) (the breakdown product of 5-HT). These subjects had a positive response to clomipramine (a 5-HT reuptake blocker) and clinical improvement correlated with decreasing CSF 5-HIAA levels after treatment. Goodman *et al.* (1989a) also found that CSF 5-HIAA levels decreased after treatment with fluvoxamine, another 5-HT reuptake blocker. However, CSF 5-HIAA levels could predict neither outcome nor response to medication treatment.

Provocative Agents

Another method of analysing the neuropharmacology of a disorder is to monitor symptoms pre- and post-exposure to a challenge agent. The 5-HT agonist *m*-chlorophenylpiperazine (*m*-CPP) is a metabolite of the antidepressant trazadone and directly stimulates 5-HT receptors. Some studies have demonstrated that oral *m*-CPP 0.5 mg/kg selectively and transiently increases obsessive thinking and rituals and blunts prolactin rise in OCD subjects compared with controls (Zohar *et al.*, 1987; Hollander *et al.*, 1988). This neuroendocrine blunting can be abolished by pretreatment with the 5-HT reuptake blockers clomipramine or fluoxetine. The *m*-CPP-induced increase in obsessions can also be blocked by metergoline, a 5-HT antagonist (Zohar *et al.*, 1987). Thus 5-HT manipulation can acutely effect the phenomenology and neuroendocrinology of OCD.

Changing the CNS dopamine system also produces differences in OCD. Insel *et al.* (1983) and later Joffe *et al.* (1991) demonstrated that acute oral administration of 30 mg dextroamphetamine transiently improves OCD symptoms. Surprisingly, this effect was not observed with 40 mg oral methylphenidate (Joffe *et al.*, 1991). Conversely, long-term treatment with dopamine agonists such as methylphenidate can result in tics and OCD-like behaviour.

Treatment Agents

The final domain implicating specific neurotransmitters involves OCD's response to treatment. Beginning with the discovery that obsessive-compulsive symptoms responded to treatment with the antidepressant clomipramine (Montgomery, 1980), several newer agents have been developed to combat OCD (fluoxetine, fluvoxamine, sertraline). All share the feature of blocking the reuptake of 5-HT in the neural cleft. Antidepressants without 5-HT activity have not proven useful in treating OCD. All of the 5-HT blockers are effective in treating OCD, with some patients responding to one but not the other agent. One study comparing the anti-obsessive efficacy of fluoxetine with clomipramine found no difference between the two agents (Pigott *et al.*, 1990).

There is a high rate of relapse if these drugs are removed, and many patients do not fully respond to a given agent. In such cases, numerous additive regimens have been developed which are proving effective (George, 1992). Many of these share the feature of altering dopamine. Dopamine thus appears to have a role in modulating OCD behaviour. For example, George *et al.* (1991d) recently demonstrated that sulpiride monotherapy reduces OCD symptoms in patients with concurrent OCD/GTS.

Summary: Known Effects of 5-HT and Dopamine

Thus 5-HT-acting agents can transiently worsen or effectively reduce OCD symptoms. There also appears to be a minor but significant role for dopamine agonists and antagonists as either additive or single agents in treating OCD.

Table 4. Provocative and therapeutic agents in OCD

Neuro-transmitter	Agent	Action	OCD effect	Reference
5-HT	*m*-CPP	5-HT agonist	Transiently worsen	Hollander *et al.* (1988)
	Fluoxetine Clomipramine Fluvoxamine Sertraline	5-HT reuptake blockade	Improve	George (1992) (for review)
Dopamine	Dextroam-phetamine	Increase dopamine release	Improve	Insel *et al.* (1983); Joffe *et al.* (1991)
	Methyl-phenidate		No effect	Joffe *et al.* (1991)
	Sulpiride	Dopamine D2 blockade	Slightly improve	George *et al.* (1991d)

Results from CSF examination, challenge studies and treatment trials demonstrate the vital role of 5-HT in OCD. These studies also implicate, to a lesser degree, that dopamine is an important ancillary neurotransmitter.

Functional Neuroimaging: A Description of the Methods and Review of Findings in OCD and Related Disorders

Description of PET and SPECT Methodologies: Methods and Measures

The basic idea behind medical radionuclide imaging involves linking a radionuclide to a specific pharmaceutical or vehicle for transport into the appropriate body tissue (Phelps *et al.*, 1986; George *et al.*, 1991a). Then, by detecting the amount of radiation coming from a specific region, one can infer the function of that region. Thus functional neuroimaging with PET and SPECT differs from conventional imaging in that the radiation source stems from radionuclides that have been injected into the body and *emit radiation out* toward a waiting camera. Conventional imaging such as X-ray or CT involves *transmitting radiation from an external source* to the patient and then monitoring its effect as it passes through the body.

There are two broad categories of radionuclides: (1) single-photon emitters, and (2) positron emitters. Single-photon emitters are used in SPECT and predominately give off gamma or X-rays. Positron emitters, used in PET, issue positrons which behave like positive electrons. Once emitted, positrons travel a short distance before they collide with a neighbouring electron in an annihilation reaction. This reaction then produces two gamma rays travelling in opposite directions. Thus, both PET and SPECT rely on the detection of gamma rays to produce an image of brain function.

Once the gamma rays have been emitted, they are detected by rotating cameras surrounding the head. In PET, a gamma ray is included for final analysis only if there is another gamma ray detected simultaneously 180° away. This coincidence event of the other gamma ray emanating from the annihilation reaction allows one to construct exact image lines and precisely identify where the annihilation event occurred. This physical fact accounts for PET's current advantage in localization compared with SPECT. In SPECT, image lines, and thus localization of the gamma rays' origin, are defined by high-resolution collimaters placed in front of the cameras. Therefore, only gamma rays travelling in a straight path will make it through the collimator and be included for analysis.

Once the gamma rays have been detected in three-dimensional space by the appropriate cameras, computers can then reconstruct the image to provide two-dimensional traditional views of the brain (e.g. sagittal, axial, coronal slices), using technology similar to that used in CT scanning.

The two modalities (PET and SPECT) differ in important ways and place advantages and limitations on their appropriate use. The positrons used in PET allow for higher image resolution (due to the annihilation reaction) and are easier to couple to pharmaceuticals and organic compounds such as oxygen or carbon. They are inherently unstable, however, and thus require that a full-time active cyclotron be located near the camera for the quick manufacture of positrons. SPECT simply requires gamma radiation to enter the brain, and these radionuclides are available in kits for wide distribution to hospitals and research centres. As a disadvantage, many of the SPECT compounds traditionally used to transport radionuclides are too large and complex to cross the blood–brain barrier. Thus, SPECT imaging is freed from the necessity of having an expensive cyclotron at each site, but is limited in terms of the available radionuclide–vehicle combinations which will cross the blood–brain barrier in a sufficient way to allow for appropriate imaging. At present, SPECT has poorer image resolution than PET, although high-resolution cone collimators are decreasing this difference. Also, SPECT now has only limited CNS compounds, although this is an active area of research and development.

The easiest function to measure with PET or SPECT is *cerebral blood flow*. After injecting the radionuclide in the peripheral venous blood, it travels to the brain in the blood and thus gives a representative picture of regions with relatively increased or decreased blood flow. Currently, the most popular SPECT radionuclide for imaging cerebral blood flow is [99Tc]-labelled hexamathyl propylene amine oxime (HMPAO). The PET tracers [15O]- or [18F]-labelled deoxyglucose (fluorodeoxyglucose; FDG) both give reasonable approximations of blood flow, although [15O] is more precisely connected to short-term changes in blood flow. Serendipitously, in most people under most condi-

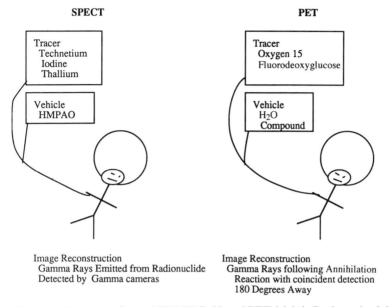

SPECT   PET

Figure 2. A relative comparison of SPECT (left) and PET (right). Both methodologies involve injecting a radiopharmaceutical into a peripheral vein and then collecting the emitted gamma radiation with cameras surrounding the head. PET initially uses unstable positrons, which are easier to couple to organic tracers such as oxygen or glucose. Positrons collide with electrons in an annihilation reaction and emit gamma radiation. SPECT employs more stable but more complex tracers to penetrate the blood–brain barrier and emit radiation. SPECT is less expensive, but has tracer limitations and, at present, less resolution. Both have been useful in understanding the pathophysiology of OCD

tions, *brain metabolism is coupled to brain blood flow* (Sokoloff, 1977). That is, brain regions that increase their metabolic activity also receive increased blood flow. Taking advantage of this lucky, yet logical, phenomenon, one can cautiously infer back from blood flow to brain metabolism. Thus a brain area demonstrating increased gamma radiation on PET or SPECT flow scanning probably has increased blood flow there *because* that region is metabolically more active. This reasoning is the bedrock beneath functional imaging and is important to remember when interpreting functional scans, either individually or in group studies. There are certain clinical situations where this coupling of flow and metabolism may not hold (e.g. infections affecting blood–brain barrier permeability such as a vasculitis, unusual patterns of blood flow such as arteriovenous malformations, or obvious blood leaks such as haemorrhages). These conditions should be screened for with conventional structural neuroimaging (CT or MRI).

In addition to examining global and regional cerebral blood flow, one can now image specific neurotransmitter subsystems using more selective radionuclides. ^{123}I-labelled iodobenzamide IBZM (dopamine), ^{123}I-labelled ketanserin (5-HT), and ^{123}I-labelled flumanezil (benzodiazapine/γ-amino butyric acid) have been used with SPECT. Similarly, newer PET ligands can demonstrate dopamine, 5-HT, opiate or benzodiazepine receptors. This field of novel PET and SPECT ligands is rapidly expanding, allowing imaging of neurotransmitters and possibly second and third messenger systems. These will undoubtedly pioneer a new wave of understanding about *in vivo* human brain function in both health and disease.

The field of functional neuroimaging is currently struggling with several methodological issues involving (1) the reproducibility of scanning in a single patient over time, (2) how to localize important structures on PET and SPECT scans and then compare activity in these regions in the same patient at different scanning times and across patients, and finally (3) how to deal with the complicated statistics involved in making repeated and multiple comparisons of many brain regions.

Scan-to-scan variability   The living brain is never inactive. At all times, including sleep, different brain regions are working at relative levels. There is no such thing as a 'resting' scan. That is, someone with their eyes open will perhaps daydream on one occasion and compute their taxes on another. One can decrease scan-to-scan variability by requiring the subject to perform the same functions during each scan. Most centres now employ continuous performance tasks (CPT) while scanning. These consist of simple auditory or visual tasks that nevertheless require concentration and attention and prevent the subjects' minds from wandering. Even with CPTs, the scan of an individual will vary somewhat from day to day. Thus, the most robust data from functional neuroimaging studies employ large numbers of subjects to reduce this problem.

Localization of regions and structures   A functional PET or SPECT image is not a picture of the brain like a CT scan. Investigators thus employ one of three general methods of localizing brain structures. One can define *regions of interest* by, either visually or with the aid of a computer, placing these regions over the appropriate region and getting a count of the radiation in that region. This method generally has the highest level of inherent error. Alternatively, one can obtain both a structural (CT or MRI) and functional (PET or SPECT) image and then *overlay* the two images. Then one uses the structural image to define the appropriate region and then obtain radiation counts from the superimposed functional image. This is probably the gold standard in addressing this problem, but is expensive. A new and novel method is to *fit* the functional image onto a predetermined 'ideal' brain or atlas. For example, Friston and colleagues (1989) at the Hammersmith hospital in London have developed a software package known as Statistical

Parametric Mapping (SPM), which stretches or shrinks each individual brain to the Talairach brain atlas. This package is useful in group studies but makes the assumption that there is no gross pathology in the brain (that is, each brain roughly corresponds to the ideal). This package is less precise in diseases with obvious focal atrophy or damage. SPM also represents an advance in the complicated area of the statistics of cross-comparing multiple brain regions across multiple patients. This area of defining regions that covary and function as neural networks remain a challenging problem for the field.

This brief overview of PET and SPECT methodology and limitations helps one better focus and interpret the functional neuroimaging studies so far carried out in OCD (Table 5). These studies, conducted in different centres with both PET and SPECT and using different neuroligands (HMPAO, FDG), have consistently found *abnormalities in the orbital frontal white matter and basal ganglia, which normalize with pharmacological or behavioural treatment.* This is one of the more remarkable and consistent findings in the recent history of biological psychiatry.

A clear anatomy of OCD emerges when one combines the results of these functional neuroanatomy studies with the neuropharmacological and neuroanatomical studies reviewed above.

At least five FDG PET studies of OCD have now shown similar but not identical results. Baxter and colleagues (1987) at UCLA used FDG PET to image 14 OCD subjects, 14 unipolar depressed subjects and 14 controls. Compared with controls or subjects with unipolar depression, OCD subjects showed increased metabolism in the left orbital frontal gyrus and both caudate nuclei. Although it was in the normal range while ill, the caudate/hemisphere ratio increased uniformly and bilaterally with improvement in OCD symptoms after drug treatment. In a follow-up study designed to improve on design flaws in the 1987 study (unequal gender distribution, co-morbid depression in OCD subjects), Baxter *et al.* (1988) imaged ten OCD subjects with FDG PET and found increased absolute metabolic rates in the heads of the caudate nuclei and orbital gyri when compared with ten controls matched for age, sex and handedness. A similar study at the National Institute of Health (NIH) in Washington, DC, by Nordahl *et al.* (1989) revealed increased metabolic rates in the orbital gyri of eight OCD subjects compared with controls. Also at the NIH, Swedo and colleagues (1989b) studied 18 subjects with onset of symptoms prior to age 18. Compared with age and sex-matched controls, OCD subjects had elevated glucose metabolism in the left orbital frontal, right sensory motor and bilateral prefrontal and anterior cingulate regions. A significant positive correlation emerged between right orbital glucose metabolic rate and OCD severity. More recently, Martinot and colleagues (1990) compared 16 non-depressed OCD subjects with 8 normal controls using FDG PET. Contrary to the US findings,

Table 5. PET and SPECT studies in OCD and related disorders

Study type	Reference	Subjects	Significant findings
FDG PET	Baxter *et al.* (1987)	14 OCD 14 depressed 14 controls	Increased metabolism in both caudate heads and left orbital gyrus. Increased caudate/hemisphere ratio in OCD responders versus OCD non-responders
	Baxter *et al.* (1988)	10 OCD 10 controls	Increased metabolism in bilateral caudate and orbital gyri in OCD versus controls
	Nordahl *et al.* (1989)	8 OCD 30 controls	Increased orbital gyri metabolism
	Swedo *et al.* (1989b)	18 OCD 18 controls	Increased right prefrontal/global ratio in OCD Increased left anterior cingulate/global ratio in OCD
	Martinot *et al.* (1990)	16 OCD 8 controls	Decreased whole cortex (absolute) Decreased lateral prefrontal cortex (normalized)
	Swedo *et al.* (1991)	10 females with trichotillo-mania 20 controls	Increased global, cerebellar metabolism Negative correlation between frontal metabolism and improvement with drug treatment
Oxygen-15 PET	Sawle *et al.* (1991)	6 obsessional slowness 6 controls	Orbital frontal, premotor hypermetabolism
Dopamine PET	Sawle *et al.* (1991)	5 obsessional slowness 6 controls	No difference with controls
HMPAO SPECT	Machlin *et al.* (1991)	10 OCD	Increased right orbital frontal metabolism
	George *et al.* (1991c)	20 GTS 8 controls	Increased right frontal metabolism

they observed decreased whole cortex metabolism along with decreased normalized lateral prefrontal cortex. Methodological differences may explain their variation in findings.

The PET findings above have now been extended to HMPAO SPECT. Machlin and colleagues (1991) used high-resolution SPECT to find right orbital hypermetabolism in ten OCD subjects compared with controls.

In addition to studying OCD subjects while ill, functional neuroimaging has been used to monitor how the brain changes as subjects improve with pharmacological and behavioural treatment. These studies simultaneously provide insight into both the anatomy of OCD and the mechanism of action of antiobsessional drugs and behavioural therapy. Baxter *et al.* (1987) originally noted that OCD subjects, after 6 weeks of treatment with trazadone, had decreased basal ganglia metabolism compared with baseline. Benkelfat *et al.* (1990) found in eight OCD subjects that 12 weeks of clomipramine treatment decreased metabolism in the orbital frontal cortex and left caudate nucleus. Those subjects with the most marked improvement on medication also tended to show the greatest brain metabolic changes over baseline. From these preliminary studies it might appear that there is a gradual progression of regional brain improvement over time, involving first the caudate nuclei, and later the orbital frontal regions. This interesting hypothesis needs further study. In a case report that may be relevant to this issue, Hoehn-Saric *et al.* (1991a) reported decreased frontal metabolism on HMPAO SPECT in an OCD subject who developed a frontal lobe syndrome (apathy, indifference) while taking high doses of fluoxetine. This led the authors to speculate that the 5-HT reuptake blockers work by decreasing frontal metabolism, with some patients on high doses of these drugs going to an extreme and losing other frontal lobe functions.

Preliminary data from Baxter and colleagues at UCLA now stand to confirm what clinicians have long known. That is, behaviour therapy for OCD produces normalization of brain metabolic changes in the caudate much as drugs do. These preliminary PET findings may be the first demonstration of long-term brain metabolic changes induced by a behavioural, cognitive or even psychotherapeutic treatment (Baxter, unpublished data).

Studies from a variety of neuroimaging sources and groups are beginning to find important similarities and differences in the brain metabolic picture of OCD-related disorders. Swedo *et al.* (1991) used FDG PET to study 10 women with *trichotillomania* compared with 20 age-matched controls. Contrary to the pattern in primary OCD, trichotillomania subjects had increased global and normalized right and left cerebellar and right superior parietal glucose metabolic rates. Interestingly, much as in primary OCD, clomipramine-induced improvement correlated with decreases in anterior cingulate and orbital frontal metabolism. George *et al.* (1991a) used HMPAO SPECT to study 20 subjects with GTS. Compared with eight controls, GTS subjects had elevated right frontal activity.

Finally, Sawle *et al.* (1991) have demonstrated the power of functional neuroimaging to understand the OCD-related disorder, *obsessional slowness* (OS), where patients exhibit extreme slowness in the execution of everyday tasks such as washing and eating. They studied six OS subjects using ^{15}O PET and found focal hypermetabolism in orbital frontal, premotor and midfrontal cortex. The midfrontal and premotor findings emphasize the movement aspects of this disorder, while the orbital frontal hypermetabolism corresponds to the functional picture seen in primary OCD. In some ways OS resembles Parkinsonism and the authors speculated that there might therefore be pathological dopamine involvement in OS. However, using ^{18}F-labelled dopa and PET, the authors found no differences from age-matched controls. Thus it does not appear that the slowness in OS is related to damaged nigro-striatal dopaminergic neurons.

George and colleagues (1991b) at the Middlesex Hospital in London used ^{123}I-labelled IBZM SPECT to examine dopaminergic pathways in patients with GTS. Drug-naive GTS subjects showed decreased initial tracer binding compared with controls. These studies display the power of functional neuroimaging to examine specific hypotheses concerning neurotransmitter dysregulation in neuropsychiatric diseases.

A Psychopharmacological Neuroanatomy of OCD: The Current Picture

At least four different and independent areas can now be assimilated to provide a functional neuroanatomical map of OCD. This map is still incomplete and will undoubtedly be expanded and changed with new psychopharmacological details. The new functional neuroimaging methodologies (PET and SPECT) have extended this map further. PET and SPECT promise to provide a simultaneous understanding of the pathophysiology of OCD, how the normal brain works to make decisions concerning the limits of grooming and checking, and the mechanisms of action of 5-HT reuptake blockers and behavioural therapy. These are summarized in Figure 3.

A functional OCD loop probably involves orbital frontal white matter, the caudate, putamen and globus pallidus, the thalamus and the cingulate gyrus. There are numerous known interconnections between these structures. Figure 3 is an attempt to demonstrate how these structures may function cohesively, such that damage at any point may produce changes in other regions. Figure 3 also provides some idea of the relative role of the important neurotransmitters dopamine and 5-HT in each of these regions, and the probable direction of information flow.

It is highly probable that the primary pathology in OCD lies somewhere within this neural net. Exactly which site is primary and which others react in concert is little more than speculation at this point. Baxter has formulated an interesting idea that the phenomenology in a genetically predisposed patient

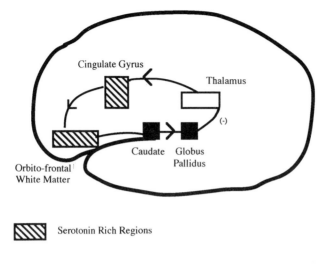

    Serotonin Rich Regions

    Dopamine Rich Regions

Figure 3. A sagittal picture of the brain with pertinent brain regions outlined. This functional loop of OCD pathology combines information from structural neuroimaging studies (CT or MRI), psychosurgery, secondary causes of OCD and neuropharmacological studies of OCD. Integrating these findings with the emerging PET and SPECT studies yields this composite picture. When OCD symptoms are at their worse, there is increased activity in the frontal white matter and caudate. These regions normalize with treatment. At present it is unclear if these regions are the primary cause of OCD, or are compensatory reactions within this functional loop

of OCD, OCD with tics, or GTS, depends on where along the circuit the pathology resides (Baxter, 1990). Those with OCD, particularly where obsessions highlight the clinical picture, would be expected to have more frontal pathology. Conversely, those with more tics, or pure GTS, would have more caudate pathology. This fascinating hypothesis has unfortunately not been confirmed by functional neuroimaging studies to date.

Obviously these and other (Modell *et al.*, 1989) neural network theories of OCD are tentative and subject to constant refinement as more data emerge. However, the exciting aspect of this proposed neuroanatomy is that it is subject to experimental confirmation or rejection in the near future using testable hypotheses with PET and SPECT.

Conclusion

An incomplete but ever-expanding picture of the likely neuropathology of OCD emerges. SPECT and PET have confirmed other studies of OCD structural changes to produce an interesting anatomy of OCD. Recent PET and SPECT studies also integrate nicely with secondary causes of OCD to further delineate this regional network. The advances made in the understanding of OCD in the last decade demonstrate the remarkable impact of a new technology and new methodology on unlocking the secrets of the brain.

Acknowledgements

The author is grateful to Drs Michael Trimble and Howard Ring for their helpful discussions concerning many of the issues and areas discussed in this chapter.

References

Alexander, R.C. (1991). Fluoxetine treatment of trichotillomania. *J. Clin. Psychiatry,* **52**, 88.
Baxter, L.R. (1990). Brain imaging as a tool in establishing a theory of brain pathology in obsessive compulsive disorder. *J. Clin. Psychiatry,* **51(s)**, 22–5.
Baxter, L.R., Phelps, M.E., Mazziotta, J.C., Guze, B.H., Schwartz, J.M., and Selin, C.E. (1987). Local cerebral glucose metabolic rates in obsessive-compulsive disorder. *Arch. Gen. Psychiatry,* **44**, 211–18
Baxter, L.R., Schwartz, J.M., Mazziotta, J.C. *et al.* (1988). Cerebral glucose metabolic rates in non-depressed patients with obsessive-compulsive disorder. *Am. J. Psychiatry,* **145**, 1560–3.
Baxter, L.R., Schwartz, J.M., Guze, B.H., Bergman, K., and Szuba, M.P. (1990). PET imaging in obsessive compulsive disorder with and without depression. *J. Clin. Psychiatry,* **51**, 61–9.
Bear, D.M., and Fedio, P. (1977). Quantitative analysis of inter-ictal behavior in temporal lobe epilepsy *Arch. Neurol.,* **34**, 454–67.
Benkelfat, C., Nordahl, T.E., Semple, W.E., King, A.C., Murphy, D.L., and Cohen, R.M. (1990). Local cerebral glucose metabolic rates in obsessive-compulsive disorder. *Arch. Gen. Psychiatry,* **47**, 840–8.
Brady, K.T., Austin, L., and Lydiard, R.B. (1990). Body dysmorphic disorder: The relationship to obsessive-compulsive disorder. *J. Nerv. Ment. Dis.,* **178**, 538–40.
Brickner, R.M., Rosner, A.A., Munroe, R. (1970). Physiological aspects of the obsessive state. *Psychosomatic Medicine,* **2**, 369–383.
Bridges, P.K., Goktepe, E.O., Maratos, J., Browne, A., and Young, L. (1973). A comparative review of patients with obsessional neurosis and with depression treated by psychosurgery. *Br. J. Psychiatry,* **123**, 663–74.
Cambier, J., Masson, C., Benammou, S., and Robine, B. (1988). La graphomanie, activite graphique compulsive manifestation d'un gliome fronto-calleux. *Rev. Neurol.,* **144**, 158–64.
Comings, D.E. (1990). *Tourette Syndrome and Human Behavior,* Duarte, CA: Hope Press.
Cummings, J.L., and Frankel, M. (1985). Gilles de la Tourette syndrome and the neurological basis of obsessions and compulsions. *Biol. Psychiatry,* **20**, 1117–26.
Ellinwood, E.H. (1967). Amphetamine psychosis. *J. Nerv. Ment. Dis.,* **144**, 273–83.
Fallon, B.A., Liebowitz, M.R., Hollander, E., Schneider, F.R., Campeas, R.B., Fairbanks, J., Papp, L.A., Hatterer, J.A., and Sandberg, D. (1990). The pharmacotherapy of moral or religious scrupulosity. *J. Clin. Psychiatry,* **51**, 517–21.

Frankel, M., Cummings, J.L., Robertson, M., Trimble, M.R., Hill, M.A., and Benson, D.F. (1986). Obsessions and compulsions in Gilles de la Tourette syndrome. *Neurology*, **36**, 378–92.

Friston, K.J., Passingham, R.E., Nutt, J.G. *et al.* (1989). Localization in PET images: Direct fitting of the intercommisural (AC–PC) line. *J. Cereb. Blood Flow Metab.*, **9**, 690–5.

Garber, H.J., Ananth, J.V., Chiu, L.C., Griswold, V.J., and Oldendorf, W.H. (1989). Nuclear magnetic resonance study of obsessive-compulsive disorder. *Am. J. Psychiatry*, **146**, 1001–5.

George, M.S. (1992). Obsessive-compulsive disorder. *Int. Clin. Psychopharmacol.*, **65**, 57s–68s.

George, M.S., Taylor, R., Seay, A.R., and Hogan, E.L. (1987). Sydenham's chorea: A disease on the increase? *J SC Med. Assoc.*, **83**, 523–7.

George, M.S., Kellner, C.H., and Fossey, M. (1989). Obsessive-compulsive disorder in a patient with MS. *J. Nerv. Ment. Dis.*, **177**, 304–5.

George, M.S., Ring, H.A., Costa, D.C., Ell, P.J., Kouris, K., and Jarritt, P. (1991a). *Neuroactivation and Neuroimaging with SPET*, London: Springer-Verlag.

George, M.S., Robertson, M.M., Costa, D.C., and Ell, P.J. (1991b). D2 Receptor activity in Tourette syndrome (GTS). *APA New Res. Program*, **NR33**, 56 (Abstract).

George, M.S., Robertson, M.M., Costa, D.C., Trimble, M.R., and Ell, P.J. (1991c). HMPAO SPECT scans of co-morbid OCD/GTS patients. *APA New Res. Program*, **NR34**, 57 (Abstract).

George, M.S., Trimble, M.R., and Robertson, M.M. (1991d). A pharmacologic (5HT vs D2) probe of patients with comorbid OCD and Gilles de la Tourette syndrome. *Biol. Psychiatry*, **29**, 444s (Abstract).

George, M.S., Melvin, J.A., and Kellner, C.H. (1992). Obsessive-compulsive symptoms in neurologic disease: A review. *Behav. Neurol.*, **5**, 19–30.

Gilles de la Tourette, G. (1885). Etude sur une affection nerveuse caracterisée par de l'incordination motrice accompagnée d'echolalie et de copralalie. *Arch. Neurol.*, **9**, 19–42 (Abstract).

Goodman, W.K., Price, L.H., and Charney, D.S. (1989a). Fluvoxamine in obsessive compulsive disorder. *Psychiatr. Ann.*, **19**, 92–6.

Grimshaw, L. (1964). Obsessional disorder and neurological illness. *J. Neurol. Neurosurg. Psychiatry*, **27**, 229–31.

Grindlinger, H.M., and Ramsay, E. (1991). Compulsive feather picking in birds. *Arch. Gen. Psychiatry*, **49**, 857.

Hamlin, C.L., Swayne, L.C., and Liebowitz, M.R. (1989). Striatal IMP–SPECT decrease in obsessive-compulsive disorder, normalized by pharmacotherapy. *Neuropsychiatry Neuropsychol. Behav. Neurol.*, **2**, 290–300.

Hoehn-Saric, R., Harris, G.J., Pearlson, G.D., Cox, C.S., Machlin, S.R., and Camargo, E.E. (1991a). A fluoxetine-induced frontal lobe syndrome in an obsessive compulsive patient. *J. Clin. Psychiatry*, **52**, 131–3.

Hoehn-Saric, R., Pearlson, G.D., Harris, G.J., Machlin, S.R., and Camargo, E.E. (1991b). Effects of fluoxetine on regional cerebral blood flow in obsessive-compulsive patients. *Am. J. Psychiatry*, **148**, 1243–5.

Hollander, E., Fay, M., Cohen, B., Campeas, R., Gorman, J.M., and Liebowitz, M.R. (1988). Serotonergic and noradrenergic sensitivity in obsessive-compulsive disorder: Behavioral findings. *Am. J. Psychiatry*, **145**, 1015–17.

Hollander, E., Liebowitz, M.R., Winchel, R., Klumker, A., and Klein, D.F. (1989). Treatment of body-dysmorphic disorder with serotonin reuptake blockers. *Am. J. Psychiatry*, **146**, 768–70.

120 *M. S. George*

Husby, G., van de Ryn, I., Zabriskie, J.B. et al. (1976). Antibodies reacting with cytoplasm of subthalamic and caudate nuclei neurons in chorea and rheumatic fever. *J. Exp. Med.,* **144**, 1094–1110.

Hymas, N., Lees, A.J., Bolton, D., Epps, K., and Head, D. (1991). The neurology of obsessional slowness. *Brain,* **114**, 2203–33.

Insel, T.R. (1988). Obsessive-compulsive disorder: A neuroethological perspective. *Psychopharmacol. Bull.,* **24**, 365–9.

Insel, T.R., Hamilton, J.A., Guttmacher, L.B., and Murphy, D.L. (1983). D-Amphetamine in obsessive-compulsive disorder. *Psychopharmacology,* **80**, 23–6.

Jelliffe, S.E. (1927). *Postencephalitic Respiratory Disorders,* Washington: Nervous and Mental Publishing.

Jellife, S.E. (1932). *Psychopathology of Forced Movements and the Oculogyric Crises of Lethargic Encephalitis,* Washington: Nervous and Mental Publishing.

Jenike, M.A. (1989). Obsessive compulsive and related disorders. *N. Engl. J. Med.,* **8**, 539–41.

Jenike, M.A., Baer, L., Ballantine, T., Martuza, R.L., Tynes, S., Giriunas, I., Buttolph, L., and Cassem, N.H. (1991). Cingulotomy for refractory obsessive-compulsive disorder. *Arch. Gen. Psychiatry,* **48**, 548–55.

Joffe, R.T., Swinson, R.P., and Levitt, A.J. (1991). Acute psychostimulant challenge in primary obsessive-compulsive disorder. *J. Clin. Psychopharmacol.,* **11**, 237–41.

Kafka, M.P., and Coleman, E. (1991). Serotonin and paraphilias. *J. Clin. Psychopharmacol.,* 223–4.

Kellner, C.H., Jolley, R.R., Holgate, R.C., Austin, L., Lydiard, R.B., Laraia, M., and Ballenger, J.C. (1991). Brain MRI in obsessive-compulsive disorder. *Psychiat. Res.,* **36**, 45–9.

Kurlan, R., Kersun, J., Ballantine, H.T., and Caine, E.D. (1990). Neurosurgical treatment of severe obsessive-compulsive disorder associated with Tourette's syndrome. *Movement Disord.,* **5**, 152–5.

Laplane, D., Widlocher, D., Pillon, B., Baulac, M., and Binoux, F. (1981). Comportement compulsif d'allure obsessionnelle par necrose circonscrite bilaterale pallidostriatale. *Rev. Neurol.,* **137**, 269–76.

Laplane, D., Levasseur, M., Pillon, B. et al. (1989). Obsessive-compulsive and other behavioural changes with bilateral basal ganglia lesions. *Brain,* **112**, 699–725.

Lees, A.J., Robertson, M.M., Trimble, M.R., and Murray, N.M.F. (1984). A clinical study of Gilles de la Tourette syndrome in the United Kingdom. *J. Neurol. Neurosurg. Psychiatry,* **47**, 1–8.

Luxenberg, J.S., Swedo, S.E., Flament, M.F. et al. (1988). Neuroanatomic abnormalities in obsessive-compulsive disorder with quantitative X-ray computed tomography. *Am. J. Psychiatry,* **145**, 1089–93.

Machlin, S.R., Harris, G.J., Pearlson, G.D., Hoehn-Saric, R., Jeffrey, P., and Camargo, E.E. (1991). Elevated medial–frontal cerebral blood flow in obsessive-compulsive patients: A SPECT study. *Am. J. Psychiatry,* **148**, 1240–2.

Maclean, P.D. (1990). *The Triune Brain in Evolution: Role in Paleocerebral Functions,* New York: Plenum Press.

Marks, I.M. (1987). *Fears, Phobias and Rituals,* New York: Oxford University Press.

Martinot, J.L., Allilaire, J.F., Mazoyer, B.M., Hantouche, E., Huret, J.D., Legaut-Demare, F., Deslauriers, A.G., Hardy, P., Pappata, S., Baron, J.C., and Syrota, A. (1990). Obsessive-compulsive disorder: A clinical, neuropsychological and positron emission tomography study. *Acta Psychiatr. Scand.,* **82**, 233–42.

McKeon, J., McGuffin, P. and Robinson, P. (1984). Obsessive-compulsive neurosis following head injury: A report of four cases. *Br. J. Psychiatry,* **144**, 190–2.

Mitchell-Heggs, N., Kelley, D., and Richardson, A.E. (1977). Stereotactic limbic leucotomy: Clinical, psychological and physiologic assessment at sixteen months. In: Sweet, W.H., and Obrador, S. (eds), *Neurosurgical Treatment in Psychiatry, Pain and Epilepsy*, Baltimore: University Park Press, pp. 367–79.

Modell, J.G., Mountz, J.M., Curtis, G.C., and Gredin, J.F. (1989). Neurophysiologic dysfunction in basal ganglia/limbic striatal and thalamocortical circuits as a pathogenetic mechanism of obsessive-compulsive disorder. *J. Neuropsychiatry Clin. Neurol.*, **1**, 27–36.

Montgomery, S.A. (1980). Clomipramine in obsessional neurosis. *Pharmacol. Med.*, **1**, 189–92.

Nordahl, T.E., Benkelfat, C., Semple, W.E. *et al.* (1989). Cerebral glucose metabolic rates in obsessive-compulsive disorder. *Neuropsychopharmacology*, **2**, 23–8.

Pauls, D.L., and Leckman, J.F. (1986). The inheritance of Gilles de la Tourette syndrome and associated behaviors. *N. Engl. J. Med.*, **315**, 993–7.

Pauls, D.L., Leckman, J.F., Towbin, K.E., Zahner, G.E., and Cohen, D.J. (1986a). A possible genetic relationship exists between Tourette's syndrome and obsessive-compulsive disorder. *Psychopharmacol. Bull*, **22**, 730–3.

Pauls, D.L., Towbin, K.E., Leckman, J.F., Jahner, G.E.P., and Cohen, D.J. (1986b). Gilles de la Tourette's syndrome and obsessive-compulsive disorder: Evidence supporting a genetic relationship. *Arch. Gen. Psychiatry*, **43**, 1180–2.

Phelps, M., Mazziotta, J.C., and Schelbert, H. (1986). *Positron Emission Tomography and Autoradiography: Principles and Applications for the Heart and Brain*, New York: Raven Press.

Pigott, T.A., Pato, M.T., Bernstein, S.E., Grover, G.N., Hill, J.L., Tolliver, T.J. *et al.* (1990). Controlled comparison of clomipramine and fluoxetine in the treatment of obsessive-compulsive disorder. *Arch. Gen. Psychiatry*, **47**, 926–32.

Pitman, R.K. (1989). Animal models of compulsive behavior. *Biol. Psychiatry*, **26**, 189–98.

Rapoport, J.L. (1990). Obsessive compulsive disorder and basal ganglia dysfunction. *Psychol. Med.*, **20**, 465–9.

Rasmussen, S.A., and Eisen, J.A. 1990). Epidemiology of obsessive compulsive disorder. *J. Clin. Psychiatry*, **51**, 10–15.

Sacks, O. (1982). *Awakenings*, London: Picador.

Sawle, G.V., Hymas, N.F., Lees, A.J., and Frackowiak, R.S.J. (1991). Obsessional slowness: Functional studies with positron emission tomography. *Brain*, **114**, 2191–2202.

Schilder, P. (1938). The organic background of obsessions and compulsions. *Am. J. Psychiatry*, **95**, 1397–1413.

Seibyl, J.P., Krystal, J.H., Goodman, W.K., and Price, L.H. (1989). Obsessive-compulsive symptoms in a patient with a right frontal lobe lesion. *Neuropsychiatry Neuropsychol. Behav. Neurol.*, **1**, 295–9.

Sokoloff, L. (1977). Relation between physiological function and energy metabolism in the central nervous system. *J. Neurochem.*, **29**, 13–26.

Swedo, S.E., Rapoport, J.L., Cheslow, D.L. *et al.* (1989a). High prevalence of obsessive-compulsive symptoms in patients with Sydenham's chorea. *Am. J. Psychiatry*, **146**, 246–9.

Swedo, S.E., Schapiro, M.B., Grady, C.L. *et al.* (1989b). Cerebral glucose metabolism in childhood onset obsessive-compulsive disorder. *Arch. Gen. Psychiatry*, **46**, 518–23.

Swedo, S.E., Rapoport, J.L., Leonard, H.L., Schapiro, M.B., Rapoport, S.I., and Grady, C.L. (1991). Regional cerebral glucose metabolism of women with trichotillomania. *Arch. Gen. Psychiatry*, **48**, 828–33.

Tan, E., Marks, I.M., and Marset, P. (1971). Bimedial leucotomy in obsessive-compulsive neurosis: A controlled serial enquiry. *Br. J. Psychiatry,* **118**, 155–64.

Thoren, P., Asberg, M., Bertilsson, L. *et al.* (1980). Clomipramine treatment of obsessive-compulsive disorder: Biochemical and clinical aspects. *Arch. Gen. Psychiatry,* **37**, 1289–94.

Tippin, J., and Henn, F.A. (1982). Modified leukotomy in the treatment of intractable obsessional neurosis. *Am. J. Psychiatry,* **139**, 1601–3.

Tonkonogy, J., and Barriera, P. (1989). Obsessive-compulsive disorder and caudate–frontal lesion. *Neuropsychiatry Neuropsychol. Behav. Neurol.,* **2**, 203–9.

Trimble, M.R. (1989). Psychopathology and movement disorders: A new perspective on the Gilles de la Tourette syndrome. *J. Neurol. Neurosurg. Psychiatry* (Suppl.), 90–5.

Von Economo, C. (1931). *Encephalitis Lethargica: Its Sequelae and Treatment,* Oxford: Oxford University Press.

Ward, C.D. (1988). Transient feelings of compulsion caused by hemispheric lesions: three cases. *J. Neurol. Neurosurg. Psychiatry,* **51**, 266–8.

Weilburg, J.B., Mesulam, M., Weintraub, S., Buonanno, F., Jenike, M., and Stakes, J.W. (1989). Focal striatal abnormalities in a patient with obsessive-compulsive disorder. *Arch. Neurol.,* **46**, 233–5.

Wohlfart, G., Ingvar, D.H., and Heilberg, A. (1961). Compulsory shouting (Benedek's 'Klazomania') associated with oculogyric spasms in chronic epidemic encephalitis. *Acta Psychiatr. Scand.,* **36**, 369–77.

Zohar, J., Mueller, E.A., Insel, T.R. *et al.* (1987). Serotonergic responsivity in obsessive-compulsive disorder: Comparison of patients and healthy controls. *Arch. Gen. Psychiatry,* **44**, 946–51.

8
The Experimental Investigation of Human Eating Behaviour

Peter J. Rogers

*Consumer Sciences Department, AFRC Institute of Food
Research, Reading, UK*

Importance of the Measurement of Human Eating Behaviour

Over the past 25 years the experimental investigation of human eating behaviour has become a very active field of research. During this time a variety
of techniques and approaches have been developed to assess different aspects
of eating and food choice, from the recording of the microstructure of chewing movements in individual subjects to the measurement of dietary patterns
in national surveys. A major impetus in this work has been the concern to
understand and treat obesity, and more recently the recognition of the desir-
ability of reducing the proportion of fat (particularly saturated fat) consumed
in the diet. Both these factors have important implications for physical health,
including coronary heart disease, stroke and certain cancers (Department of
Health, 1992).

It has proved to be remarkably difficult to demonstrate, even in the most
careful studies, that obese people overeat compared to lean people, which
has led to the claim that there is an underlying metabolic 'defect' in obesity.
However, recent studies on energy balance have not found a reduced energy
requirement associated with obesity, and it is now more certain that increased intake is the primary aetiological factor in obesity (Prentice *et al.*,
1989). The failure to find evidence of elevated food intake is probably due
mainly to a greater tendency in obese subjects to under-report the amount
eaten, and also because the maintenance energy requirement for obese
people is not that much larger than for lean people. There are few if any
reliable data on long-term food intake during the spontaneous development
of obesity in humans, owing to the many problems in making such measurements (see below).

Human Psychopharmacology, Vol. 4. Edited by I. Hindmarch and P. D. Stonier
© 1993 John Wiley & Sons Ltd

Important as these realizations are, it must be said that it is far from clear what aspects of appetite control differ between lean and obese people, although a role for dietary fat is implicated by various results including, for example, a positive correlation between the proportion of calories eaten as fat and body fatness (reviewed by Rogers, 1990a). In any case, it is widely agreed that approaches to the treatment of obesity should comprise strategies to increase energy expenditure as well as reduce energy intake. Pharmacological treatments have been developed along both of these lines, and include appetite suppressants with central and/or peripheral actions and thermogenic agents. Comprehensive reviews of the clinical pharmacology of appetite and treatment of obesity are available elsewhere (e.g., Blundell *et al.*, 1990; Bray and Inoue, 1992), and this material is not repeated here. Instead, the present chapter examines the structure and control of human eating behaviour, before going on to consider issues of measurement and experimental design relevant to the pharmacological manipulation of appetite. In particular, the discussion will focus on the different processes controlling eating, the associated subjective experiences and the measurement of those experiences.

Palatability, Satiety and Cognition in the Control of Food Intake

Structure of Eating

Eating in humans occurs in bouts called meals, and food intake can vary according to the number and/or size of meals eaten. ('Snacks' are probably best considered as small meals, since this appears to be a distinction based mainly on social convention rather than any substantial differences in the processes controlling eating.) The meal, therefore, can be considered the basic unit for the analysis of eating behaviour which, in turn, may be divided into three distinct phases: namely, the initiation, maintenance, and termination of eating.

Meal initiation is identified with appetitive states such as hunger and food cravings which direct behaviour towards eating and perhaps particular foods. Internal cues related to, for example, the dynamics of blood glucose can provide a reliable stimulus for the initiation of eating both in rats and humans (Campfield and Smith, 1986; Smith *et al.*, 1992); however, the role of energy depletion in meal initiation appears to have been overemphasized compared with the effects of external cues. Eating usually occurs in anticipation of nutritional requirements rather than in direct response to low-energy availability (Collier, 1986), and can be motivated by the sight and smell of food and learned contextual cues such as location and times of day (Weingarten, 1985; Weingarten and Cowans, 1991).

Once the meal begins, eating is controlled by the action of both stimulatory and inhibitory influences. These influences, as depicted in Figure 1, combine to give a cumulative intake curve similar to that observed in studies of the microstructure of human eating (Spiegal and Jordan, 1978; Westerterp-Plantenga *et al.*, 1990). Of course, identical curves can be obtained with stimulatory and inhibitory influences varying in a number of different ways; so, for instance, there may be some decline in the strength of positive feedback during the meal (see below). Positive feedback from eating probably plays an essential role in keeping behaviour 'locked in' to eating. Simulations show that without positive feedback there is a tendency for behaviour to oscillate or dither between activities (Houston and Sumida, 1985; McFarland, 1971).

The operation of negative feedback during normal eating is illustrated by the results of studies on sham feeding. Rats fitted with a chronic gastric fistula eat (drink) vastly increased amounts when the liquid food is allowed to drain out of the open fistula, compared with when the fistula is closed (Smith *et al.*,

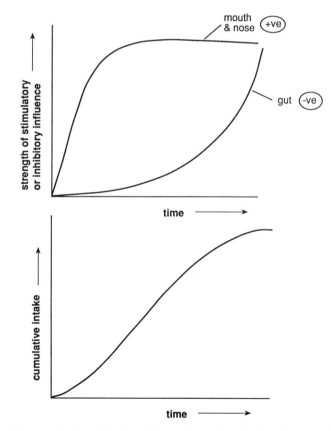

Figure 1. Hypothetical model of positive and negative feedbacks operating on eating during a meal. Top: stimulatory and inhibitory effects of sensory and gut-mediated signals. Bottom: resulting cumulative amount of food eaten across the meal

1974). In other words, satiety does not occur if ingested food fails to distend the stomach or enter the small intestine—thus excluding taste, other oral stimuli, pharyngeal and oesophageal movements, and the contact of food with the gastric mucosa as potent stimuli for satiety. (Although the sham-fed rat does eventually stop eating, this is likely to be due to fatigue or the effects of the digestion and absorption of a portion of the ingested nutrients (Sclafani and Nissenbaum, 1985).)

Results from sham feeding experiments also indicate that learning contributes to satiety and the control of meal size. A large increase in meal size is not seen on the first occasion that rats are sham fed. Instead there is a suppression of eating during initial sham feeds due to learned satiety (Weingarten and Kulikovsky, 1989). During normal feeding the sensory properties of the food become associated with the post-ingestive effects experienced, and this provides anticipatory control of meal size. On the first sham feed, meal size is modulated according to the 'expected' post-ingestive effects, but with continued sham feeding this learning extinguishes and meal size increases. There is, however, also a direct influence of the post-ingestive and post-absorptive effects of food ingestion (filling of the gastrointestinal tract, release of regulatory hormones such as cholecystokinin, the detection of nutrients absorbed into the systemic circulation, etc.) on meal size, as well as on the maintenance of satiety in the post-meal interval (Blundell *et al.*, 1990). The anticipatory control of meal size is a refinement which is needed because the post-ingestive and post-absorptive effects of food are delayed relative to the moment of eating.

The positive feedback effect is assumed to arise from sensory (mainly olfactory and gustatory) contact with food. This stimulation of eating by eating would appear to be consistent with subjective experience—l'appétit vient en mangeant (appetite comes with eating). In addition, there are behavioural data which support the existence of such an effect. A good example comes from Wiepkema's (1971a, 1971b) detailed analysis of feeding in the mouse. At the beginning of a spontaneous meal a large increase in the length of successive feeding bouts was observed, while the length of non-feeding intervals was unchanged during this part of the meal. Wiepkema (1971b) interpreted these and other findings using a model, similar to that shown in Figure 1, in which positive feedback from sensory contact with food plays a central role in the maintenance of eating during meals. Furthermore, the strength of the positive feedback effect is supposed to depend on the quality of the sensory stimuli (i.e., palatability). When bitter, less preferred food—the standard food adulterated with sucrose octoacetate—was offered the early increase in feeding-bout length was much reduced. Therefore, consumption of highly palatable foods may be expected to have a powerful positive feedback effect on eating, leading in turn to an increase in meal size and perhaps total daily food intake.

What is Palatability?

There is considerable confusion surrounding the term palatability. Sometimes its use appears to be synonymous with food intake or the vigour of ingestive responses, but in this sense palatability is merely a descriptive term which contributes little or nothing to the understanding of eating behaviour. There is, nonetheless, clearly a need for a concept which refers to the hedonic or affective quality of orosensory stimuli as experienced by the consumer (e.g., human, rat or mouse), and used in this way the concept can have explanatory value (Rogers, 1990b). However, its status as an explanatory concept (hypothetical construct) means that palatability is not itself open to direct measurement. Perhaps the best approximation can be obtained in studies of human behaviour where pleasantness ratings of food may, if interpreted carefully, indicate hedonic quality and therefore palatability.

A variety of psychobiological studies have shown that palatability is influenced by innate factors and that it can also be modified by learning (discussed in Rogers, 1990b; Rogers and Blundell, 1990). Thus certain taste preferences appear to be present at birth. The facial expressions of human newborns indicate acceptance and a positive hedonic response to sweet stimuli, while bitter stimuli evoke rejection coupled with negative expressions (Steiner, 1987). Such innate biases would seem to be adaptive: bitter tastes tend to be correlated in nature with the presence of toxins (e.g., alkaloids in plants), and sweet tastes will normally signal a ready source of energy in the form of sugars. Even more significant, the near-universally enthusiastic response to sweetness may be an important factor facilitating the infant's early acceptance of its mother's milk (Booth, 1991; see also Blass, 1991).

As for the effects of experience, it has long been established that animals learn to avoid food when consumption of that food is paired with illness and gastrointestinal upset (Garcia *et al.*, 1974). This learning can be very rapid, it can occur with long delays between food ingestion and onset of illness, and is very persistent. The occurrence of food aversions in humans has been examined in retrospective questionnaire surveys (Garb and Stunkard, 1974; Logue *et al.*, 1981), and the findings suggest that humans can acquire food aversions through the same conditioning process as other species. Following the demonstration of food aversion learning it was generally assumed that preferences could also be modified by the positive after-effects of food ingestion. It is possible, for example, that the medicinal effect of a food containing a needed nutrient could condition a positive preference for that food (Garcia *et al.*, 1974). Nonetheless, clear evidence of learned preferences was lacking until recently, when Sclafani and his colleagues (e.g., Elizalde and Sclafani, 1988, 1990) were able to demonstrate strong conditioning of preferences for flavours paired with intragastric Polycose infusions (Polycose is a partially hydrolysed corn starch). Increases in favour preference controlled by the post-ingestive effects of nutrient manipulations have also been demonstrated in humans (e.g., Birch *et al.*, 1990).

Learned preferences and aversions as discussed above appear to be characterized by alterations in the actual pleasantness or liking of the food's taste, flavour, texture, etc. (i.e., a change in palatability) (Elizalde and Sclafani, 1990). 'Conditioned aversion is a nasty taste, not merely or at all the refusal to take something which is perceived as dangerous' (p. 566, Booth, 1979). In other words, while the hedonic or pleasure response to orosensory cues during eating is in part pre-programmed, it is also modified by learning. Most importantly, this response, presumably mediated through brain reward pathways (see below), would appear to play a central role in motivating ingestive behaviour and guiding the choice and consumption of foods in relation to their biological utility. Thus clearly it is not possible to separate palatability from food composition.

One aspect of palatability over which there is considerable debate at present concerns the extent to which the hedonic value of orosensory stimuli varies as a function of immediate physiological conditions. It is often asserted that palatability is enhanced in a state of depletion and/or diminishes during repletion. There is evidence, however, suggesting that hunger and palatability may act largely independently. Thus palatability, hunger and post-ingestive satiety can be dissociated behaviourally and by pharmacological and physiological manipulations (Rogers, 1990b, and see below). This is also confirmed in recent phenomenological data. During a meal, perceived (i.e., self-reported) hunger declines and fullness increases; however, ratings of the pleasantness of the 'taste' of the food eaten remain relatively unchanged (Rogers and Blundell, 1990). This would be consistent with little or no reduction in positive feedback from eating, as depicted in Figure 1. That is, sensory contact with preferred food is always stimulatory, and never itself contributes to the development of satiation and satiety as claimed by some authors (e.g., Rolls *et al.*, 1984). One source of confusion here may have been the failure to distinguish between the pleasantness of the 'taste' of food in the mouth (influenced by palatability) and the pleasantness of eating or ingesting that food— which presumably is influenced both by palatability, and hunger and satiety (fullness of the stomach, etc.). When human subjects are asked to rate simply the pleasantness of food they are probably rating it in terms of pleasantness to eat, which does decline markedly during the courses of a typical meal (Blundell and Rogers, 1991; Rogers and Blundell, 1990).

A further way in which palatability may influence eating is by affecting the return of hunger during the post-meal interval. In a widely cited paper Hill *et al.* (1984) showed that self-reported hunger and desire to eat were greater during the consumption of preferred food compared with an equi-caloric meal of less-preferred food. Although the ratings then fell to a similar low level in the early post-meal interval, hunger and desire to eat subsequently increased more rapidly following the preferred food. The authors suggest that this 'de-layed priming effect' of palatability on hunger may have important con-sequences for the control of food intake, perhaps leading to increased inter-meal snacking or higher intake at the next main meal. The latter result was confirmed in another study reported by Rogers and Schultz (1992). While it is not yet clear what mediates these prolonged effects, one possibility is that palatability influences the strength of the cephalic phase responses, including insulin secretion. These events may then in turn alter the metabolic disposal of calories consumed in the meal and consequently the rate at which hunger recovers during the post-prandial interval (Rogers and Schutz, 1992). The same mechanism has been invoked to explain the stimulation of hunger and food intake by sweet taste (Rogers and Blundell, 1989; Tordoff and Alleva, 1990).

Implications for the Control of Food Intake and Body Weight

The longer-term effects of palatability on eating predicted from the above discussion would appear to be confirmed by studies of diet-induced obesity in animals. For example, in so-called cafeteria feeding rats given access to a variety of 'palatable' foods rich in fat and/or carbohydrate show substantially elevated food intake due mainly to an increase in meal size and an associated increase in the rate of eating. Initially there may also be some increase in meal frequency (reviewed by Rogers and Blundell, 1984). Resultant weight gains can be very substantial.

These findings are important, because they demonstrate the influence of palatability and food composition on food intake and they challenge the view that body weight or body fatness is regulated around an internal set point. This concept, which until recently has dominated much of the thinking about the biological mechanisms of appetite control, includes the notion of homeo-static behaviour. The basic idea is that behaviour is initiated in response to perturbations of the internal state. For example, eating might be triggered when the level of circulating metabolic fuels falls below a particular critical value. However, as indicated above, this fails to take into account ecological constraints. In most natural habitats food supplies are unpredictable, and accordingly certain physiological and behavioural adaptations have evolved which permit the anticipation of needs and the optimal exploitation of the resources available. Adipose tissue is an example of such an adaptation. The storage of energy in the form of body fat in times of plenty can provide a buffer against food shortages (this is taken to extremes in hibernating ani-mals). Accordingly, the appetite control system appears to be highly respon-sive to an under-supply of energy, but relatively tolerant of over-supply (i.e., overeating), with the consequence that there is more resistance to weight loss than weight gain (reviewed in Rogers, 1990a).

Emotionality, Dietary Restraint and the Cognitive Control of Eating

Finally, it is important to recognize the major role of emotional and cognitive factors in the control of food intake in humans. Stated simply, the psychosomatic view of obesity is that obesity is due to overeating that occurs in response to emotional stimuli. While the most common response to arousal states, such as anger, fear and anxiety is the loss of appetite, it is argued that some individuals react by eating excessively. Eating then modifies the emotional state; for example, it reduces anxiety. Overeating is thus a learned behaviour which can be viewed either as a coping response or as resulting from a confusion of internal cues associated with activation and stress and natural hunger cues (Kaplan and Kaplan, 1957; Bruch, 1962, Robbins and Fray, 1980). These and related ideas have been investigated extensively and have received some empirical support. For example, individuals who are overweight are more likely to report eating when depressed or anxious (Plutchik, 1976). Furthermore, both experimentally induced and naturally occurring anxiety have been shown to lead to over-consumption in the obese, whereas the same manipulations inhibited eating in lean subjects (Slochower, 1983).

   A difficulty with much of the research testing the psychosomatic hypothesis, however, is that it has failed to take into account the possible interaction between effects related to obesity and the effects of dieting (there is a high prevalence of dieting in the obese population). For instance, current dieting appears to be a better predictor of the amount eaten during depressed or dysphoric mood than is obesity (Baucom and Aiken, 1981). The consequences of dieting and dietary restraint were examined in a highly influential study by Herman and Mack (1975). They gave subjects 'preloads' of either two glasses of milkshake, one glass, or none, and then required them to rate the taste of various ice-creams. Whereas the intake of ice-cream was inversely related to the size of the preload in so-called unrestrained subjects, restrained subjects responded in a 'counterregulatory' fashion; that is, their intake of ice-cream increased as the size of the preload increased. A similar result was obtained by manipulating subjects' beliefs about the calorie content of the preload consumed while keeping its actual calorie content constant. Restrained subjects tended to overeat following a preload identified as high calorie, but ate rather little following a preload identified as low calorie (Polivy, 1976; Spencer and Fremouw, 1979). This suggests a disinhibition of behaviour. The preload, by forcing the perceived intake of calories above a critical threshold (or 'diet boundary'), causes normally restrained eaters to suspend their self-imposed restraint, thereby releasing their underlying desire to eat (due to hunger, emotional or other reasons) (Herman, 1978; Herman and Mack, 1975; Herman and Polivy, 1984). In addition to a food preload, emotional events (induction of anxiety, depression and dysphoric mood), the consumption of alcohol, the behaviour of others and even the sight and smell of palatable food have been shown to precipitate breakdown of restraint and overeating (Baucom and Aiken, 1981; Herman, 1978; Herman and Polivy, 1975; Rogers and Hill, 1989). In turn, these results would appear to implicate dieting in the aetiology of binge eating and bulimia nervosa (Hill, 1983; Polivy and Herman, 1985; Wardle and Beinart, 1981).

Measurement of Eating Behaviour and the Pharmacological Manipulation of Appetite

Methods for Recording Eating Behaviour and Food Intake

This section discusses some of the techniques that have been developed for the measurement of human eating behaviour. A detailed description of this methodology is unnecessary since this can be found in Blundell and Hill (1988). Nonetheless, it is worth indicating the range of techniques that is available. Many of the methods are quite ingenious, although none can be said to be perfect. In general there is a trade-off between precision of measurement, degree of experimental control and the ecological validity of the investigation.

Continuous monitoring of eating behaviour and food intake in the laboratory began with experiments using apparatus consisting of a reservoir of liquid food and a pump which the subject could activate to deliver the food through a 'straw' into the mouth or directly into the stomach via an intragastric tube (Jordan, 1969). This technique was used to study cumulative intakes during single meals as well as the regulation of food intake over the longer term. Of particular interest were the effects of manipulations of the caloric density of the food and how eating responses differed between lean and obese subjects (e.g., Campbell *et al.*, 1971; Spiegel, 1973). Methods developed subsequently have enabled the measurement of eating within meals under more naturalistic conditions. These methods include the Universal Eating Monitor, which consists of a concealed electronic balance for the continuous weighing of solid or liquid food remaining on the subject's plate (Kissileff *et al.*, 1980), and a device known as a Bite-Indicating Telemetering Eatometer (BITE), which operates through specially constructed spoons and forks that transmit a signal when each portion of food is placed in the mouth (Moon, 1979). Another technique relies upon the electromyographic recordings of masseter muscles, or the measurement of chewing with a strain gauge, together with detection of swallowing (Pierson and LeMagnen, 1969; Bellisle and LeMagnen, 1981). Finally, in addition to these mechanical methods, the detailed observation of the microstructure of eating behaviour either 'live' or recorded on video tape has also proved to be a valuable tool for investigating the structure of eating and the effects of experimental manipulations (e.g., Rogers and Blundell, 1979).

A variety of measures can be obtained from the analysis of data collected using these various techniques, including meal duration, number and size of mouthfuls, number of chews per mouthful, eating rate and duration of non-eating activity during the meal. The rate of change in eating rate across the meal is also of interest and, along with certain other measures, is differentially affected by the anorexic agents amphetamine and fenfluramine (Rogers and Blundell, 1979). It is fairly typical to find that the rate of eating slows as the meal progresses, giving a negatively decelerating cumulative intake curve (see Figure 1). However, obese subjects are more likely to show a linear rate of eating and perhaps a higher overall rate of eating. Although such data have been used to support the idea of an 'obese eating style', it is not at all clear that these differences are directly related to obesity (reviewed by Spitzer and Rodin, 1981). In studies where observations were made in natural settings (e.g., restaurants) the results may be confounded by the lack of control on food choice. Obese people appear to show an exaggerated response to palatability (Spitzer and Rodin, 1981), and in turn palatability has a major influence on eating rate (Bellisle and LeMagnen, 1981). Similarly, the lack of a slowing in eating rate toward the end of the meal in the obese or in dieters (Westerterp-Plantenga *et al.*, 1992) does not necessarily indicate a defect of satiety. This may be due simply to the conscious restriction of eating by these restrained subjects in an attempt to limit their intake. Thus analysis of the microstructure of eating and the cumulative intake curve may be used to identify the operation of some of the processes influencing eating; however, caution is needed in the interpretation of results and particularly in relating the measures to different theoretical constructs.

The simplest and most widely used method for investigating human eating behaviour in the laboratory is to provide subjects with a 'test meal' given at a fixed time of day. Typically this will consist of a selection of foods appropriate for the time of day and offered in excess. Subjects are instructed to eat as much or as little as they want, or until they are comfortably full. The amount eaten is recorded by weighing the food items beforehand and reweighing them after the subject has left, providing data on amount eaten, food choice and macronutrient consumption. In order to improve the degree of experimental control, subjects are asked to keep a defined routine of eating and activity for 8–24 hours before testing, although they will not usually be food restricted. Testing in the laboratory gives the advantage of a high degree of control and accuracy of measurement, and these methods are capable of detecting quite subtle effects of nutritional and pharmacological manipulations (e.g. Rogers and Blundell, 1979; 1989; Rogers *et al.*, 1991). They can also be extended by including microstructural measures (using, for example, video recording), further test meals, or by giving subjects diaries in which to record their food intake outside the laboratory. Other variants on this basic method allow subjects access to an automated vending machine (Silverstone *et al.*, 1980), or provide all of the subjects' food for several weeks from the laboratory or metabolic ward where they are resident or semi-resident for the entire duration of the study (e.g., Foltin *et al.*, 1988; Lissner *et al.*, 1987; Porikas *et al.*, 1982). In these situations the timing and frequency of meals, as well as meal size, can be free to vary.

The assessment of food intake and dietary patterns in free-living individuals and groups has a long history (see Quandt, 1987). One approach relies on subjects maintaining detailed dietary records of all foods eaten either by direct measurement of the weight or volume of items consumed, or by estimation in relation to model portion sizes. The main problem here is that the effort of recording, perhaps together with an increased awareness of what is being eaten, frequently leads to an under-reporting and distortion of normal intake and eating patterns. This distortion is probably more pronounced in certain groups such as the obese, but does not necessarily indicate a conscious bias by these subjects (Prentice *et al.*, 1989). The problem is illustrated in Table 1, which shows the results of the most recent national survey of the dietary habits of British adults. Compared with the estimated energy requirements of this population sample, this appears to have considerably underestimated energy intake, particularly for women.

Table 1. Measured energy intakes and estimated energy requirements for UK adults (mean ± SE)

	Women	Men
Daily energy intake (kcal)[a]	1680 ± 13 ($n = 1110$)	2450 ± 18 ($n = 1087$)
Estimated average requirement for energy (kcal)[b]	1935	2545

[a]*The Dietary and Nutritional Survey of British Adults* (Gregory et al., 1990).
[b]*Dietary Reference Values for Food Energy and Nutrients for the United Kingdom* (Department of Health, 1991).

Another approach is to ask subjects to recall their past food intake, usually during the previous 24 hours, or to describe their typical daily intake. Again this is open to conscious or unconscious bias and also relies on accurate memory for the foods consumed. In addition, all the methods (except where duplicate samples are collected for direct analysis) depend on tables of food composition for the conversion of dietary data to energy and nutrient intakes, which is a further source of error, especially when used on an individual basis (Paul and Southgate, 1978). Nonetheless, in certain contexts these shortcomings of dietary assessment in free-living subjects may be relatively unimportant. For example, in a double-blind, placebo-controlled trial of an anorexic agent any lack of precision in dietary recording should not normally introduce systematic bias toward one treatment over another. At worst it may be expected to contribute noise to the data, and thus reduce the sensitivity of measurement and the likelihood of detecting true treatment differences (i.e., increased probability of a type II error).

Self-report Measures of Hunger, Satiety and Palatability

Self-report scales for assessing feelings of hunger and fullness have been employed routinely in studies of human eating behaviour, and the first use of this method to examine the appetite-suppressant effects of anorexic drugs appears to have been by Silverstone and Stunkard (1968). Although the form of such scales varies considerably between laboratories (see Blundell and Hill, 1988, for details), probably the most widely used is a simple 100 mm unipolar visual-analogue scale. This consists of a horizontal 100 mm line anchored at the left-hand end with a description such as 'not at all hungry (full)' and at the right-hand end with a description such as 'hungry (full) as I have ever felt' (e.g. Rogers and Blundell, 1979). Similar scales have been used to obtain ratings of food preference and pleasantness (Rolls *et al.*, 1984), as well as in the appraisal of the sensory characteristics of foods and beverages (Mela, 1992). Food preferences can also be assessed successfully using food check-lists consisting of the names or pictures of foods representing different sensory or nutrient categories (Blundell and Rogers, 1980; Blundell and Hill, 1988; Drewnowski *et al.*, 1992a). While there are many technical reasons cited in favour of one form of scale over another (e.g., visual-analogue versus category scale), in practice it is not clear that these have any great influence on the performance of such scales. On the other hand, there are a number of important issues related to the interpretation of data collected using these instruments which are often neglected (Blundell and Rogers, 1991; Rogers, 1990b).

One of these issues was discussed above in relation to 'palatability' or pleasantness ratings. Taking another example, it is clear that the term hunger can refer to a motivational construct in scientific theory, particular feelings and bodily sensations experienced by an individual, or ratings or verbal reports made by that individual. Hunger ratings, however, are not a direct measure of either the hunger construct or hunger feelings. The latter will influence the subject's ratings, but so will his or her attributions and expectations. For instance, a high rating of hunger may be made because the subject anticipates eating a large meal. Or subjects may tailor their ratings according to what they believe ought to happen in the experiment. Of even greater importance, though, is the specificity or often the lack of specificity of changes identified by self-report ratings. A decrease in rated hunger can, with some certainty, be taken to indicate a decreased willingness to eat, and this could be due to an effect on processes controlling appetitive motivation. But, equally, the subjects may feel nauseated or may find the food less palatable. Similarly, changes in pleasantness ratings of individual foods (Hetherington *et al.*, 1989; Rolls *et al.*, 1984) or sweet solutions (Cabanac, 1971) do not provide conclusive evidence for a role of palatability in either satiety or the longer-term regulation of food intake. Thus the main issue is not the extent to which self-report measures correlate with the amount of food consumed or food choices (e.g., Mattes, 1990), but the appropriate interpretation of these measures. The examples below demonstrate that self-report measures of hunger, fullness, palatability and bodily sensations such as feelings of nausea are invaluable tools in research on appetite control and in uncovering the effects of pharmacological manipulations. However, it is generally the case that most insight is gained where there is dissociation between the different measures, because this can implicate the involvement of specific underlying mechanisms.

Case Studies

This section considers three case studies illustrating recent research on the psychopharmacology of appetite. The first of these concerns so-called carbohydrate-craving obesity. A neurochemical link between the choice and over-consumption of high-carbohydrate foods and obesity has been outlined by Wurtman and Wurtman (1989). They propose that increased carbohydrate consumption can influence brain serotinergic activity and in turn relieve depressed mood. In support of this are the results of several studies indicating elevated intake of high-carbohydrate foods (often also high in fat) associated with depression, seasonal affective disorder, premenstrual syndrome, as well as carbohydrate-craving obesity (Fernstrom *et al.*, 1987; Krauchi and Wirz-Justice, 1988; Lieberman *et al.*, 1986; Rosenthal *et al.*, 1987; Wurtman and Wurtman, 1989). Moreover, the increase in carbohydrate intake appears to be driven by an increase in preference for high-carbohydrate foods which has been termed 'carbohydrate craving' (Wurtman and Wurtman, 1989). In other words, liking for these foods may be reinforced by the mood effects of consuming carbohydrate.

Further aspects of these relationships are illustrated by a recent study (Wurtman *et al.*, 1987) where a group of obese carbohydrate cravers and a group of obese non-carbohydrate cravers were identified and compared in their responses to the drug *d*-fenfluramine (which increases serotoninergic neurotransmission). Carbohydrate craving was defined on the basis of the frequent consumption of snacks high in carbohydrate and fat, but low in protein (average of seven such snacks per day). The smaller number of non-carbohydrate cravers had a similar frequency of snacking, divided about equally between high-protein and high-carbohydrate snacks. The subjects were initially identified on the basis of self-reported eating behaviour which was confirmed by assessment in a residential laboratory. Compared with placebo, treatment with *d*-fenfluramine had a more immediate and larger effect on the frequency of snacking and snack intake in the carbohydrate cravers, although there was also a significant reduction in snacking in the non-carbohydrate cravers during the third and final month on *d*-fenfluramine. In addition, mealtime energy intake was reduced significantly by *d*-fenfluramine in carbohydrate cravers (similar reduction in intake of all macronutrients), but not in non-carbohydrate cravers. These results are broadly consistent with the hypothesis that *d*-fenfluramine decreases hunger for carbohydrates in the carbohydrate craver by mimicking the effects of carbohydrate consumption on serotoninergic functioning.

The second case study, however, is provided by work that challenges the notion of carbohydrate craving on the grounds that the preferences appear to be for foods high in both fat and (sweet) carbohydrate (Drewnowski *et al.*, 1992b). This behaviour, moreover, has been linked with activity of the endogenous opioid system rather than serotoninergic mediation (Drewnowski, 1992). There is growing evidence from studies in both humans and animals that opioid peptides play an important role in the regulation of food and fluid intake, and a consensus is emerging that opioids are involved specifically in the mediation of hedonic responses to orosensory stimuli (Drewnowski, 1992; Kirkham and Cooper, 1988; Kirkham, 1990). In studies of rats sham feeding sucrose, the opioid antagonist naloxone did not alter the latency to approach food and initiate eating, but appeared to reduce the rate of intake in a similar manner to the effect of lowering the concentration of sucrose (Kirkham and Cooper, 1988). This indicates a dissociation of hunger and palatability, and results of studies on humans (Drewnowski, 1992; Yeomans and Wright, 1991; Yeomans *et al.*, 1990; and see Hetherington *et al.*, 1991, for review) generally confirm a lack of an effect or minimal effect of opioid antagonists on self-reported hunger, while pleasantness ratings and intake of preferred foods and/ or sweet and high-fat foods are often markedly reduced. Perception of the intensity of sensory stimuli is unaffected. Following on from this, naloxone was reported to be particularly effective in reducing food intake in binge eaters, again largely due to an effect on sweet, high-fat foods such as chocolate and biscuits (Drewnowski *et al.*, 1992a). Also opioid antagonists suppress stress-induced overeating (Fullerton *et al.*, 1985). Other findings indicate that opioids are released in response to the ingestion of palatable foods (Blass, 1991; Fullerton *et al.*, 1985). In one experiment by Blass and his colleagues, 2–3-day-old human infants were given 2 ml of 12% sucrose solution to drink immediately prior to blood collection made using a heel lance. Compared with the same volume of water, the sucrose markedly reduced the initial amount and duration of crying in response to the blood collection procedure. Sweet taste rather than a direct nutritional effect is implicated in this antinociceptive and/or calming property of sucrose, since the response was very rapid and the small volume of sucrose was presumably nutritionally insignificant.

From these various results it has been suggested that overeating and reported cravings for foods high in sugar and fat may share a common mechanism

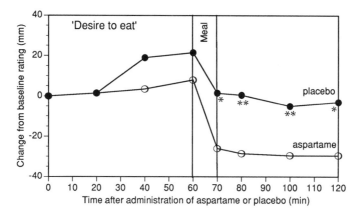

Figure 2. Self-report ratings (100 mm visual-analogue scale) of desire to eat, showing the interaction of pretreatment with capsulated aspartame and a fixed meal of milkshake. Aspartame or placebo were given immediately after the baseline rating made at time zero minutes. Treatment effects were significantly different at 70, 80, 100 and 120 minutes (*$p < 0.05$, **$p < 0.02$, 2-tail). From P.J. Rogers and S. Edwards, unpublished data

with opiate drug addiction (Drewnowski, 1992). However, although it is clear that the endogenous opioid system is important in mediating affective responses during eating, it is perhaps premature to be definite about a role for opioid-mediated effects in the development of compulsive eating and obesity.

The final case study concerns the effects on appetite of the dipeptide sweetener aspartame, which in a series of studies has been found to suppress food intake when administered in capsules (Rogers *et al.*, 1990, 1991). Compared with placebo, moderate doses of 200–400 mg aspartame inhibited food intake in a test meal by up to 14% (175 kcal). Since the aspartame was not tasted, this effect must be due to a post-ingestive action of the dipeptide or a breakdown product. The exact mechanism of action remains to be elucidated; however, an important finding is that there appeared to be little or no reduction in pre-meal hunger ratings after treatment with aspartame. This is in contrast to the effects of the anorexic drugs amphetamine and fenfluramine (Blundell and Rogers, 1980), and suggests that aspartame may act somehow to amplify the satiating capacity of food. This, in turn, is consistent with the suggestion that the 'satiety hormone' cholecystokinin may mediate the anorexic action of aspartame (Rogers *et al.*, 1991). Further recent studies have confirmed these results using a fixed meal design. Here subjects were given placebo or aspartame treatments followed 1 hour later by a fixed volume of milkshake. Ratings of desire to eat were only marginally and not significantly reduced by aspartame prior to the milkshake, but the combination of aspartame plus milkshake led to a much greater suppression of desire to eat than when the milkshake was given following the placebo (Figure 2). Additional results indicate that pleasantness ratings of foods are more or less unaffected by aspartame and that, at least at these doses, aspartame does not appear to make subjects feel nauseous or produce any other untoward effects (P.J. Rogers and S. Edwards, unpublished). The extent to which this anorexic action of capsulated aspartame can be exploited clinically remains to be established, since it is not possible to predict, for example, the anti-obesity effects of repeated administration of the aspartame from these initial acute studies. Nonetheless, the results to date indicate considerable promise for this novel treatment. This work, together with the previous examples, also illustrates very well the use of the various approaches available for the investigation of human eating behaviour and shows some of the potential benefits of basic research in this area.

References

Baucom, D.H., and Aiken, P.A. (1981). Effect of depressed mood on eating among obese and nonobese dieting and nondieting persons. *J. Pers. Soc. Psychol.,* **41**, 577–85.

Bellisle, F., and Le Magnen, J. (1981). The structure of meals in humans: Eating and drinking patterns in lean and obese subjects, *Physiol. Behav.,* **27**, 649–58.

Birch, L.L., McPhee, L., Steinberg, L., and Sullivan, S. (1990). Conditioned flavour preferences in young children, *Physiol. Behav.,* **47**, 501–5.

Blass, E.M. (1991). Suckling: Opioid and nonopioid processes in mother-infant bonding. In Friedman, M.I., Tordoff, M.G., and Kare, M.R. (eds), *Chemical Senses: Vol. 4, Appetite and Nutrition,* New York: Marcel Dekker, pp. 283–302.

Blundell, J.E., and Hill, A.J. (1988). Descriptive and operational study of eating in humans. In Binder, B.J., Chaitin, B.F., and Goldstein, R. (eds), *The Eating Disorders*; PMA Publishing, pp. 65–85.

Blundell, J.E., and Rogers, P.J. (1980). Effects of anorexic drugs on food intake, food selection and preferences, hunger motivation and subjective experiences, *Appetite,* **1**, 151–65.

Blundell, J.E., and Rogers, P.J. (1991). Hunger, hedonics, and the control of satiation and satiety. In Friedman, M.I., Tordoff, M.G., and Kare, M.R. (eds), *Chemical Senses: Vol. 4, Appetite and Nutrition,* New York: Marcel Dekker, pp. 127–48.

Blundell, J.E., Lawton, C.L., Hill, A.J., and Rogers, P.J. (1990). Psychopharmacology of hunger and satiety. In Fichter, M.M. (ed.), *Bulimia Nervosa: Basic Research, Diagnosis and Therapy,* Chichester: Wiley, pp. 180–207.

Booth, D.A. (1979). Acquired behaviour controlling energy intake and output. *Psychiatr. Clin. North Am.,* **1**, 545–579.

Booth, D.A. (1991). Protein- and carbohydrate-specific cravings: Neuroscience and sociology. In Friedman, M.I., Tordoff, M.G. and Kare, M.R. (eds), New York: Marcel Dekker, pp. 262–76.

Bray, G.A., and Inoue, S. (1992). Pharmacological treatment of obesity. *Am. J. Clin. Nutr.,* **55**, 151S–319S.

Bruch, H. (1961). *Eating Disorders,* New York: Basic Books.

Cabanac, M. (1971). The physiological role of pleasure. *Science,* **173**, 1103–7.

Campbell, R.G., Hashim, S.A., and Van Itallie, T.B. (1971). Studies of food intake regulation in man: Responses to variations in nutritive density in lean and obese subjects. *N. Eng. J. Med.*, **265**, 1402–7.

Campfield, L.A., and Smith, F.J. (1986). Functional coupling between transient declines in blood glucose and feeding behaviour. *Brain Res. Bull.*, **14**, 605–6.

Collier, G. (1986). The dialogue on the strategy between the economist and the resident physiologist. *Appetite*, **7**, 188–9.

Department of Health (1991). *Dietary Reference Values for Food Energy and Nutrients for the United Kingdom*. London: HMSO.

Department of Health (1992). *Health of the Nation*. London: HMSO.

Drewnowski, A. (1992). Food preferences and the opioid peptide system. *Trends Food Sci. Technol.*, **3**, 97–9.

Drewnowski, A., Krahn, D.D., Demitrack, M.A., Nairn, K., and Gosnell, B.A. (1992a). Taste responses and preferences for sweet high-fat foods: Evidence for opioid involvement. *Physiol. Behav.*, **51**, 371–9.

Drewnowski, A., Kurth, C., Holden-Wiltse, J., and Saari, J. (1992b). Food preferences in human obesity: Carbohydrate versus fats. *Appetite*, **18**, 207–21.

Elizalde, G., and Sclafani, A. (1988). Starch-based conditioned preferences in rats: Influence of taste, calories and CS–US delay. *Appetite*, **11**, 179–200.

Elizalde, G., and Sclafani, A. (1990). Flavour preferences conditioned by intragastric infusions: A detailed analysis using an electronic esophagus preparation. *Physiol. Behav.*, **47**, 63–77.

Fernstrom, M.H., Krowinski, R.L., and Kupfer, D.J. (1987). Appetite and food preference in depression: Effects of imipramine treatment, *Biol. Psychiatry*, **22**, 529–39.

Foltin, R.W., Fischman, M.W., Emurian, C.S., and Rachlinski, J.J. (1988). Compensation for caloric dilution in humans given unrestricted access to food in a residential laboratory. *Appetite*, **10**, 13–24.

Fullerton, D.T., Getto, C.J., Swift, W.J., and Carlson, I.H. (1985). Sugar, opioids and binge eating. *Brain Res. Bull.*, **14**, 673–80.

Garb, J.L., and Stunkard, A.J. (1974). Taste aversions in man. *Am. J. Psychiatry*, **131**, 1204–7.

Garcia, J., Hankins, W.G., and Rusiniak, K.W. (1974). Behavioural regulation of the milieu interne in man and rat. *Science*, **185**, 824–31.

Gregory, J., Foster, K., Tyler, H., and Wiseman, M. (1990). *The Dietary and Nutritional Survey of British Adults*, London: HMSO.

Herman, C.P. (1978). Restrained eating. *Psychiatr. Clin. North Am.*, **1**, 593–607.

Herman, C.P., and Mack, D. (1975). Restrained and unrestrained eating. *J. Pers.*, **43**, 647–60.

Herman, C.P., and Polivy, J. (1975). Anxiety, restraint and eating behaviour. *J. Abnormal Psychol.*, **6**, 666–72.

Herman, C.P., and Polivy, J. (1984). A boundary model for the regulation of eating. In Stunkard, A.J., and Stellar, E. (ed.), *Eating and Its Disorders*, New York: Raven Press, pp. 141–56.

Hetherington, M., Rolls, B.J., and Burley, V.J. (1989). The time-course of sensory-specific satiety. *Appetite*, **12**, 57–8.

Hetherington, M.M., Vervaet, N., Blass, E., and Rolls, B.J. (1991). Failure of naltrexone to affect the pleasantness or intake of food. *Pharmacol. Biochem. Behav.*, **40**, 185–90.

Hill, A.J. (1993). Causes and consequences of dieting and anorexia. *Proc. Nutr. Soc.*, in press.

Hill, A.J., Magson, L.D., and Blundell, J.E. (1984). Hunger and palatability: Tracking ratings of subjective experience before, during and after the consumption of preferred and less preferred food. *Appetite,* **5**, 361–71.

Houston, B.O., and Sumida, B. (1985). A positive feedback model for switching between two activities. *Anim. Behav.,* **33**, 315–25.

Jordan, H.A. (1969). Voluntary intragastric feeding: Oral and gastric contributions to food intake and hunger in man. *J. Comp. Physiol. Psychol.,* **68**, 498–506.

Kaplan, H.I., and Kaplan, H.S., (1957). The psychosomatic concept of obesity. *J. Nerv. Ment. Dis.,* **125**, 181–201.

Kirkham, T.C. (1990). Enhanced anorectic potency of naloxone in rats feeding 30% sucrose: Reversal by repeated naloxone administration. *Physiol. Behav.,* **47**, 419–26.

Kirkham, T.C., and Cooper, S.J. (1988). Naloxone attenuation of sham feeding is modified by manipulation of sucrose concentration, *Physiol. Behav.,* **44**, 491–4.

Kissileff, H.A., Klinsberg, G., and Van Itallie, T.B. (1980). Universal eating monitor for continuous recording of solid or liquid consumption in man. *Am. J. Physiol.,* **238**, R14–R22.

Krauchi, K., and Wirz-Justice, A. (1988). The four seasons: Food intake frequency in seasonal affective disorder in the course of a year. *Psychiatry Res.,* **25**, 332–38.

Lieberman, H., Wurtman, J., and Chew, B. (1986). Changes in mood after carbohydrate consumption among obese individuals. *Am. J. Clin. Nutr.,* **45**, 772–8.

Lissner, L., Levitsky, D.A., Strupp, B.J., Kalkwarf, H.J., and Roe, D.A. (1987). Dietary fat and the regulation of energy intake in human subjects. *Am. J. Clin. Nutr.,* **46**, 886–92.

Logue, A.W., Ophir, I., and Strauss, K.E. (1981). The acquisition of taste aversions in humans. *Behav. Res. Ther.,* **19**, 319–33.

Mattes, R. (1990). Hunger ratings are not a valid proxy measure of reported food intake in humans. *Appetite,* **15**, 103–13.

McFarland, D.J. (1971). *Feedback Mechanisms in Animal Behaviour.* London: Academic Press.

Mela, D.J. (1992). Sensory evaluation methods in nutrition and dietetics research. In Monsen, E.R. (ed.), *Research: Successful Approaches,* American Dietetic Association, pp. 220–47.

Moon, R.D. (1979). Monitoring human eating patterns during the ingestion of non-liquid foods. *Int. J. Obes.,* **3**, 281–8.

Paul, A.A., and Southgate, D.A.T. (1978). *McCance and Widdowson's The Composition of Foods* (4th edn), London: HMSO.

Pierson, A., and Le Magnen, J. (1969). Etude quantitative du processus de régulation des éesposes alimentaires chez l'homme. *Physiol. Behav.,* **4**, 61–7.

Plutchik, R. (1976). Emotions and attitudes related to being overweight. *J. Clin. Psychol.,* **32**, 21–4.

Polivy, J. (1976). Perception of calories and regulation of intake in restrained and unrestrained subjects. *Addict. Behav.,* **1**, 237–43.

Polivy, J., and Herman, C.P. (1985). Dieting and binging: A causal analysis. *Am. Psychol.,* **40**, 193–201.

Porikos, K.P., Hesser, M.F., and Van Itallie, T.B. (1982). Caloric regulation in normal weight men maintained on a palatable diet of conventional foods. *Physiol. Behav.,* **29**, 293–300.

Prentice, A.M., Black, A.E., Murgatroyd, P.R., Goldberg, G.R., and Coward, W.A. (1989). Metabolism or appetite: Questions of energy balance with particular reference to obesity. *J. Hum. Nutr. Diet.,* **2**, 95–104.

Quandt, S.A. (1987). Methods for determining dietary intake. In Johnson, F.E. (ed.), *Nutritional Anthropology*, New York: Alan R. Liss, pp. 67–84.

Robbins, T.W., and Fray, P.J. (1980). Stress-induced eating: Fact, fiction or misunderstanding? *Appetite*, **1**, 103–33.

Rogers, P.J. (1990a). Dietary fat, satiety and obesity. *Food Quality Pref.*, **2**, 103–10.

Rogers, P.J. (1990b). Why a palatability construct is needed. *Appetite*, **14**, 167–70.

Rogers, P.J., and Blundell, J.E. (1979). Effect of anorexic drugs on food intake and the micro-structure of eating in human subjects. *Psychopharmacology*, **66**, 159–65.

Rogers, P.J., and Blundell, J.E. (1984). Meal patterns and food selection during the development of obesity in rats fed a cafeteria diet. *Neurosci. Biobehav. Rev.*, **8**, 441–53.

Rogers, P.J., and Blundell, J.E. (1989). Separating the actions of sweetness and calories: Effects of saccharin and carbohydrates on hunger and food intake in human subjects. *Physiol. Behav.*, **45**, 1093–9.

Rogers, P.J., and Blundell, J.E. (1990). Psychobiological bases of food choice. *Br. Nutr. Found. Nutr. Bull.*, **15** (Suppl 1), 31–40.

Rogers, P.J., and Hill, A.J. (1989). Breakdown of dietary restraint following mere exposure to food stimuli: Interrelationships between restraint, hunger, salivation, and food intake. *Addict. Behav.*, **14**, 387–97.

Rogers, P.J., and Schutz, H.G. (1992). Influence of palatability on subsequent hunger and food intake: A retrospective replication. *Appetite*, **19**, 55–6.

Rogers, P.J., Pleming, H.C., and Blundell, J.E. (1990). Aspartame consumed without tasting inhibits hunger and food intake. *Physiol. Behav.*, **47**, 1239–43.

Rogers, P.J., Keedwell, P., and Blundell, J.E. (1991). Further analysis of the short-term inhibition of food intake in humans by the dipeptide L-aspartyl-L-phenylalanine methyl ester (aspartame). *Physiol. Behav.*, **49**, 739–43.

Rolls, B.A., Duijvenvoorde, P.M., and Rolls, E.T. (1984). Pleasantness changes and food intake in a varied four course meal. *Appetite*, **5**, 337–48.

Rosenthal, N.R., Genhart, M., Jacobson, F.M., Skwerer, R.G., and Weht, T.A. (1987). Disturbances of appetite and weight regulation in seasonal affective disorder. *Ann. NY Acad. Sci.*, **499**, 216–23.

Sclafani, A., and Nissenbaum, J.W. (1985). Is gastric sham feeding really sham feeding? *Am. J. Physiol.*, **248**, R387–R390.

Silverstone, J.T., and Stunkard, A.J. (1968). The anorectic effect of dexamphetamine sulphate. *Br. J. Pharmacol.*, **33**, 513–22.

Silverstone, T., Fincham, J. and Brydon, J. (1980). A new technique for the continuous measurement of food intake in man. *Am. J. Clin. Nutr.*, **33**, 1852–5.

Slochower, J.A. (1983). *Excessive Eating*, New York, Human Sciences Press.

Smith, F.J., Campfield, L.A., and Rosenbaum, M. (1992). Human hunger: Is there a role of blood glucose dynamics? *Proceedings of the First Independent Conference of the Society for the Study of Ingestive Behaviour*, Princeton, June 1992.

Smith, G.P., Gibbs, J., and Young, R.C. (1974). Cholecystokinin and intestinal satiety in the rat. *Fed. Proc.*, **33**, 1146–1149.

Spencer, J.A., and Fremouw, W.J. (1979). Binge eating as a function of restraint and weight classification. *J. Abnorm. Psychol.*, **88**, 262–7.

Spiegel, T.A. (1973). Caloric regulation of food intake in man. *J. Comp. Physiol. Psychol.*, **84**, 24–37.

Spiegel, T.A., and Jordan, H.A. (1978). Effects of simultaneous oral–intragastric ingestion on meal patterns and satiety in humans. *J. Comp. Physiol. Psychol.*, **92**, 133–41.

Spitzer, L., and Rodin, J. (1981). Human eating behaviour: A critical review of studies in normal weight and overweight individuals. *Appetite*, **2**, 293–329.

Steiner, J.E. (1987). What the neonate can tell us about umami. In Kawamura, Y., and Kare, M.R. (eds), *Umami: a Basic Taste*, New York: Marcel Dekker, pp. 97–123.

Tordoff, M.G., and Alleva, A.A. (1990). Oral stimulation with aspartame increases hunger. *Physiol. Behav.*, **47**, 555–9.

Wardle, J., and Beinart, H. (1981). Binge eating: A theoretical review. *Br. J. Clin. Psychol.*, **20**, 97–109.

Weingarten, H.P. (1985). Stimulus control of eating: Implications for a two-factor theory of hunger. *Appetite*, **6**, 387–401.

Weingarten, H.P., and Cowans, S.E. (1991). Sensory control of eating: The meal as a stream of sensations. In Getchell, T.V. (ed.), *Smell and Taste in Health and Disease*, New York: Raven Press, pp. 381–9.

Weingarten, H.P., and Kulikovsky, O.T. (1989). Taste-to-postingestive consequence conditioning: Is the rise in sham feeding with repeated experience a learned phenomenon? *Physiol. Behav.*, **45**, 471–6.

Westerterp-Plantenga, M.S., Westerterp, K.R., Nicolson, N.A., Mordant, A., Schoffelen, P.F.N., and ten Hoor, F. (1990). The shape of the cumulative food intake curve in humans, during basic and manipulated meals. *Physiol. Behav.*, **47**, 569–76.

Westerterp-Plantenga, M.S., van den Heuvel, E., Wouters, L., and ten Hoor, F. (1992). Diet-induced thermogenesis and cumulative food intake curves as a function of familiarity with food and dietary restraint in humans. *Physiol. Behav.*, **51**, 457–65.

Wiepkema, P.R. (1971a). Behavioural factors in the regulation of food intake. *Proc. Nutr. Soc.*, **30**, 142–9.

Wiepkema, P.R. (1971b). Positive feedbacks at work during feeding. *Behaviour*, **39**, 266–73.

Wurtman, J., Wurtman, R., Reynolds, S., Tsay, R., and Chew, B. (1987). Fenfluramine suppresses snack intake among carbohydrate cravers but not among noncarbohydrate cravers. *Int. J. Eating Disord.*, **6**, 687–99.

Wurtman, R.J., and Wurtman, J.J. (1989). Carbohydrates and depression. *Sci. Am.*, **260**, 50–7.

Yeomans, M.R., and Wright, P. (1991). Lower pleasantness of palatable foods in nalmafene-treated human volunteers. *Appetite*, **16**, 249–59.

Yeomans, M.R., Wright, P., Macleod, H.A., and Critchley, J.A.J.H. (1990). Effects of nalmafene on feeding in humans: Dissociation of hunger and palatability. *Psychopharmacology*, **100**, 426–32.

9

Psychopharmacology of Memory Components

*Hervé Allain, †Alain Lieury and ‡Jean-Marc Gandon

*Laboratoire de Pharmacologie Clinique, Faculté de Médecine,
†Laboratoire de Psychologie Expérimentale, Université de
Rennes II, 35043 Rennes, and ‡Biotrial S.A., Drug Evaluation
and Pharmacology Research, Technopole Atalante—Villejean,
35000 Rennes, France*

Introduction

For a century, experimental psychology has provided classic neurological diagnostic examinations with the possibility of assessing with more precision anomalies in neuropsychological or cognitive performance (Mesulam, 1985). The tendency today is to define patterns of competence or cognitive disorders (Table 1) in relation to a given neurological or psychiatric illness. Such patterns are tentatively correlated, in anatomico-pathological studies or thanks to the advance in imagery, with cerebral structural localizations or identified neurotransmission circuits (Levin and Benton, 1984; Lieury et al., 1990).

For example, in psychiatry, depression is commonly associated with a right hemisphere dysfunction, or certain schizophrenic forms, or to a left lobe dysfunction. This cognitive approach is a valued tool since some forms of illness, especially psychiatric, are not accompanied by visible anatomical lesions that could be analysed by standard medical means. Likewise, to pharmacologists, the issue of the cognitive impact of drugs is crucial, enabling the possibility of improving functions or cognitive components that had so far been considered as 'untouchable' (Allain et al., 1990a; Sarter, 1991), and, most of all, the possibility of predicting deleterious repercussions for a given drug. These observations are highly relevant to human psychopharmacology, the drug concretely appearing as a therapeutic tool complementing any approach to mental illness, particularly the cognitive or psychotherapeutical ones. Qualitative rather than quantitative handling of cognitive functionings is definitely the most urgent challenge to psychopharmacology.

Human Psychopharmacology, Vol. 4. Edited by I. Hindmarch and P. D. Stonier
© 1993 John Wiley & Sons Ltd

Table 1. Cognitive test disabilities

Orientation and remote memory	Early dementia Recovery after stroke Amnesic syndromes
Attention–vigilance	Head injury Toxic conditions Epileptic disorders
Reaction time (RT)	Simple RT: level of arousal Complex RT: decision making response Selection capacity to shift attention
Learning memory	Short term, 30 sec Long term (above 30 sec) Verbal and non-verbal tests
Visual/auditory perception	Capacity to process and integrate visual or auditory information
Abstract reasoning and problem solving	Capacity to form concepts Ability to shift strategies in problem solving
Constructional praxis	Drawing, constructing block model
Language functions	Naming, word association, sentence repetition Token test

Without falling into excessive systematization or hierarchization of the higher functions, our team of psychopharmacologists have tackled this issue from the perspective of mnestic information processing (Allain *et al.*, 1990b; Lieury, 1990, 1992) with a view to modifying at will some of its components by resorting to various drug classes (cognitive enhancers, antidepressants, anti-anxiety drugs, etc.). The diversity, complexity and abundance of literature data on this subject are a true handicap and justify making a theoretical and methodological detour before presenting formal data that can be used therapeutically.

An Exploded View of Memory

General Principles

Human memory appears to be a complex combination of data-processing modules which communicate through interfaces (Figure 1).

Schematically, memory could be described as a modular hierarchy whose function is to code information using increasingly abstract codes, from ephemeral sensory codes (visual or 'iconic' memory lasts a mere half second at the most) to symbolic codes such as verbal memory and image memory. Verbal memory appears to be essentially constituted (beside the first steps of graphic/phonological coding) by a lexical system (morphological unit of a word without its meaning) and a semantic system (semantic memory). Like-

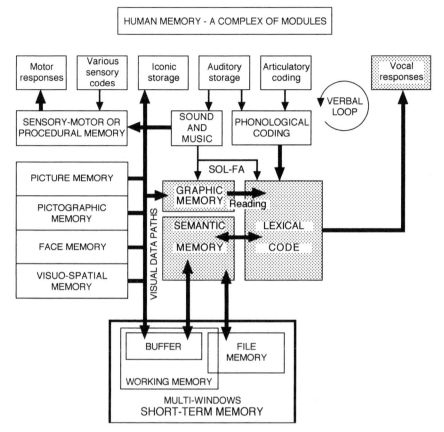

Figure 1. A modular view of memory components

wise, the visual system is complex and includes a storage system for familiar faces, and other systems, pictographic (ideograms to Asians, but also 'road signs' to Westerners), or visuo-spatial (spatial visualization factor in factor studies of intelligence, mental rotation, etc., corresponding to the spatial memory tests of Benton, Kohs, etc.).

These systems are akin to dedicated computers interconnected by communication links (visual information) and interfaces. The lexical system is thought to be the interface of various ports of graphic, auditive inputs and articulate output, while the semantic system would mainly interface with the verbal and the imaged system. All these systems operate in the short or in the long term.

Multi-windowing of Short-term Memory

Short-term memory is not a simple structure either, but it can be conceived as the bulk of circulating data, akin to the central processing unit of a computer, displayed in a multi-windowing mode similar to that of certain computer file management displays.

Allan Baddeley, whose work on short-term memory is profuse (Baddeley, 1988a, 1988b), was the first to propose breaking down the monolith of short-term memory, in its acceptance as a working memory. From his work on cognitive competition, this author showed that the main tasks (verbal or visuo-spatial) are hampered only by other tasks of the same type; from that he formulated a theory of working memory that would include a central processor and two slave systems: the articulate loop and a visuo-spatial system. These components probably do not represent all of short-term memory, which to us also comprises other functions, in particular the short-term activation and the file memorization functions. The 'short-term' activation function has to be evoked to explain the short-term functioning of any sensory memory (iconic, tactile) or even semantic, since semantic identification is very rapid. Short-term memory also operates as a memory file for retrieval processes, by short-term storage of only retrieval indices (e.g., a category index to retrieve the sub-words within a category).

Plurality of Memory

Mishkin and Appenzeller (1987) discovered in primates two main memory systems. One corresponds to the usual definition of memory and can be qualified as 'episodic' according to Tulving (1972) (or declarative memory according to some authors (Squire, 1986)), which involves different areas of the cortex and the hippocampus; the other system involves the nigrostriatal system and concerns 'procedural' memory, or procedure learning, in particular motor-sensory learning. This distinction was confirmed in man by the fact that amnesic subjects who fail the episodic memory tests do succeed in procedure learning, whereas Parkinson's disease alters the latter (Saint-Cyr *et al.*, 1988).

Since the fruitful distinction between episodic memory and semantic memory was made, episodic memory has been seen as encased in semantic memory (Lieury, 1979), itself being encased in procedural memory (Tulving, 1985). However, episodic memory, as a storage memory of data in context, probably relies on multiple memories: semantic, phonetic, auditive, etc. In a variant of the 'failure to recognize cued words' technique (Tulving and Thomson, 1973), Tiberghien and Lecocq (1983) demonstrated that when encoding is phonetic (verger–berger (*shepherd*)) (rhymed cue and target words), recognition in semantic associations (the link word being 'mouton' (sheep)) is markedly lower (34%) than in the converse, i.e. when encoding is semantic (saddle–horse) and recognition associations are phonetic (47%) (e.g., the associating word is 'chenal'). Cued recall is the same in both cases, and when calculating the proportion of words that were not recognized but were recalled (cued recall) the results show that there are almost twice as many (53% versus 32%) when encoding was phonetic. A simple interpretation of these results could be that in this case phonetic encoding induced storage in a phonetic (or lexical) module different from that of the semantic memory. Only a part of the data will have been 'transferred' into the semantic memory, permitting recognition in the semantic context. Semantic encoding does not induce as much of that effect, since phonetic encoding probably precedes the semantic code, resulting in storage in both modules.

Another technique, developed by Juan de Mendoza (1988), is based on a combination of the hemi-field visual presentation technique—to stimulate split-brain processing—and the use of different retrieval modes. Presentation of words printed in lower case is achieved in the right or left visual hemi-field, but the retrieval mode is changed. When the visual format of recognition is the same (lower case), presentation in either hemi-field is the same, but the more different the retrieval format—different graphics (upper case), word auditive recognition or even free verbal recall—the wider the deviation between the presentation hemi-fields. The words therefore pass through recording phases which predominantly involve the left hemisphere, probably including lexical recording for auditive recognition and semantic recording for verbal recall.

Thus there would be not just one, but several episodic memories; each coding module—graphic, auditive, lexical, imaged, semantic—corresponds to as many 'separate memories' which require to go from one to the other, transcoding with some data loss. Lastly, as will be seen, factor analysis of the various memory tasks (Lieury *et al.*, 1991) and, in pathology, various patterns of mnestic decline (Moss *et al.*, 1986; Lieury *et al.*, 1990) strongly suggest that there is a multi-module structure in memory. The issue for human psychopharmacology is whether these transcoding modules can be modified selectively, either by illness or by drugs.

Methods

Evaluating the Memory Components

To assess the various mechanisms of memory, a test was developed and named SM9 (Score of Memory), which includes nine mnestic scores involving: verbal/image coding; free recall; recognition recall; pictures/faces. The battery of tests takes the form of four standardized 16-item modules for comparison purposes: Words (M16), Pictures (D16), Organization (O16) and Faces (V16). This test, which has now been assessed on more than 500 individuals, is perfectly adapted to elderly subjects, to the depressed or anxious, as well as to clinical trial requirements. Technical specifications can be found in previous studies based on this assessment battery (Lieury *et al.*, 1990, 1991; Allain *et al.*, 1992).

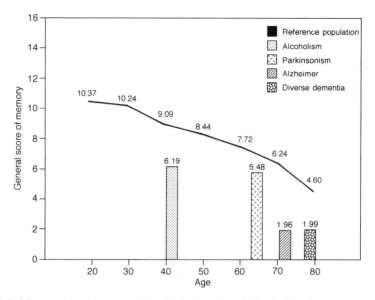

Figure 2. Memory loss for normal (solid line) and pathological ageing

A synopsis of the results obtained with this battery indicates that the overall score of memory (on the nine scores of SM9) relates to two gradients (normal or pathological ageing) which are predictors of the pathological character of memory deficit (Figure 2).

The SM5 Battery

SM5 is a mini-test extracted from the SM9 battery and which retains the scores most saturated with the factors of factorial analysis of all the 17 scores of the battery, and involving around 100 subjects (Lieury *et al.*, 1991). In an analysis which involved a larger number of subjects ($n = 324$), only one of the five factors (answer checking) was not expressed. The other four factors appeared quite stable: Verbal coding, Picture storage, Word storage and Face storage; in addition, we found a subdivision of the 'Verbal coding' factor into 'saturated with immediate recall' and 'saturated with delayed recall', which shows that they can be linked to the mechanisms of short or long-term memory (Table 2). The SM5 (five memory scores) thus features the five fundamental and independent measures of memory, in a rapid transfer form.

(1)   D16 presentation module (Pictures).
(2)   M16 presentation module (Words).
(3)   Immediate recall of words.
(4)   V16 presentation module (Faces).

Table 2. Correlation matrix with the five memory factors extracted from the SM9 test and the scores which are mainly saturated (n = 274 young healthy subjects; Lieury, Allain, Pichon, Van Acker and Gandon, unpublished). Note: correlations below 30 are not reported, for readability

	Verbal coding		Information storage		
	STM	LTM	Picture	Word	Face
Immediate recall (word)	0.89	0.36	–	–	–
Delayed recall (word)	0.35	0.89	–	–	–
Recognition (picture)	–	–	0.98	–	–
Recognition (word)	–	–	–	0.94	–
Recognition (face)	–	–	–	–	0.96

(5) Delayed recall of words.
(6) General recognition D + M.
(7) Face recognition.

Dual Coding

Three of the five factors (Table 2) were interpreted (Lieury *et al.*, 1991) as reflecting data-specific primary storage systems, similar to specialized libraries (words, pictures, faces). SM5 is therefore more a test for memory primary storage (and short-term memory). Tests are therefore necessary to evaluate dynamic aspects, such as Sternberg's paradigm. Nevertheless, this is not easily reproduced in the elderly, owing to their very slow and variable response time. This gave us reason for developing a paradigm of Word/Picture doubling code speed—a more robust and reliable 'dual coding' test. Previous research (Paivio and Csapo, 1969; Lieury and Calvez, 1986) had shown that picture memorization involved dual coding, both imaged and verbal. This verbal coding requires additional time, so that it 'breaks up' at speeds less than 500 ms in young subjects. It is likely that such speed-coding processes require complete mobilization of all the brain's biological and biochemical resources, and should therefore be very sensitive to the biochemical action of pharmaceutical products.

This appeared to be the case for a molecule we tested,* and whose action on neuronal metabolism and blood flow redistribution may lead to improved information processing in the elderly. This was a double-blind versus placebo, double Latin square study, involving 18 individuals aged 60–80 years (66.6 ± 3.8). Relative to the placebo group (Figure 3a), where the critical double-dose threshold appeared to be reached only after 960 ms presentation time (between 250 and 500 ms in the young), dose 1 and dose 2 treatments (with no difference between doses) seemed to permit double coding after 480 ms, which may indicate an improvement of the picture-transcoding speed in verbal code (Figure 3).

---

*EGB761, Ipsen, France.

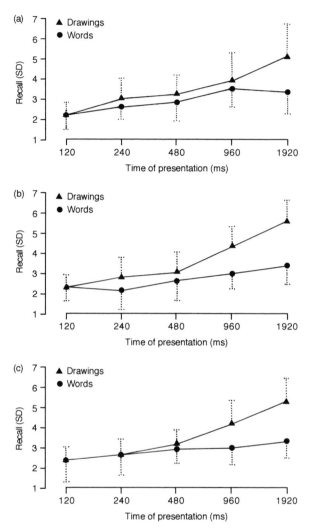

Figure 3. Effect of a nootropic drug at two dosages on dual coding: a) placebo; b) first
dose x; c) second dose 2x

Other Cognitive Parameters

Cognitive interactions (motivation, vigilance, attention, fluidity, etc.) exist,
which for instance account for the repercussion on mnestic performance of
isolated vigilance deficiency, and hence its effect on specifically mnestic test
scores. Memory tests are therefore systematically complemented with validated
and known tests that explore other cognitive states: critical flicker fusion point
(CFF), simple and complex reacting times (SRT, CRT), and possibly other

Table 3. Main psychometric tests used in evaluation

(1)	Memory (declarative/episodic/procedural)	Digit span
		Benton's visual retention test
		Buschke's task
		Associated pair learning test
		Word list learning task
		Posner's memory test
		Dual coding task
		SM9 battery
		SM5 battery
		Toronto/Hanoi tower test
(2)	Attention, vigilance cortical awareness	Continuous performance task (CPT)
		Phasal alert task
		Divided attention task
		Tracking task
		CFF
		CRT
		DSST
		SCT
		KT
(3)	Anxiety, inhibition, stress	DRL task
		Gonogo's task
		Stroop's task

techniques—waiting capability test (DRL), procedural tests (Toronto tower)—all these techniques being computerized and compatible with the chronological (timing) requirements of pharmacological studies (Table 3).

Search for Factors which Influence Mnestic Performance

General

One of the characteristics of memory studies is the heterogeneity of performance, which sometimes presents wide variations. It is therefore important that psychopharmacological studies detect those factors which influence mnestic performance, in order to obtain absolute and homogeneous baseline values. Educational level, age and underlying pathology are the most relevant parameters, even if other factors deserve to be investigated, such as sex, for example (Harshman *et al.*, 1983). Compilation or summation of these parameters may lead to misleading clinical patterns (e.g., pseudo-dementia in the depressed elderly).

Educational Level

The SM9 battery, aimed at evaluating the various memory performance scores, was applied to 274 young individuals (aged between 17 and 24) with

H. Allain et al.

Table 4. Educational level and memory performance in the young

	Postgraduate n = 22	Young workers n = 19	General secondary n = 210	Technology school n = 23
	12.6 ± 2.1	11 ± 3.1	12.1 ± 2.7	8.9 ± 2.8
		p < 0.10		p < 0.001
Mean overall score (16 items)	10.4	9.7	10	9.5

Note: There was no difference in the other memory components.

different educational levels, as assessed from the type of studies followed: higher education, general secondary education, technology school, young workmen's hostel. It clearly appeared that at the 0.05 threshold, besides semantic organization, there was no significant difference (Table 4). In practice, therefore, any group of young subjects could be taken as a reference, except for semantically organized words.

Age

Considering the often wide age differences in pharmacological trials, and relative to the current theories that emphasize the role of age on mnestic performance (Light, 1991) (failure of retrieval processes, opposition of automatic and controlled processes), it appeared urgent to assess the SM9 battery according to age bracket, in healthy individuals. To us, it appears that cerebral ageing is also reflected by a differentiated decline of memory components, memory not being affected as a whole. Most scores gradually decrease with each decade (recall, word and face recognition), except image storage of pictures (objects, animals), which is well sustained (Figure 4).

Pathology

In various pathologies (weaned alcoholism, Parkinson's disease, Alzheimer's disease, etc.), specific profiles of mnestic impairment can be noted (Figures 2 and 4). For instance, Parkinson's disease induces a moderately decreased performance in verbal information (recall and recognition, Figure 4a) while visual information processing remains identical to that of healthy subjects of the same age (27). In contrast, the difference between alcoholics and Alzheimer's patients is striking: while alcoholic patients have subnormal scores for verbal information, relative to demented patients (low or null scores), the converse is true for visual information (picture or face recognition). Such complex results bolster the multi-module concept, whose systems are impaired differently according to the neurological pathology. It

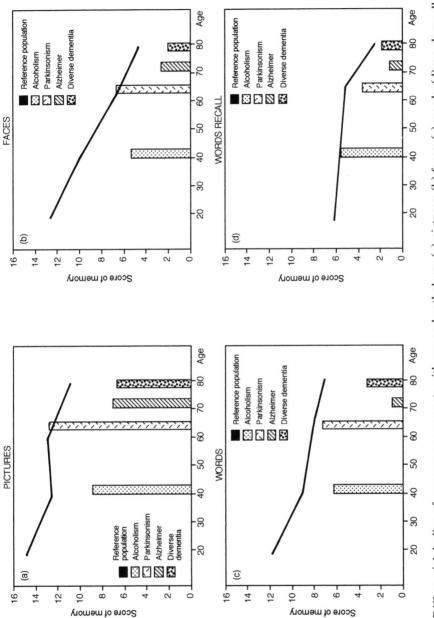

Figure 4. Differential decline of memory components with age and pathology: (a) pictures; (b) faces; (c) words; (d) words recall

seems highly probable that similar results may be obtained in psychiatry, thus making it possible to define mnestic patterns according to the disease characterized.

Pharmacology of Memory Components

Antidepressants

Rapp, in a recent editorial (1991), raised the issue of justification of a large number of antidepressants that are available. While it is clear that most of them have the same antidepressant potency, these drugs are clearly different in their levels of tolerance or acceptability. Cognitive repercussions, in this perspective, are a crucial issue. In a recent publication, Thompson (1991) tried, from published literature data, to evaluate the impact of antidepressants on memory, and underlining at the same time the classic methodological difficulties: negative effect of depression on memory, variable effectiveness on health volunteers or depressed subjects, or depending on acute or chronic administration of treatment, or whether or not the timing of cognitive tests is related to the pharmocokinetics of the product under study, or whether or not the various components of cognition (sedation, vigilance) are analysed separately, etc. In a recent comparative study (Allain et al., 1992), we studied the cognitive impact of three anti-depressant drugs, whose mechanisms of action are radically different in a population of young and depressed (28 years; Montgomery–Asberg Depression Rating Scale (MADRS) > 20) highly educated individuals who were treated and followed up for 42 days. Drugs were administered in doses considered as therapeutic, according to a double-blind protocol: maprotiline (150 mg per day, quadricyclic substance with anticholinergic properties); viloxazine (300 mg per day, agonist of β-adrenoceptors); moclobemide (450 mg per day, reversible) monoamineoxydase inhibitor (IMAO-A). The three molecules evaluated had the same antidepressant effect, but produced different cognitive profiles, only the IMAO-A coming out as slightly and steadily beneficial to mnestic performance (SMg general score), with D0 as a baseline reference (Figure 5a). However, the overall score is merely indicative, due to the multiplicity of memory components. The promnestic effect is explained by the improvement in two scores: word delayed recall (where viloxazine and moclobemide had a beneficial effect; Figure 5b) and face recognition (Figure 5a). Maprotiline had no or only transient effect, which may be due to its central anticholinergic mechanism of action (Figure 5).

   Such a trial therefore demonstrated the interest of trying to analyse specifically the memory components: delayed recall and face recognition are generally more fragile (as in ageing or pathology, for instance), probably because they involve multiple transcodings.

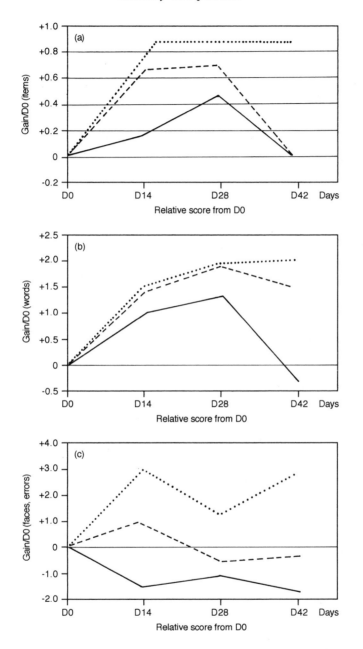

Figure 5. Comparative effect on memory of three antidepressant drugs—moclobemide, viloxazine, maprotiline: (a) general memory score; (b) words delayed recall; (c) familiar faces recognition; · · · moclobemide; - - - maprotiline; —— viloxazine

Anti-anxiety Drugs

What precedes applies particularly well to anti-anxiety drugs, or 'anxio-lytics', either benzodiazepines (BZD) or non-benzodiazepines (Curran *et al.*, 1987; Rodrigo and Lusiardo, 1988; Hindmarch, 1990); it appears useful, methodologically, to illustrate with regard to this class of drugs the crucial importance of posology on the various cognitive parameters (Wittenborn, 1988). Within this framework, we undertook a randomized, double-blind trial to compare in parallel groups three acute doses of bromazepam versus placebo (1.5, 3 and 6 mg). Seventy-two healthy male volunteers (4 × 18 students) were selected from their mnestic scores. The cognitive parameters, recorded over 12 hours, were the following: declarative memory tests (four-trial learning of a 21-item list); procedural memory test (Toronto/Hanoi tower test); and procedural activity (DRL and GO/NO-GO procedure) (Table 5). Repeated blood samplings provided concurrent plasma bromazepam levels. It appeared that the 6 mg dose alone impairs the declarative and procedural memories, correlatively with the blood levels measured (Figure 6). Conversely, the 3 mg dose significantly altered Logan's test (GO/NO-GO) and the DRL, which reflects the disinhibitor effect and the reduction in waiting capacity induced by this posology Figures 7 and 8). This work thus illustrates the fact that different psychopharmacological effects (memory, disinhibition) may be obtained with the same drug, depending on the single doses used; selective cognitive effects may simply depend on posology.

Table 5. Effect of three dosages of acute bromazepam (15, 3, 6 mg) versus placebo in young healthy volunteers (4 × 18 subjects), showing a deleterious effect of the highest dosage on memory as well as a disinhibition at the two lowest dosages (statistically different performances versus placebo)

Paradigm	Drug dosage inducing an effect	Timing of maximum effect	Effect
Declarative memory	6 mg	1.5–5 h	Words (−50%)
Procedural memory (Toronto tower)	6 mg	1st learning	Manipulations (+10%)
Logan procedure (GO/NO-GO) (inhibition)	1.5 mg, 3 mg	–	% Correct stops
DRL procedure (capacity to delay)	Placebo < 3 mg < 1.5 < 6 mg	–	Time (counting)

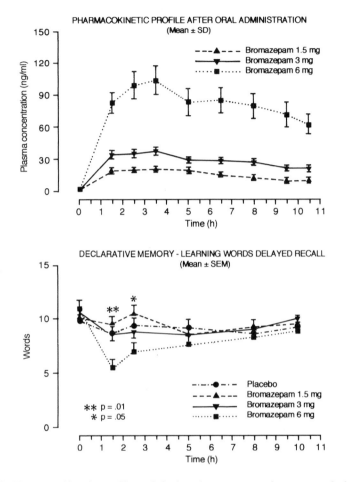

Figure 6. Pharmacokinetic profile and declarative memory after acute administration of three dosages of bromazepam (1.5 mg; 3 mg; 6 mg) in healthy volunteers

Neuroleptics

Since the 1950s, the deleterious effect of antipsychotic drugs on memory and cognitive functions has been suspected (Daston, 1959; Tune *et al.*, 1982a; Calev *et al.*, 1987). There again, the role of anticholinergic substances, classically associated with neuroleptics (Tune *et al.*, 1982b; Perlick *et al.*, 1986; Fennig *et al.*, 1986), has to be underlined, as well as the repercussion of the illness itself on memory components (Cutting, 1979). The example of the drug class is instructive, because it highlights not only the differences of cognitive impact according to the drug in question, but also those resulting from

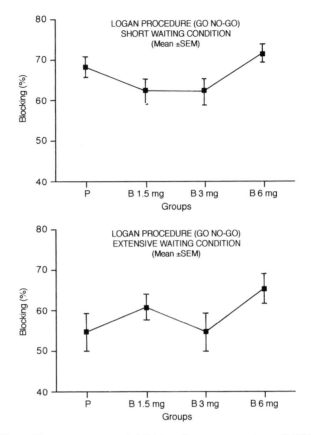

Figure 7. Effect of bromazepam on inhibition (Logan procedure: GO/NO-GO test).
P = placebo; B = bromazepam

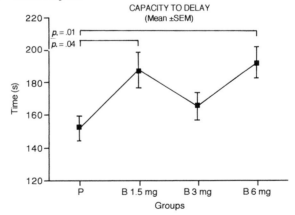

Figure 8. Effect of bromazepam on the capacity to delay. P = placebo;
B = bromazepam

treatment duration. Eitan *et al.* (1992) could, on such criteria, differentiate between four neuroleptics in adult schizophrenic subjects (19–46 years). Thioridazine and chlorpromazine, after cumulative administration, impair story recollection (20 phrases, categorization); conversely, haloperidol and trifluoropurazine improved the scores on the same test. Concentration capacities were not impaired (digit span test). The authors' interpretation is consistent with the hypothesis that anticholinergic neuroleptics have a deleterious role, aggravated by chronic administration; the beneficial effect of haloperidol and trifluoropurazine is hardly explained, except by the fact that low doses were used (4×2 mg and 4×5 mg, respectively). Lastly, none of the other memory tests used in this experiment (orientation, picture recall, digit repetition) was altered by treatment.

Nootropics

Many compounds have been developed or marketed with a view to improve cognitive functions, and in particular memory in the elderly. It is striking to note that an often misguided habit is to use global assessment scales, which provide little information on memory proper, even when they have been validated Minimental Status Examination—MMSE: 3 memory items among 30, 10%; Alzheimer's Disease Assessment Scale—ADAS: 27 of 70, 30%; Syndrom–Kurz Test—SKT: 9 of 27, 33%). The most specific criteria, in most of these trials, appear in secondary assessment criteria (Table 6) (Allain *et al.*, 1988, 1992a, 1992b) and are always characterized by very heterogeneous values, hardly sensitive to pharmacological agents, and sometimes sensitive to placebo and learning effect. Such criticisms have recently been voiced by Eagger *et al.* (1992) about tetrahydroaminoacridine (THA) in Alzheimer's disease. These negative experiences can only argue for the development and implementation of specific tests for the multiple components of memory, to help identify both the disorder and the effect of a given drug. By using adapted tests (reversed word reading, Braille), we have identified in 16 Parkinsonians a marked impairment of procedural memory (–61%), associated with impaired episodic memory (SM5 = –28%); in a similar manner, Reid *et al.* (1992) also revealed the deleterious effect of anticholinergic drugs (benzhexol) on short-term storage, verbal learning and sustained attention, in Parkinsonians. Such approaches are now routinely used in neurology (Galloway *et al.*, 1992), thus establishing a bridge between a given neurotransmission system, cognitive impairment and a drug (Milon *et al.*, 1992).

Lastly, nootropics, whose action on cognitive and mnestic functions is thought to have been proven, could be used as psychopharmacological tools to study the impact that the improvement of these functions may have on the outcome and evolution of psychiatric illness. Indeed it cannot be ruled out that promnestic drugs may optimize the effects of most psychotropic drugs currently available.

Table 6. Effect of different compounds on cognitive functions

Drug	Published (P) or not (N)	Target symptom	Population (mean age)	Dosage	Main assessment criterion	Duration (number of subjects per group)	Main problem
Dihydroergocristine/ Raubasine (nootropics) (Allain et al., 1992b)	P	Cognitive complaint	Elderly (62)	40 mg/d	Global Scale from L. Israel	3 months (55)	Strong placebo effect
Selegiline (IMAO-B)	N	Memory complaint	Elderly (70)	5; 10 mg/d	DNBC[a] scale from MacNair	3 months (55; 62)	Ceiling effect at inclusion
Exifone (Scavenger) (Allain et al., 1988)	P	Cognitive deficit	Parkinson's disease (67)	600; 1200 mg/d	MMS global scale from L. Israel	3 months (15; 15)	Hetero-geneity at inclusion
Exifone (Scavenger)	N	Memory loss	Alzheimer's disease (69)	600 mg/d	MMS	6 months (30)	Accuracy of diagnosis
Apomorphine (D_1/D_2 agonist)	N	Cognitive complaint	Parkinson's disease (64)	1 s.c. injection (2.5 mg)	DNBC[a]	Acute (9)	No control group
Cebaracetam (piracetam-like compound) (Allain et al., 1992c)	P	Cognitive deficit	Slight cognitive decline in elderly (75)	1.500 mg/d	MMS	4 weeks (15)	Too small sample treated

[a]DNBC: déficit neurobiologique de la cinquantaine—subjective global scale from Steru et al. (1988).

Effect Potency and Signification

The issue of the potency of the observed effect, and its relevance or significance to patients, has been frequently raised; answers are either evasive or expressed as all or nothing. Engel and Satzger (1992) recently tackled the problem with regard to the drugs studied in senile dementia, and underscored the following points: modification of at least half the standard deviation of the main criterion; in chronic treatment, modification of the recognized evolutive slope of the treated disorder; correlation with the subject's global evaluation, life quality and daily activities. To our team, the answers to the question result from the parametering (calibration) of the various tests on offer, any deviation induced by the drug in comparison with placebo and in relation to those considered normal for a given age bracket (return to normal, performance increase or decrease) being considered as a therapeutically relevant drug effect. Note that this approach is symmetrical to the work of Crook *et al.* (1986), who proposed the term age-associated memory impairment (AAMI), based on isolated mnestic deficit quantization. Standardization of these tests makes them usable in the early phases of drug development, precisely when effects on memory are customarily investigated. Obviously, the indirect benefit of such pharmacologically induced memory improvements on various pathologies remains to be assessed and quantified; in psychiatry, such a benefit can intuitively be foreseen (Rogler *et al.*, 1992).

Conclusion

Psychopharmacology of memory has long been confronted with the difficulty of finding reliable, reproducible and drug-sensitive assessment methods. Currently, tools are adapted to research in cognitive pharmacology. They provide proof of the deleterious or beneficial action of several compounds on the components of mnestic processes. The cognitive issue may now enter into the choice and comparison of products. The therapeutic consequences of pharmacologically induced memory changes have taken increasing importance and led to greater rationalization of psychotropic drug usage. As regards research, such a systematization of memory component distinction and analysis provides instructive correlations with either underlying neurochemical mechanisms, or the brain structures involved, as identified by *in vivo* imaging.

Summary

The possibility now available of modulating human cognitive functions with different drugs constitutes one of the main avenues in human pharmacology, with memory as one of the most important targets. In this perspective, it is urgent to give priority to the standardization of the methods required for that objective. On the basis of the theoretical multi-mode model of cognitive memory, the factors which modulate memory have to be described: age, educational level, sex and underlying pathology. Moreover, memory component analysis must be systematically combined with the assessment of other functions (vigilance, attention, fluidity, etc.) determinant to overall performance scores. Such an approach clearly shows that antidepressants can have different patterns of action on these mnestic components, that the impact of anti-anxiety drugs on memory is highly dose dependent, and that major tranquillizers can be widely different compounds according to the study. Finally, it is worth assessing the effect of nootropic drugs on disease evolution, on the assumption that cognitive improvement could be beneficial in psychiatry. Such an approach is highly relevant to the improvement and optimization of psychotropic drug use. Qualitative rather than quantitative improvement of the memory process could be the coming challenge to pharmacology.

Acknowledgements

We are grateful to Ch. Boujon, F. Le Coz, I. Gueho, G. Guidon, J.P. Martinet, Ph. Pichon, P. Raoul, J.M. Reymann, R. Thirion, P. Trebon and Ph. Van Acker for their cooperation in study implementation and evaluations, and to Mrs C. Maillard and Philip Cunningham for their patient and valued assistance in the preparation and translation of the manuscript.

References

Allain, H., Denmat, J., Bentue-Ferrer, D., Milon, D., Pignol, P., Reymann, J.M., Pape, D., Sabouraud, O., and Van Den Driessche, J. (1988). Randomized double-blind trial of exifone versus cognitive problems in Parkinson's disease. *Fundam. Clin. Pharmacol.*, **2**, 1–12.

Allain, H., Bentue-Ferrer, D., and Decombe, R. (1990a). Choosing a target for cognitive enhancers. *Clin. ther.*, **12**, 108–14.

Allain, H., Lieury, A., Reymann, J.M., Martinet, J.P., Trebon, P., Decombe, R., Bentue-Ferrer, D., and Gandon, J.M. (1990b). Le développement des médicaments promnésiants *Ann. Med. Interne*, **4** (suppl. 1), 19–25.

Allain, H., Lieury, A., Brunet-Bourgin, F., Mirabaud, Ch., Trebon, P., Le Coz, F., and Gandon, J.M. (1992a). Antidepressants and cognition: Comparative effects of moclobemide, viloxazine and maprotiline. *Psychopharmacology*, **106**, S56–S61.

Allain, H., Carraro, J.C., Morel, G., and Authier, M. (1992b). Etude comparative contre placebo de l'association raubasine-dihydroergocristine dans la plainte cognitive. *Psychol. Med. (Paris)*, in press.

Allain, H., Llull, J.B., Morel, G., and Gandon, J.M. (1992c). Phase I study of a new nootropic compound cebaracetam (ZY 15119) in the elderly. *VIth Congress on Clinical Pharmacology and Therapeutics*, Yokohama, July 1992.

Baddeley, A.D. (1988a). Imagery and working memory. In Denis, M., Engelkamp, J., and Richardson, J.T.E. (eds), *Cognitive and Neuropsychological Approaches to Mental Imagery*, Dordrecht: Martinus Nijhoff, in cooperation with NATO Scientific Affairs Division, pp. 169–80.

Baddeley, A.D. (1988b). Measuring memory. In Hindmarch, I., and Ott, H. (eds), *Benzodiazepine, Receptor Ligands, Memory and Information Processing,* Berlin: Springer-Verlag, pp. 12–22.

Calev, A., Berlin, H., and Lerer, B. (1987). Remote and recent memory in long hospitalized chronic schizophrenics. *Biol. Psychiatry,* **22**, 79–85.

Crook, T., Bartus, R., Ferris, S.H., Whitehouse, P., Cohen, G.D., and Gershon, S. (1986). Age-associated memory impairment: Proposed diagnostic criteria and measures of clinical change. Report of National Institute of Mental Health Work Group. *Dev. Neuropsychol.,* **2**, 261–78.

Curren, V., Allen, D., and Lader, M. (1987). The effects of single doses of alpidem and lorazepam on memory and psychomotor performance in normal humans. *J. Psychopharmacol.,* **2**, 81–9.

Cutting, J. (1979) Memory in functional psychosis. *J. Neurol. Neurosurg. Psychiatry,* **42**, 1031–7.

Daston, P.G. (1959). Effects of two phenothiazine drugs on concentrative attention span of chronic schizophrenics. *J. Clin. Psychol.,* **15**, 106–9.

Eagger, S., Morant, N., Levy, R., and Sahakian, B. (1992). Tacrine in Alzheimer's disease: Time courses of changes in cognitive function and practice effects. *Br. J. Psychiatry,* **160**, 36–40.

Eitan, N., Levin, Y., Ben-Artzi, E., Levy, A., and Neumann, M. (1992). Effects of antipsychotic drugs on memory functions of schizophrenic patients. *Acta Psychiatr. Scand.,* **85**, 74–6.

Engel, R., and Satzger, W. (1992). Methodological problems in assessing therapeutic efficacy in patients with dementia. *Drugs Aging,* **2**, 79–85.

Fennig, S., Levine, Y., Naisberg, S., and Elizur, A. (1986). The effect of trihexiphemdyl (Artane) on memory in schizophrenic patients. *Prog. Neuropsychopharmacol. Biol. Psychiatry,* **11**, 71–8.

Galloway, P., Sahgal, A., McKeith, I., Lloyd, S., Cook, J., Ferrier, I., and Edwardson, J. (1992). Visual pattern recognition memory and learning deficits in senile dementias of Alzheimer and Lewy body types. *Dementia,* **3**, 101–7.

Harshman, R.A., Hampson, E., and Benbaum, S.A. (1983). Individual differences in cognitive abilities and brain organization. Part 1: Sex and handedness differences in ability. *Can J. Psychol.,* **37**, 144–92.

Hindmarch, I. (1990). Alpidem and psychological performance in elderly subjects. *Pharmacopsychiatria,* **23**, 124–8.

Juan de Mendoza, J.L. (1988). Spécialisation hémisphérique et mémoire verbale: effet des variations d'indices entre l'endocage et la restitution. *L'Année Psychol.,* **88**, 169–78.

Levin, H.S., and Benton, A.L. (1984) Neuropsychologic assessment. In Baker, A.B. (ed.), *Clinical Neurology,* Philadelphia: Harper & Row.

Lieury, A. (1979). La mémoire épisodique est-elle emboîtée dans la mémoire sémantique? *L'Année Psychol.,* **79**, 123–42.

Lieury, A. (1990). *Manuel de Psychologie Générale,* Paris: Dunod.

Lieury, A. (1992). *La Mémoire: Théories et Résultats* (4th edn), Brussels: Mardaga.

Lieury, A., and Calvez, F. (1986). Le double codage des dessins en fonction du temps de présentation et de l'ambiguité. *L'Année Psychol.,* **86**, 45–61.

Lieury, A., Raoul, P., Gandon, J.M., Decombe, R., Reymann, J.M., and Allain, H. (1990). Profil des capacités mnésiques dans les maladies de Parkinson et d'Alzheimer. *Psychol. Med (Paris),* **22**, 1210–17.

Lieury, A., Raoul, P., Boujon, Ch., Bernoussi, M., and Allain, H. (1991). Le vieillissement des composants de la mémoire: Analyse factorielle de 17 scores de mémoire. *L'Année Psychol.,* **91**, 169–86.

Light, L.L. (1991). Memory and aging: Four hypotheses in search of data. *Ann. Rev. Psychol.,* **42**, 333–76.

Mesulam, M.M. (1985). *Principles of Behavioral Neurology,* Philadelphia: FA Davis.

Milon, D., Gandon, J.M., Lieury, A., Boujon, C., Allain, H., Malledant, Y., and Saint-Marc, C. (1993). Mémoire et anesthésie. *J. Fr. Anesth. Reanim.,* in press.

Mishkin, M., and Appenzeller, T. (1987). The anatomy of memory. *Sci. Am.,* **256**, 62–71.

Moss, M.B., Albert, M.S., Butters, N., and Payne, M. (1986). Differential patterns of memory loss among patients with Alzheimer's disease, Huntington's disease and alcoholic Korsakoff's syndrome. *Arch. Neurol.,* **43**, 239–46.

Paivio, A., and Csapo, K. (1969). Concrete image and verbal memory codes. *J. Exp. Psychol.,* **80**, 279–85.

Perlick, D., Stastny, P., Katz, I. *et al.* (1986) Memory deficits and anticholinergic levels in chronic schizophrenics. *Am. J. Psychiatry,* **143**, 230–2.

Raoul, P., Lieury, A., Decombe, R., Chauvel, P., and Allain, H. (1992). Déficit mnésique au cours de la maladie de Parkinson. *Press. Med (Paris),* **21**, 69–72.

Rapp, M.S. (1991) Antidepressants: Too many choices? *Can. J. Psychiatry,* **36**, 615–16.

Reid, W.G.J., Broe, G.A., and Morris, J.G.L. (1992). The role of cholinergic deficiency in neuropsychological deficits in idiopathic Parkinson's disease. *Dementia,* **3**, 114–20.

Rodrigo, G., and Lusiardo, M. (1988). Effects on memory following a single oral dose of diazepam. *Psychopharmacology,* **95**, 263–7.

Rogler, L.L., Malgady, R., and Tryon, W. (1992). Evaluation of mental health: Issues of memory in the diagnosis interview schedule. *J. Nerv. Ment. Dis.,* **180**, 215–22.

Saint-Cyr, J.A., Taylor, A.E., and Lang, A.E. (1988). Procedural learning and neostriatal dysfunction in man. *Brain,* **111**, 941–59.

Sarter, M. (1991). Taking stock of cognition enhancers. *Trends Pharmacol. Sci.,* **12**, 456–61.

Squire, L.R. (1986). Mechanisms of memory. *Science,* **232**, 1612–19.

Steru, L., Crevier, B., Lancrenon, S., Sevestre, M., Thabuy, P., and Vetel, J.M. (1988). Pourquoi une nouvelle population, pourquoi une nouvelle échelle, définition et mesure d'un nouveau syndrome: Le déficit neurobiologique de la cinquantaine. *Rev. Prat. (Paris),* **38** (Suppl.), 45–8.

Thompson, P.J. (1991). Antidepressants and memory: A review. *Hum. Psychopharmacol.,* **6**, 79–80.

Tiberghien, G., and Lecocq, P. (1983). *Rappel et Reconnaissance: Encodage et Recherche en Mémoire,* Lille: Presses Universitaires.

Tulving, E. (1972). Episodic and semantic memory. In Tulving, E. and Donaldson, W. (eds), *Organization of Memory,* New York: Academic Press, pp. 333–371.

Tulving, E. (1985). How many memory systems are there? *Am. Psychol.,* **40**, 385–98.

Tulving, E., and Thomson, D.M. (1973). Encoding specificity and retrieval processes in episodic memory. *Psychol. Rev.,* **80**, 352–73.

Tune, L.E., Strauss, M.S., Lew, M.D. *et al.* (1982a). Serum levels of anticholinergic drugs and impaired recent memory in chronic schizophrenic patients. *Am. J. Psychiatry,* **139**, 1460–2.

Tune, L.E., Lew, M.F., Bretlimger, E., and Coyle, J.T. (1982b). Serum levels of anticholinergic drugs and impaired recent memory in chronic schizophrenic patients. *Am. J. Psychiatry,* **139**, 1460–2.

Wittenborn, J.R. (1988). Assessment of the effects of drugs on memory. In: Hindmarch, I., and Ott, H. (eds), *Benzodiazepine Receptor Ligands, Memory and Information Processing. Psychometric, Psychopharmacological and issues,* Berlin, Heidelberg, Springer-Verlag, pp. 67–78.

10

Measuring Drug–Alcohol and Drug–Drug Interactions of Psychotropic Drugs on Human Skilled Performance

*Mauri J. Mattila, *Marja E. Mattila and †Esko Nuotto

Department of Pharmacology and Toxicology, and †National Medicines Control Laboratory, University of Helsinki, Finland

Introduction

Results from epidemiological field studies, supervised driving, and particularly from laboratory tests have indicated that agents depressing the central nervous system (CNS) dose-dependently impair human skilled performance related to driving and various occupational tasks (Seppälä *et al.*, 1979; Nicholson and Ward, 1984; O'Hanlon and deGier, 1986). The research literature of this field is so vast that even its subtopics, drug–alcohol and drug–drug interactions, cannot be adequately treated in this chapter. Since the general principles and practice concerning experimentation with psychotropic drugs are important, we first outline the constituents of the interaction studies on performance and then treat briefly the research results of theoretical or practical interest. This chapter reflects the experiences of our own group, after having carried out drug interaction studies for two decades. A specific review of drug–ethanol interactions on performance exists (Starmer and Bird, 1984).

The word *'interaction'* needs to be defined because it is often misused. An interaction of two agents refers, strictly, to their combined action that deviates from the expected additive effect, and either potentiation or antagonism may then occur. In order to analyse and illustrate the combined actions

Human Psychopharmacology, Vol. 4. Edited by I. Hindmarch and P. D. Stonier
© 1993 John Wiley & Sons Ltd

of two drugs, isoboles have been constructed (Curry, 1977) but such analyses are uncommon in human studies. Thus, alleged interactions affecting the CNS, such as decremental combined effects of drugs and alcohol on skill performance in man, have not been fully documented for various reasons.

Minor impairments of performance by low doses of anxiolytics, hypnotics and antidepressants are difficult to assess, and their combined effects may suggest mild interactions which can have promotional but not clear clinical consequences. Ethical reasons preclude the use of high doses of drugs for mere experimental purposes. If conclusive evidence for mild to moderate potentiating or antagonistic interactions of centrally active drugs is not furnished, the term 'combined effect' would remain the most appropriate in these cases. For brevity and convenience the word 'interaction' is often used in a broad sense, but the results should be always defined more exactly in terms of addition, potentiation or antagonism.

Pharmacokinetic interactions result from the alterations in the plasma and tissue concentrations of the agents concerned—one or both of them—alterations that can also modulate drug effects. Inhibition of the metabolism of the ultra-short-acting benzodiazepines triazolam and midazolam by non-sedative agents like macrolide antibiotics (Warot *et al.*, 1987; Aranko *et al.*, 1991) is such an example. This kind of combined effect is non-specific and, as such, a clear issue unless peculiar deviations resulting from the dose-dependent pharmacokinetics cloud it. The consequences of pharmacokinetic interactions depend on the rate(s) of elimination of the agent(s) concerned, on their volume of distribution, and certainly on their effects and therapeutic safety margins.

Pharmacodynamic interactions refer to the altered effects of the agent(s) on receptor level without essential changes in their plasma concentrations. Even then, pharmacokinetic changes can occur on the tissue level, beyond the usual non-invasive techniques used for the drug sampling, particularly if the kinetic state of the drug(s) is unsteady. Such a complex situation is not uncommon in single-dose studies where the distribution and redistribution of drugs render the relationship between the plasma concentrations of drugs and their central effects very complex (Ellinwood and Nikaido, 1987; Dingemanse *et al.*, 1988). Sometimes the interactions recorded have both kinetic and dynamic components (Sellers *et al.*, 1972, 1980), and the final combined effects can be difficult to predict. Since the practical implications between drugs and alcohol are often important, overwhelming amounts of research reports exist and numerous reviews cover separate aspects of the interactions of drugs and ethanol in neural and non-neural tissues (for references see Sellers and Holloway, 1978; Moscowitz, 1981; Ciraulo and Barnhill, 1986; Mattila, 1990).

Strategies and Methods for Measurement of Psychotropic Drug Interactions

Experimental Design

The design, the numbers of subjects, and the tests selected for psychopharmacological research (Klebel, 1981) also apply to drug interaction studies (Starmer and Bird, 1984) and much depends on the problems to be solved. Effects of acute intake of ethanol during a prolonged treatment with medicinal drugs (H_1-antihistamines, antihypertensives, anxiolytics, antidepressants, etc.) often raise the question of whether or not the medicine enhances alcohol effects on human performance, or vice versa. As a rule, the results and the conclusions are applied to target the driving fitness of motorists in traffic. To allow such implications, the effects of alcohol on performance should be measured with adequate double-blind tests during the randomized cross-over maintenance treatments with placebo and active drug which have reached the steady kinetic state. Comparisons of the effects of active drug with placebo, and ethanol + active drug with ethanol + placebo can then be made easily. The ethanol effects are evaluated by comparing the responses to ethanol and placebo drink during the maintenance with placebo. Relevant pharmacokinetic measurements, without exaggeration, belong to the trial rules.

It is desirable to complete the above design by measuring the responses to the first dose of the drug, along and/or in combination with alcohol. This procedure may furnish information of tolerance which might develop during the maintenance. However, the inclusion of such initial interaction tests to the protocol provides an extra burden of work, and they are usually omitted so as not to render the whole trial too strenuous. Such single-dose studies sometimes replace maintenance doses if a prolonged treatment with medicinal drugs, such as neuroleptics given to healthy subjects, gives rise to ethical concern, or if the primary interest lies in the comparison of several combined actions and their time courses in one trial (Mattila *et al.*, 1988a, 1989). Interesting or clinically significant findings may then be re-evaluated in further studies with prolonged administration of drugs.

When looking for the time courses of interactions, possible clockwise or counter-clockwise hysteresis curves of the agents during the test session must be taken into account when estimating the additive or supra-additive nature of the interaction. Clockwise hysteresis refers to development of acute tolerance, characteristic of single doses of diazepam and some hypnotics. Counterclockwise hysteresis, characteristic of cannabis and lorazepam for example, is uncommon and refers to sensitization and enhanced responses to given concentrations of the drug that develop with time during the session. There are arguments about the real background of these phenomena (Ellinwood and Nikaido, 1987; Dingemanse *et al.*, 1988), and the type of hysteresis can also depend on the variable measured.

Four comparative treatments are the minimum in an interaction study: two interactive agents alone and in combination, and placebo. The inclusion of placebo is essential because it covers non-pharmacological sources of variation, and allows an estimation of intersubject and intrasubject variances of the test(s) used. The few exceptions to the placebo rule include patient studies where the use of placebo could prove impracticable, or raise ethical concerns, as is often the case with maintenance studies in depressive outpatients. In these cases, inclusion of more than one dose of the test drug(s) or an extra active drug may prove necessary to evaluate the degree of the combined action concerned.

At least one of the single agents given must produce a clear effect to confirm that the tests work properly, and to provide a quantitative comparison for the drugs under study. The question of whether this positive control ('verum') should be an approved standard drug is debatable. The verum should be safe, and its effects should resemble fairly closely those of the study drug qualitatively and quantitatively. Since psychotropic drugs may differently affect various modalities, and since the combined effects can even be unpredictable, sufficient doses of the study drugs can serve as verum. Ethanol is the natural verum in drug–alcohol interaction studies, but another verum, a psychotropic drug, would be desirable as well. Since ethanol affects the brain as a non-specific solvent, it should not be used as an extra comparator for the effects of drugs and their combinations on performance unless there are reasons for it (Volkerts *et al.*, 1987; Mattila *et al.*, 1988a).

Inclusion of more than one dose of interactive agent(s) increases the number of comparative treatments (Linnoila and Mattila, 1973; Seppälä *et al.*, 1982a; Mattila *et al.*, 1986a) to an extent which can be problematic for the statistical handling of the data, and two placebo sessions are sometimes used to improve evaluation of the results. The number of sessions in single-dose studies can be reduced by administering both alcohol and drug to the same subject in the same session, alcohol intake being postponed until the first measurement of drug effects has been done (Strömberg and Mattila, 1987). Alternatively, two trials or more may prove necessary (Laisi *et al.*, 1979). The number of subjects needed depends on the number of treatment groups, the reliability of the tests in terms of their intersubject and intrasubject variances, on the doses of the agents used, and also on the question to be answered to make certain statements. The treatments which are to be compared with each other should be defined before the final analysis.

More subjects are needed to prove the equality of the treatments (drug + alcohol combination does not differ from alcohol alone) than to document their inequality (drug, alcohol and their combination all separately differ from placebo). The numbers of subjects needed can be calculated when the trial constituents are known. The need and justification for the exact (and often promotional) statements, such as 'the active treatment equals placebo' seems doubtful for two reasons. Firstly, that statement may not be true if applied to people other than the self-selected trial subjects, who may, for example, differ from the larger age-matched population in their personality variable (Pieters *et al.*, 1992). Secondly, exact statements require the exposure of considerable numbers of subjects to a new drug or drug combination although the implications of the results were untrue. As to drug studies in healthy volunteers, we prefer the use of fewer subjects—just enough to document significant actions and interactions that allow sound conclusions and fair but not exaggerated implications, applied with common sense, to the life situation. Adequate statistical advance planning is essential.

Statisticians regularly prefer clear-cut comparisons between parallel groups treated with active drug and placebo. Since the number of groups to be compared in interaction trials is four or more, the puristic view requires large numbers of subjects—perhaps 20 subjects for each group (Linnoila and Mattila, 1973). This is often impracticable and it may raise ethical concern if robust effects are to be expected from drug combinations. Cross-over design is then preferable to reduce variation between groups, numbers of subjects exposed to new drugs and, perhaps, non-Gaussian distributions of drug responses. Intervals between testing days should be from the usual one week up to one month (Laisi *et al.*, 1978), depending on the drugs given. For single-dose studies, we have found it useful if the subjects had minor pretrial experience of the effects of drugs of the same group, just to reduce the extra variation created by (behavioural?) tolerance which may develop to the effects of, for example, benzodiazepines given to drug-naive subjects (File and Lister, 1983).

To reduce non-pharmacological variation (weather, common cold, etc.) we test all our subjects ($n = 10$–15) on the same day if possible, starting the rounds of consecutive tests at regular intervals. Such a 'conveyor belt' design carries some extra arousal that can modify the results (Cohen *et al.*, 1984), and the recognition of alcohol intake by the other subjects not receiving it. However, the subjects themselves easily recognize alcohol from its effects, and tricks to disguise ethanol drinks seem unnecessary if doses of ethanol are 0.5 g/kg or more. The role of chronopharmacology in the actions and interactions on performance awaits further research.

The conventional view favours using absolute values of test functions for statistical handling, avoiding the use of changes from respective baseline (Δ-values) although these represent the actual drug responses in single-dose studies. The use of Δ-values is complicated by deviating baselines, but as the performances of trained subjects are known, the baselines can be repeated if major deviations appear. Their main cause may be the subject's inadequate compliance with the trial rules, including proper rest before coming to the test session. Routine breath testing at the baseline does not, unfortunately, reveal these rule violations. We pay the subjects for their time but not for the scores, although the latter might sensitize some tests to drug or alcohol effects.

As to statistics, repeated-measures three-way (subjects × drug × order) ANOVA and split-split plot ANOVA are well suited to the data analysis in cross-over trials, completed with other parametric or non-parametric tests according to the design and problems of the study. Sets of several tests carried out are problematic because they are burdened by an 'alpha-inflation' which refers to type I errors. This derives from the large number of analyses from many parallel tests within the limited number of test subjects. It can be reduced by defining the few primary test variables from the set used, by avoiding unnecessary tests for significance, and perhaps by applying G-analysis to the pooled data of more than one test.

Subjects

Although the tests and testing designs as such are adequate, intersubject and intrasubject variations in the results recorded much depend on the abilities and motivation of the test subjects. Subjects can choose different strategies in performing the test, and also change them due to the learning process during the test (Broadbent, 1984). The role of the test subjects if often ignored and criticism addressed to the methods only. Similar or even greater intersubject variations of skill performance may exist in real life, and intersubject variance in performance tests can never match the small variance seen in chemical laboratory assay methods.

The fundamental follow-up study by Häkkinen (1976) on the 100 Helsinki city bus drivers showed that the inadequate performance in three to four relevant laboratory tests revealed the drivers' inability to control complex situations and that this characteristic correlated positively with their traffic accident records collected from an 8-year period. The worse half of the drivers in the test had twice as many accidents as compared to the better half. They thus revealed their accident proneness (Shaw and Sichel, 1971). The accident coefficient was most strongly saturated (0.52) on the attention factor determined primarily in the driving apparatus and in expectancy reaction tests. Another characteristic with high (0.47) loading of accident proneness was the lowered involuntary control of motor function (hastiness, susceptibility to disturbances, motor restlessness), whereas eye-to-hand coordination, and especially intelligence and simple reaction time, were invalid predictive tests. Accident proneness measured in the baseline study remained similar during the follow-up of the drivers' accident records collected during several further years (Häkkinen, 1976).

The contribution by subjects to overall variation, particularly in the interaction studies, is regularly seen when analysing the data, e.g. with multivariant ANOVA, and it can be reduced by employing cross-over designs and trained subjects where possible and relevant. Our simulated driving test (Mattila *et al.*, 1989) was easier to learn for driving instructors than for the age-matched students, suggesting that the drivers had better coordination and anticipation of events. However, the groups needed the same amount of practice to learn a strenuous central and peripheral attention test (Mattila, 1988, unpublished). In Häkkinen's (1976) study the test subjects' driving experience did not much modify their performance in the driving apparatus test. As a whole, parallel groups of untrained subjects are less likely to produce stable results with Gaussian distribution than the trained subjects do in the cross-over tests.

The subjects' *age* contributes to the decremental effects of benzodiazepines on psychomotor performance, the impairment increasing with age. Theoretically this could result from altered distribution of psychotropic drugs according to the well-known altered body constitution of the elderly (reduced muscle mass and water space, increased body fats). That may be the case with alcohol, since it is distributed in the water space, and blood alcohol concentrations (BACs) produced by the standard dose of alcohol are usually higher in the elderly. However, the drug-induced impairment increasing with age results mainly from the poor baseline performance of the elderly subjects, while the actual responses to moderate doses of nitrazepam (Castleden and George, 1979), diazepam (Palva *et al.*, 1982), chlormethiazole (Fagan *et al.*, 1990) or amitriptyline (Mattila *et al.*, 1988b; 1989) are roughly similar in old and young subjects. The combined effects of ethanol and lorazepam on performance have been shown to be similar in young and middle-aged subjects (Seppälä *et al.*, 1986). On the whole, young subjects may be more sensitive than older ones to subjective sedation.

In order to avoid excessive training and refusals, the performance tests administered to aged subjects should not be too complex and data-paced, and the manual dexterity needed should be moderate only. Effects of drug combinations may be more unpredictable than the effects of single agents, yet clear evidence of this is scanty. To play safe, it is unwise to conduct interaction studies with aged subjects for merely experimental purposes, as they can be subject to polypharmacy due to several ailments. If aged subjects are to be recruited for drug–alcohol or drug–drug interaction studies, the expected lack of important adverse effects must be obvious, and the effects of the drugs and the subjects' health must be carefully checked. The ethical aspects are different for patients who are actually treated with several agents: the experimental drugs are part of their treatment, and the extra measurements are not only indicated but also appreciated, provided the methods are practicable and fitted to the patient's condition. This principle suits, of course, younger patients as well (Aranko *et al.*, 1985a). For general updated guidelines on the ethics in volunteer research see Haynes and Webb (1991).

Placebo-controlled cross-over single-dose studies of psychotropic agents in healthy young subjects are often criticized as being irrelevant. With regard to healthy subjects versus patients, the actions of anxiolytic (Saario *et al.*, 1976) and antidepressant (Seppälä *et al.*, 1978) drugs during 2 weeks' treatment of fairly young patients were similar to those we have measured for healthy subjects in our laboratory. Patients with joint pains who received multiple doses of oral dextropropoxyphen and amitriptyline in combination (Saarialho-Kere *et al.*, 1989) responded about similarly as did young subjects to comparable acute combinations. With more severe diseases and/or with acquired tolerance to benzodiazepines in particular (Aranko *et al.*, 1983, 1985a), psychomotor responses are very different from those measured in drug-naive subjects. In any case, the conclusions drawn from the results must take these similarities and differences into account.

Silverstone (1988) has reviewed the relative contribution of psychiatric disease and its treatment to driving performance. The patients have a higher than expected rate of involvement in road traffic accidents, but not all types of psychiatric patients are hazardous. Elderly patients with failing cognitive powers run a greater risk, and patients with frank dementia do so even more. Manic-depressive disease carries probably a greater risk than schizophrenia. Anxiety is an important issue because the number of patients treated with benzodiazepine hypnotics and anxiolytics is large. Anxiolytic drugs may increase the likelihood of involvement in road traffic accidents, but the exact role of drugs in this increase remains unsolved thus far (Silverstone, 1988). As to the drug interaction studies of hypnotics, healthy subjects may well be suited to them because a fair number of hypnotic consumers are basically healthy people who take hypnotics for social and occupational reasons. A contribution by the non-pathological personality of the individuals (Pieters *et al.*, 1992) to their drug responses may exist, but this matter has been under debate (Klebel, 1981) and is not discussed here.

Performance Tests

Although the neural basis of impaired performance produced by drugs and their combinations is complex and not fully understood (Linnoila *et al.*, 1986; Rohrbauch *et al.*, 1987), adequate methods must be used to document the drug-induced alterations of human performance objectively and subjectively. Methods range widely from electroencephalogram (EEG) analysis (Greenblatt *et al.*, 1989; Bührer *et al.*, 1990) to driving well-equipped test cars on the road in real traffic (O'Hanlon, 1984; Volkerts *et al.*, 1987). The dominating group are the sets of performance tests carried out in the laboratory; they lie between the two extremes mentioned above and represent a preferable alternative for many purposes. The physiological background of the methods used to measure information processing is inadequately known, and the theoretical views of psychologists often clash with the practical views of pharmacologists, especially when concerning the act of driving and its impairment by drugs and their combinations (Sanders, 1986; Sanders and Wauschkuhn, 1988; Koelega, 1988; Linnoila *et al.*, 1986, Nicholson, 1988).

The fast-Fourier-transformed *EEG power spectra* are elegant and sensitive to detect dose dependently the effects of, for example, benzodiazepines (BZDs) on the CNS, and for modelling the concentration/effect relationships of drugs (Dingemanse *et al.*, 1988; Bührer *et al.*, 1990). The techniques do not need much active contribution by the test subject, thus providing an objective measure for drug effects. However, their sensitivity, in terms of the BZD effects related to respective plasma levels (Greenblatt *et al.*, 1989; Bührer *et al.*, 1990), is no better than that of good performance tests. Further, alterations in the EEG indicate effects on the neural tissue without indicating which functions are impaired or improved, unless they are concomitantly measured with performance tests. The EEG mappings and their changes are often used qualitatively to classify psychotropic drugs showing predominantly anti–psychotic, antidepressant or anxiolytic characteristics (Saletu *et al.*, 1989). Those EEG analyses are not suitable for drug interaction studies because the interactive agents, either alone or together, may have several (non-specific?) actions on the EEG, and the combinations thus cloud the analysis. With regard to alcohol effects, it is well known that peak inebriation after acute intake of ethanol correlates positively with BACs and impairment of skill performance, but does not coincide with definite EEG changes, which rather coincide with late subjective sedation.

Real driving of the test car in traffic is a relevant test to reveal unwanted drug actions and interactions on driving fitness. The long duration of the test (1 hour or more) renders it vulnerable to potential pharmacokinetic changes (distribution and redistribution) during the trial after single doses of certain drugs. Multiple dosing or even steady kinetic state of the drug is therefore mandatory. It is useful to consider the records of the total drive in consecutive sections according to the dynamic and kinetic time courses of the agent(s) given. Short-lasting performance tasks (not EEG) suitably done during the driving session may also prove useful in making the test more versatile and extending the implications of the results, not only to road traffic but also to occupational 'man–machine interactions' linked with both hazardous and ordinary tasks. The last-mentioned implication may become more important with ever-increasing occupational demands and stress, and because a motorist can take a bus but cannot escape from the work.

Performance tests in the laboratory well represent the daily tasks in jobs (book-keepers, bank assistants, cashiers in shops, etc.) which need keen attention for varying time periods, and adequate manual skill on a computer keyboard. These tests may also provide significant prediction of the drug-induced decrements in driving fitness on the road. Performance tests vary greatly from complex, extensive and expensive simulators to varying sets of separate laboratory tests (Hindmarch, 1980; Borland and Nicholson, 1984; Moscowitz, 1984;

Starmer and Bird, 1984; Mattila *et al.*, 1988a; Irving, 1988) which are mainly based on computerized electronics but can be simple pencil and paper tests as well. The attention–arousal state, choice reactive and coordinative skills, and cognitive functions are fundamental variables when the effects of agents on psychomotor function are assessed objectively, but they still much depend on the subjects' real motivation. Incorporation of these variables in one complex test is desirable, but not mandatory, and sets of tests can be valuable as well (Häkkinen, 1976; Broadbent, 1984; Nicholson, 1988). Divided attention (Moscowitz, 1984) and risk-taking behaviour are two important variables where alcohol and driving are concerned. Qualitative or semi-quantitative rating scales may provide some information about risk taking and its alteration by drugs.

The duration of individual tests and the environmental levels of arousal have been debatable issues, and moderate to high environmental arousal has, for example, rendered healthy subjects objectively and subjectively less responsive to the central effects of diphenhydramine (Cohen *et al.*, 1984). The full divided-attention test (Moscowitz, 1984) lasts for 1 hour, and long-lasting lonely tests have been considered mandatory (Sanders, 1986; Koelega, 1988). That may be true when applying the test results to quiet driving in low-density traffic, but it is exaggerated for cases where active conversation, listening to the radio, and talking on the phone while driving increase the arousal, particularly in busy city traffic. Long-lasting tests are not suitable for estimation of the time-course of drug action after single doses unless the records are studied in sections. When applying the results to occupational tasks, short-lasting tests in a moderately vigilant environment seem relevant if not preferable for prediction of the decremental actions and interactions of drugs on human performance.

The primary objective tests in our laboratory at present comprise short-lasting simulated driving with and without a simultaneous mixed reaction task (5 minutes), and the sustained digit symbol substitution test (3 minutes) using pencil and paper or computer. These are supplemented with other tests (flicker fusion, Maddox wing, central and peripheral attention, body sway, etc.) according to the drugs and combinations to be tested. This battery is well suited for drug interaction studies (Mattila *et al.*, 1988a, 1989) where ethanol readily impairs the ability to recognize the number of digits substituted and prolongs reaction times. Simple tracking is not clearly impaired by ethanol at BACs below 0.7 mg/ml, although it is definitely impaired by 1–2 mg lorazepam. Fagan *et al.* (1987) found similar limited sensitivity to ethanol but not to drugs in their test battery including the continuous attention test. Our test battery contains the same elements, but not the same tests as those used by Häkkinen (1976) in his studies on accident proneness.

Ideal methods should adequately reveal both impairments and improvements of performance (e.g. diazepam, alcohol, amphetamine and their combinations). Interpretation of the real mode(s) of action drugs may be difficult. For instance, digit symbol substitution, much used as a cognitive test, also contains a clear motor component. Alcohol and BZDs importantly affect not only cognition but also the motor component, and that must be resolved by using other tests. Since sets of performance tests vary from laboratory to laboratory, they should be defined precisely enough to help critical readers judge the data and justification of the conclusions. Even a declarative manual of the tests would be desirable (Parrott, 1991). The International Committee on Alcohol, Drugs and Traffic Safety (ICADTS) has now taken the initiative to produce a manual where relevant aspects of drug effects on performance related to driving safety will be harmonized with epidemiological data (Ferrara and Giorgetti, 1992).

The clinical test for drunkenness (CTD) comprises a set of *motor* (walking with eyes open and closed, gait in turning, finger to finger, collecting small objects), *vestibular* (Romberg with eyes open and closed, nystagmus) and *mental* (subtraction backwards, orientation as to time) subtests. It was developed for the assessment of driving fitness of persons arrested by the police for violating alcohol and driving rules, and was used before the era of breath tests and other quick BAC assays. Tolerance to alcohol reduces the value of the CTD. Since this test is used in Finland at present, we have compared it with our regular performance tests in drug interaction studies (Kuitunen *et al.*, 1990, 1990b). The CTD proved less sensitive than performance tests in revealing impaired performance after BZDs and antidepressants, but detected the decremental effects of drug–alcohol and drug–drug combined on fitness. In a double-blind pilot study, two of the subtests of CTD (subtraction backward; finger to finger, eyes closed) revealed the combined action of diazepam 10 mg + ethanol 0.5 g/kg, which also modified coordinative and reactive skills in the machine tests (Linnoila and Mattila, 1973, unpublished).

The drug-induced *subjective* actions and interactions are an important aspect in human psychopharmacology, but they are often neglected or globally noted as 'sedation' of varying degree. For brevity that simple word is commonly used even this chapter. Some conservative authorities even consider that drug-induced sedation, as it is vaguely indicated in ordinary trials, and common sense are enough to predict drug actions and interactions on driving fitness, and no further objective tests are needed. If that opinion was followed up, the minimum requirement would be to evaluate the character of sedation by using suitable visual analogue scales (VAS) (Bond and Lader, 1974) or representative rating scales.

Subjective sedation recorded on the VAS scales or by scoring can be distinguished from objective impairment of performance as demonstrated, for example with buspirone (Seppälä *et al.*, 1982a) and with mianserin and alcohol (Strömberg and Mattila, 1987). Non-specific 'unpleasant' sedation occurring after intake of various psychotropic drugs has been attributed to their central H_1-antihistamine and anti-α_1-adrenergic properties (Linnoila *et al.*, 1986). Other types of sedation are associated with BZDs ('pleasant drowsiness') and centrally acting α_2-agonists such as clonidine or dex-medetomidine (Mattila *et al.*, 1991). Buspirone, having complex 5-hydroxy-tryptamine (serotonine (5-HT_{1A})) partial agonist and mixed dopamine agonist–antagonist properties (Eison and Temple, 1986; Yocca, 1990), exhibits clear sedation without significant impairment of performance (Seppälä *et al.*, 1982a).

Since most psychotropic drugs often exhibit more than one type of action, the sedative effects of drug combinations leave little space for mechanistic speculations. Some combinations impair the objective performance relatively more than the subjective variables on visual analogue scales (Mattila *et al.*, 1989). Drug-induced lowering of the flicker fusion threshold is commonly regarded as an objective measure of drowsiness, but this assumption does not apply to all psychotropic drugs and drug combinations, partly owing to modulation of retinal circulation.

Interactions of Ethanol with Psychotropic Drugs

Ethanol represents an anxiolytic agent with pharmacokinetics subject to alterations by various drugs and procedures (Mattila, 1990). In inebriating doses producing BACs of 0.5 mg/ml (11 mM) or more, ethanol disturbs the lipid bilayers of the neural cell membranes ('increased fluidity'), thus interfering with synaptic functions. It inhibits cell membrane ATPase, impairs the function of cholinergic muscarinic receptors, and may reduce cytoplasmic Ca^{2+} concentrations. The net effects of ethanol on the release of neuro-transmitters are difficult to interpret owing to interactions of neural pathways, synaptic feedback mechanisms, and the phase of alcohol intoxication—whether rising, falling or withdrawal—which greatly modify the finding. Ethanol may also activate the γ-aminobutyric acid (GABA)–BZD receptor complex (see Samson and Harris, 1992), thus enhancing the inward chloride flux and depolarizing the neuronal membrane. Although it remains uncertain whether that mechanism is important for the actions of ethanol in man, it nevertheless renders the ethanol–BZD interaction especially interesting. Enhanced body sway with the eyes open or closed, and the reduced angle of horizontal gaze nystagmus, are two characteristic neural effects of alcohol; this nystagmus is very sensitive to alcohol but less sensitive or insensitive to psychotropic drugs. For a review on the actions and interactions of alcohol on performance tests see Nuotto and Mattila (1990) and Hindmarch *et al.* (1991). The actions and interactions of psychotropic drugs on memory and learning are mainly omitted in the present chapter.

Ethanol and Hypnotics

The fatal hypnotic–ethanol intoxications remain beyond the scope of this chapter but deserve a comment. The combined toxicity of barbiturates and ethanol is additive only. The ethanol effect dominates that of short- and long-acting barbiturates, whilst the intermediate-acting barbiturates are unpredictably toxic by themselves (see Mattila, 1990). The development of tolerance to both agents in prolonged use reduces the lethal toxicity of combinations to behavioural toxicity, as is well known among alcoholics and barbiturate addicts.

With low to moderate doses of hypnotics taken with ethanol, increased sedation and impaired skills performance is to be expected. Chloral hydrate is reduced by erythrocytes to its active hypnotic metabolite trichloroethanol, which is a substrate and competitive inhibitor of alcohol dehydrogenase. The interaction also works in man. The combined sedative effect of ethanol and chloral hydrate is anecdotally strong ('knock-out drops'), assumed to result from both pharmacodynamic and simple pharmacokinetic interaction. The case is kinetically more complex, and Sellers *et al.* (1972) failed to document either an altered rate of ethanol elimination or a knockout effect when giving chloral hydrate 15 mg/kg together with 0.5 g/kg ethanol. Enhanced impairment of skilled performance and increased BAC levels were recorded.

Interactions of hypnotics and ethanol in the absorption phase often lead to unpredictable plasma concentrations of drugs (Curry, 1977) resulting from modulated pyloric opening rates, the presence of food, and the characteristics (solubility, first-pass metabolism) of the hypnotic concerned. Life-threatening major changes sometimes occur when treating ethanol withdrawal symptoms with oral chlormethiazole in therapeutic doses. The bioavailability of this drug is normally low (8–10%) but much improved in the presence of cirrhotic liver damage and ethanol in combination (Neuvonen *et al.*, 1981). Although moderate doses of ethanol increase the bioavailability of chlormethiazole in healthy subjects much less, that mechanism may modify and enhance the central pharmacodynamic interaction in performance studies. Chlormethiazole much resembles the ultra-short-acting BZD hypnotics (triazolam, midazolam); it could replace them in many cases, and new interest in chlormethiazole has recently been shown (Fagan *et al.*, 1990). In the presence of alcohol, this drug is to be used with great care in reduced oral doses. With parenteral dosing the drug avoids first-pass metabolism and is therefore safer. Diazepam does not share the kinetic drawback of chlormethiazole and its use is preferable at ethanol withdrawal.

Ethanol and Benzodiazepines

The acute toxicity of conventional 1,4-BZDs is low, but intravenous midazolam, an ultra-short-acting imidazole-BZD, depresses respiration more than thiopentone does (Keats, 1985). In chronic abusers of ethanol and drugs, high BACs (3–3.5 mg/ml) in combination with high plasma diazepam levels (2.5–3.5 µg/ml) produced behavioural toxicity but were less toxic than expected (Schmidt and

Bösche, 1981), obviously owing to the development of a high degree of tolerance. The therapeutic doses of various BZDs mostly but not always are decremental to skilled performance (Linnoila, 1983), and more so in combination with ethanol (Linnoila and Mattila, 1973; Sellers *et al.*, 1980), thus risking traffic and occupational safety. These aspects have been reviewed by our group (Seppälä *et al.*, 1979; Mattila, 1984) and by others (e.g. Sellers and Busto, 1982; Ciraulo and Barnhill, 1986); see also O'Hanlon and de Gier (1986).

Conventional 1,4-BZDs (diazepam, lorazepam, etc.) differ from 3,4-BZDs (tofisopam) and perhaps from 1,5-BZDs (clobazam) both in potency and in efficacy. Short-acting triazole and imidazole derivatives of 1,4-BZDs (triazolam, midazolam) are rapidly metabolized, and the concomitant use of fair amounts of ethanol might enhance and prolong their effects. The pharmacokinetic interaction of triazolam and ethanol is, however, not important (Dorian *et al.*, 1985; Kuitunen *et al.*, 1990), and the late cognitive impairments reported to have occurred after taking these BZDs with ethanol (Subhan and Hindmarch, 1983) may be pharmacodynamic in nature. The concept of Ω-receptor agonists (Langer and Arbilla, 1988) refers to drugs (zolpidem, alpidem, zopiclone, suriclone, β-carbolines, etc.) which act on the GABA$_A$–BZD receptor complex though deviating structurally from BZDs. This new concept has recently been realized by separation and cloning of 15 different GABA$_A$ receptor subunits, much by Seeburg's group (see Burt and Kamatchi, 1991). These subunits can, in turn, combine with each other, theoretically producing about 500 different heterogeneous receptors.

Some Ω-agonists may differ in their receptor kinetics and effects from the standard BZDs (different GABA$_A$ receptor subtypes?), and their interactions with ethanol thus could be quantitatively and perhaps qualitatively different. Such a variation could in principle explain, for example, the odd inverse interaction of ethanol and the triazolo-1,4-BZD loprazolam (McManus *et al.*, 1983). However, Linnoila *et al.* (1990a) reported that adinazolam, a triazolo-1,4-BZD with anxiolytic and antidepressant actions, dose-dependently (15 and 30 mg) impaired several variables of performance and showed additive effect with ethanol 0.8 g/kg. Diazepam 10 mg impaired performance subjectively more than objectively and acted additively with ethanol. Linnoila's group reported similar results when comparing alprazolam, another triazolo-1,4-BZD, in doses of 0.5 and 2 mg with 10 mg diazepam, each alone and in combination with ethanol (Linnoila *et al.*, 1990b). It seems that alcohol interactions with individual BZDs are rather similar. If differences between them exist, the use of several 'equipotent' doses for each BZD is needed to document them.

Although the combined actions of BZDs and alcohol are often believed to being potentiative, such a supra-additive effect has been documented only occasionally, if ever. Linnoila and Mattila (1973) found a clear potentiation when comparing diazepam (5 and 10 mg) and ethanol (0.5 and 0.8 g/kg) alone and in several combinations against placebo in untrained young subjects, who even improved their performance in response to small doses of diazepam. These results might represent a combined effect at the lower end of the dose–response graph, where an additive effect looks as though it were a potentiation. The lack of true potentiation does not argue against the view that a part of the ethanol action takes place via the $GABA_A$–BZD receptor complex, because two agents acting on the same receptor seldom potentiate each other. In cross-over experiments with low oral single doses of alcohol (0.5 g/kg) and diazepam (5–10 mg) at weekly intervals, an adaptation to diazepam actions minimized or cancelled the additive action of these agents on skilled performance (Palva *et al.*, 1979).

In general, pharmacodynamic combined actions outweigh ethanol-induced altered kinetics of diazepam. One study from our laboratory demonstrated that impaired performance measured after diazepam–ethanol combinations correlated with BACs better than with plasma diazepam levels (Laisi *et al.*, 1979). Raised plasma diazepam concentrations after a concomitant ethanol intake result from the inhibition of diazepam metabolism. This does not lead to major dynamic consequences because the formation of nordiazepam is retarded by ethanol. This was demonstrated by Sellers *et al.* who injected diazepam intravenously and gave ethanol orally several times to maintain BACs at about 0.8–1 mg/ml (Sellers *et al.*, 1980). In this study, clear additive impairment of performance by diazepam and ethanol was measured. The same group has suggested (1978, 1980) that a proper analysis of the ethanol–diazepam interaction requires the parallel assay of plasma diazepam and its free fraction since diazepam is bound to plasma proteins. Acute ingestion of ethanol elevates the levels of plasma triglycerides, which in turn can modify protein binding and the actions of diazepam. But the clinical relevance of this postulated mechanism is uncertain and the whole procedure rather complex to be carried out in standard interaction studies.

The time course of the combined actions of ethanol and BZDs has been inadequately analysed but could be important. The clearest effect might be seen when ethanol is given before diazepam so that their concentrations in the blood are rising at the same time (Laisi *et al.*, 1979; Sellers *et al.*, 1980). If moderate doses (10–20 mg) of diazepam are given well before ethanol (0.8–1 g/kg) the rapid peak concentration of plasma diazepam may not coincide with rising BACs and inebriation, and the combined effect could be less than expected. However, when giving diazepam or lorazepam orally well before ethanol, they still produced with alcohol an enhanced impairment of skills over many hours (Aranko *et al.*, 1985b). Although treatment intervals (1 month versus 1 week) and subjects were different in the studies of Laisi *et al.* (1979) and Aranko *et al.* (1985b) and might have contributed to the diazepam–alcohol interaction, the timing of the intake of these agents might not be decisive.

Palva and co-workers (1982) found that after oral single doses of diazepam young students and middle-aged policemen and army officials (42–58 years) responded similarly to oral 10 mg diazepam given alone and in combination with 0.5 g/kg ethanol. The overall poorer performance of the older subjects after diazepam or diazepam + ethanol was related to their poorer baseline performance in spite of extensive training, rather than to their actual responses to diazepam which produced similar drug concentrations in the plasma of old and young subjects. The age aspects have been discussed above.

Ethanol, Antidepressants and Antipsychotics

Scandinavian regulations state that antidepressants and neuroleptics are *possibly* dangerous when driving, whereas hypnotics, BZDs and opioids are *designated* as dangerous. The combined effects of antidepressants and alcohol have been rather extensively investigated; for details and references see the articles reviewing the psychomotor effects of antidepressants in general (Seppälä and Linnoila, 1983) and of the selective inhibitors of 5-HT reuptake (Strömberg, 1988).

Amitriptyline represents sedative tricyclic antidepressants (TCAs), which inhibit the reuptake of both noradrenaline and 5-HT. It also has clear-cut antimuscarine, H_1-antihistamine and local anaesthetic actions. An oral single dose of 50 mg amitriptyline impairs skilled performance and learning acquisition, the latter obviously resulting from the antimuscarinic action of amitriptyline, and it additively augments ethanol effects. This interaction may have a pharmacokinetic component because ethanol retards the metabolism of amitriptyline (Dorian et al., 1983). Concerning other TCAs, imipramine and chlorimipramine might impair performance to a similar extent or less than amitriptyline does. In a recent study controlled with placebo (Strömberg et al., 1991), simple psychomotor tests were administered to healthy subjects after their 2 weeks maintenance (50 mg b.d.) with imipramine or amitriptyline. Either drug alone failed to impair choice reaction times or digit symbol substitution, as compared with respective records during the placebo period, but both active drugs clearly enhanced the decrement caused by ethanol (1 g/kg) on digit substitution. It is presumable, but not exactly known, that those actions and interactions are stronger in the patients treated with larger doses of TCAs.

Among atypical antidepressants mianserin has a wide profile of actions (antihistamine, anti-adrenergic, antiserotonin, weak inhibitor of the reuptake), it is sedative and adds to the effects of ethanol (Seppälä and Linnoila, 1983). The same applies (Hindmarch and Subhan, 1986) to trazodone, which is a mixed amine reuptake inhibitor and produces a direct 5-HT agonist metabolite. Contrary to mianserin, trazodone and maprotiline (Strömberg et al., 1988), the 'dopaminergic' drugs nomifensine and bupropion are stimulant and they may, indeed, even counteract the effects of ethanol (Parrott *et al.*, 1982; Peck and Hamilton, 1983). We have failed to antagonize alcohol effects significantly with two dopaminergic agents: bromocryptine or amantadine (Nuotto and Mattila, 1982).

Selective inhibitors of the reuptake of 5-HT neither impair performance nor add to the effects of ethanol (Strömberg, 1988; Allen and Lader, 1989). They can occasionally counteract the cognitive decrement recorded after ethanol, but that anti-alcohol effect remains debatable. The novel inhibitor of monoamine oxidase (MAO), which inhibits selectively and competitively the activity of (MAO_A) isoenzyme, has impaired the psychomotor performance of patients treated with moclobemide for 4 weeks. The parallel group treated with maprotiline (a sedative tetracyclic antidepressant inhibiting predominantly noradrenaline uptake) produced roughly similar impairment (Classen and Laux, 1989). Another parallel group maintenance study, carried out in healthy subjects without proper placebo control, showed that moclobemide (200 mg t.i.d.) + ethanol (peak BAC 0.6 mg/ml) impaired performance less than clomipramine (25 mg b.i.d.) + alcohol (Berlin *et al.*, 1990).

Studies on the effects of antipsychotic drugs (neuroleptics) on human skilled performance are rare. Outpatients who are on long-term maintenance with low doses of neuroleptics should be studied because many of them may drive, and schizophrenia as a whole carries an accident risk (Silverstone, 1988). Grüber-Mathyl (1986) compared the cognitive performance of age-matched groups of healthy controls and patients who were on maintenance with neuroleptic monotherapy. As expected, the healthy subjects' performance was better than that of the patients subjected to continuous stress and time pressure. The patients were mindful of errors and that partly compensated for their poorer cognition. The test data did not correlate with the doctor's evaluation of their driving fitness (Grüber-Mathyl, 1986).

Neuroleptics are often combined with ethanol during the weekend breaks taken by long-term psychiatric patients. The combined toxicity is hard to estimate, but moderate to strong inebriation with BACs of 1–1.5 mg/ml in the presence of moderate antipsychotic maintenance treatment has often occurred without major hazards. Chlorpromazine inhibits alcohol hydrogenase activity *in vitro* and *in vivo*, and its administration with ethanol results in a combined sedative effect. These effects are probably non-specific since chlorpromazine prolongs the half-lives of some other drugs as well, and since it has strong H_1-antihistamine and anti-adrenergic actions.

We have measured skilled performance of healthy subjects after single doses of 100 mg remoxipride and 0.8 g/kg ethanol (Mattila *et al.*, 1988a). This benzamide blocks predominantly dopamine D_2-receptors, with minor effects on the poorly defined σ-receptors. It produced drowsiness, clumsiness and mental slowness, and impaired digit substitution without important decrements in simulated driving. Its combination with ethanol proved detrimental to objective and subjective performance, the impairment lasting for several hours. Ethanol alone produced clumsiness and mental slowness but objective impairment at 90 minutes only. There was no pharmacokinetic interaction, nor did ethanol alter the increase of plasma prolactin induced by remoxipride.

Various Psychotropic Drugs and Alcohol

Cannabis is a non-medicinal psychotropic drug, and its non-addictive derivatives (nabilone, levonantradol) have been used as anti-emetics in cancer chemotherapy. On the road, the use of cannabis is associated with one-vehicle accidents, while alcohol is associated more with multi-vehicle accidents, being dangerous in heavy traffic and at road crossings in particular. Accordingly, both of these agents impair reactive and cognitive processes in performance tests, but cannabis mainly impairs vigilance while ethanol is more detrimental to peripheral divided attention (Moscowitz, 1984). The cannabis-induced decrement in attention at peripheral signals might be less in chronic cannabis users than in non-users, thus indicating a test-selective development of tolerance to cannabis-induced impairment (Marks and McAvoy, 1989). It is possible that the counter-clockwise hysteresis curve (sensitization during the session) characteristic of cannabis action plays some role in its interactions with ethanol which may be potentiative and multidimensional, as shown by Attwood *et al.* (1981) when reporting the results of their airfield driving experiments. For further details and references see also Starmer and Bird (1984) and Perez-Reyers *et al.* (1988).

Sedative H_1-antihistamines, such as diphenhydramine and hydroxyzine, have previously been used and again recommended for the treatment of neurotic disorders. The central decremental effect of chlorpheniramine is attributable to its (+)-D-isomer (Nicholson et al., 1991) whereas central depressant effects of hydroxyzine could be linked with serotonergic pathways (Levander *et al.*, 1984). Centrally active antihistamines impair performance and may add to alcohol effects on performance (Seppälä *et al.*, 1979), while modern non-sedative antihistamines in regular doses do not. (Moser *et al.* (1978) showed that terfenadine did not add to alcohol or diazepam effects on performance.

As to *opioids*, ethical aspects restrict studies on opioid–alcohol interactions in healthy subjects, and acquired tolerance is a confounding factor that restricts the conclusions. There is no doubt that opioids such as methadone and pethidine given in robust doses to drug-naive subjects impair performance. Moscowitz and co-workers have maintained ex-addicts on methadone for several months and found that even high doses (60–80 mg) of methadone failed to impair performance in a representative set of tests, including divided attention. However, a slowing of information processing was evident. Alcohol interaction studies with opioids are rare. Codeine 50 mg given to drug-naive healthy conscripts increased the number of collisions in simulated driving; in combination with 0.5 g/kg ethanol an additive increase in collisions was found, associated with a subjective impairment (Linnoila and Häkkinen, 1973). Also 25 mg codeine showed a weak additive effect with ethanol. For discussion on analgesics see Starmer (1986).

'*Anti-alcohol drugs*' is a much used but poorly defined title since it covers both the alcohol motivation and ways of reducing the effects of alcohol intoxication. Several research groups (see Linnoila and Mattila, 1981) have tried to counteract ethanol effects on psychomotor performance but with meagre success. The candidates tested for antagonizing ethanol comprise noradrenergic and dopaminergic agents—amphetamine included—methylxanthines, doxapram, pyritinol, thyreoliberin, ACTH analogues, BZD inverse agonists and naloxone, which all seem to antagonize ethanol in rodents but not in man.

Drug–Drug Interactions of Psychotropic Drugs

Rational psychotropic drug therapy favours monotherapy whenever possible, but moderate polypharmacy often proves mandatory, mainly resulting from the coexistence of somatic disorders, diagnostic problems and the treatment of 'target symptoms' with additional drugs. Non-specific control of anxiety in depressive and psychotic disorders is rather common, and the use of BZDs with other sedative and non-sedative drugs can be regarded as an everyday event (Ochs *et al.*, 1987). Scientific aspects on the important psychotropic drug–drug interactions, together with the requirements of the regulatory bodies, have activated the measurement and analysis of such interactions on skilled performance. However, the literature on drug–alcohol interactions outweighs that on drug–drug interactions.

Depressant Drug–Drug Combinations

In the laboratory, the serotoninergic *anxiolytic* buspirone (15 mg) proved inactive objectively but matched diazepam (0.3 mg/kg) subjectively; a dose-related objective impairment was seen with diazepam (0.15 and 0.3 mg/kg) in healthy subjects. In combinations, buspirone prolonged the diazepam-induced sedation, and objectively added to the diazepam effects in Maddox wing and letter cancellation tests. It was inert on coordinative and reactive skills and tended to antagonize diazepam effects on attention (Mattila *et al.*, 1986a). In terms of the visual analogue scales, buspirone perhaps counteracted diazepam when shifting the assessment scores towards antagonistic. Respective clinical interactions have not been analysed.

An H_1-antihistamine, diphenhydramine, sometimes used as a sedative in neurotic disorders, did not add to the subjective or objective decrements caused by diazepam (0.3 mg/kg) given to healthy subjects during their maintenance with diphenhydramine (50 mg b.d.) or placebo (Mattila *et al.*, 1986b). Tolerance to diphenhydramine, in terms of its effects related to plasma concentrations, was acquired during maintenance. The first dose of diphenhydramine (100 mg) produced drowsiness, reduced the number of digits substituted and lowered flicker fusion threshold without impairments in tracking or choice reactions. Diphenhydramine opposed diazepam in the Maddox wing test (extraocular muscle balance)—a variable which is very sensitive to diazepam.

As to the *neuroleptics*, diazepam (15 mg) in combination with remoxipride produced a prolonged subjective and objective impairment in performance tests, learning acquisition excluded. The combination outweighed the respective effects of either drug alone and was considered to be additive rather than potentiative (Mattila *et al.*, 1988a). Pharmacokinetic interactions were not seen. Interestingly, diazepam + remoxipride increased body sway only with the eyes closed, while ethanol + remoxipride produced considerable sway irrespective of the eyes being open or closed. This suggests that diazepam affects compensatory visual pathways at the cortical or, perhaps, retinal level.

In another study (Mattila *et al.*, 1988c) small anxiolytic doses (1 and 2 mg) of racemic flupentixol proved more or less in objective performance tests, 15 mg diazepam impaired performance less than 2.5 mg, and the combination of diazepam + 1 mg flupentixol did not differ from diazepam alone. In a patient study, Aranko *et al.* (1985a) did not find attenuated responses in performance tests to the test dose of 3 mg lorazepam given to patients who were on maintenance with neuroleptics or antidepressants, while marked attenuation was seen in patients who regularly received moderate or robust doses of BZDs.

As to the *sedative antidepressants*, single doses of 15 mg diazepam combined with 50 mg amitriptyline or 15 mg Org 3770, an analogue of mianserin, produced definite and long-lasting decrements in reactive, coordinative and cognitive performance (Mattila *et al.*, 1989). Diazepam produced moderate subjective and mild objective impairment, while Org 3770 (inert on simulated driving) and amitriptyline proved detrimental subjectively and objectively, not necessarily in the same tests. The combined effects were additive (including learning acquisition) or supra-additive (simulated driving, digit substitutes) but subjectively less than additive. No important pharmacokinetic alterations were seen. The CTD showed impairment with the drug combinations but not with any drug alone. Patat *et al.* (1988) reported additive or supra-additive impairments of performance by the combination amitriptyline 75 mg + diazepam 10 mg. For further references see Patat *et al.* (1988).

Antidepressants and neuroleptics are increasingly administered to support the effects of *opioids* in the relief of severe or chronic pain. Our group has carried out a series of placebo-controlled cross-over human studies to find out possible significant interactions in this field; for details see Saarialho-Kere (1988). Performance was measured subjectively and objectively, and respiratory depression was used as a reference to check that opioids (buprenorphine, codeine, dextropropoxyphene, pentazocine, nalbuphine) were really acting.

Briefly, orally administered codeine (100 mg) and pentazocine (75 + 75 mg) failed to affect objective performance, but subjectively they reversed the sedation induced by diazepam (0.25 mg/kg). Buprenorphine (0.4 mg sublingually) and pentazocine (30–40 mg intramuscularly) impaired sensory processes but left motor skills intact. Subacute amitriptyline did not enhance the effects of opioids on performance but enhanced opioid-induced respiratory depression. Nalbuphine (0.15 mg/kg intramuscularly) transiently impaired coordination, whereas cognitive dysfunction and cortical depression persisted longer. Haloperidol did not enhance the ventilatory actions of nalbuphine. In rheumatoid patients, oral dextropropoxyphene (130 mg) impaired vigilance and had additive psychomotor effects with amitriptyline (25 mg). Plasma μ-opioid concentrations measured with the radioreceptor assay were considerable for nalbuphine but lower for other opioids used. In summary, amitriptyline and haloperidol in the doses commonly used as adjuvants for pain relief did not importantly enhance the effects of opioids on skilled performance even in drug-naive healthy subjects.

Traditional *anticonvulsants* phenytoin and carbamazepine suppress repetitive discharges, thus counteracting the generalization of focal bursts to the cerebral cortex, and they may impair motor performance (Trimble, 1987). As carbamazepine and BZDs support each other in controlling seizures, the same could apply to skilled performance as well. An additive combined impairment by oral single doses of 7.5 mg zopiclone and 600 mg carbamazepine has been found (Kuitunen *et al.*, 1990) in several performance tests. Different time courses and certain test selectivity of the individual drugs complicated the issue. Also the CTD gave positive results with drug combinations but not with either drug alone. Tolerance and cross-tolerance to different BZDs has been a problem in the treatment of epilepsy and tolerance develops to impaired psychomotor performance as well. Our group has recently evaluated the responses (digit substitution, flicker fusion, saccadic eye movements) to oral diazepam (0.25 mg/kg) in epileptic patients on maintenance with carbamazepine or sodium valproate. Occasional extra maintenance with clonazepam did not attenuate diazepam responses, thus resembling nitrazepam, which has not produced measurable tolerance to lorazepam in our studies. Valproate-treated patients showed perhaps enhanced responses to diazepam (K. Aranko, unpublished data).

Antagonistic Interactions

It is well known that *flumazenil,* a specific BZD receptor antagonist, cancels the effects including impaired skilled performance caused by BZD agonists (see Brodgen *et al.*, 1988), and it even ameliorates hepatic encephalopathy considered to result from the effects of endogenous BZD receptor ligands. Flumazenil might not equally antagonize the effects of all BZDs and Ω-agonists in all of their different effects (motor skills versus memory), and the issue still awaits further studies.

A non-sedative antidepressant, *nomifensine*, an inhibitor of dopamine re-uptake, has proved inactive on psychomotor and cognitive functions and on psychological parameters, while the 1,5-BZD clobazam proved sedative. The combination of these two drugs did not modify objective performance but improved self-rated anxiety (Parrott *et al.*, 1982). *Bupropion*, another 'dopaminergic' antidepressant (Peck and Hamilton, 1983), has proved inert on skilled performance, while (+)-amphetamine improved and amitriptyline impaired them after single doses to healthy volunteers. Diazepam (2.5–5 mg) produced drowsiness and impaired auditory vigilance, which were antagonized by 100 mg bupropion given concomitantly.

The interactions of *methylxanthines* and centrally acting *sympathomimetics* with BZDs have been discussed earlier (Mattila, 1984). Briefly, caffeine and theophylline have antagonized BZD effects on performance in most but not all the tests administered. The doses, order and time lapses when administering the interacting drugs may modify the net results. In our laboratory, caffeine prevented diazepam-induced drowsiness and impaired digit substitution in a study where drugs were given together to parallel groups of untrained subjects, who much improved their performance during the placebo session (Mattila and Nuotto, 1983). A robust dose of caffeine (10 mg/kg) did not prevent diazepam (0.3 mg/kg) effects on these variables when given 1 hour before diazepam to trained subjects in a randomized cross-over study (Mattila *et al.*, 1988d). An α_2-antagonist, yohimbine (0.8 mg/kg), also failed to antagonize diazepam.

Caffeine has been reported to bind to brain adenosine receptors at low concentrations; at high concentrations beyond normal coffee consumption it could bind to BZD receptors, reversing the effects of BZDs (Marangos *et al.*, 1979). Enprophylline, a phosphodiesterase antagonist without adenosine blocking action, does not antagonize diazepam effects, thus suggesting that caffeine acts via the adenosine receptors (Niemand *et al.*, 1984). Oddly enough, zopiclone 7.5 mg has counteracted 300 mg caffeine better than caffeine antagonized zopiclone (Mattila *et al.*, 1992). These results were obtained from parallel groups of untrained subjects; the ranked changes from the baseline were analysed with parametric tests, and caffeine alone clearly improved several variables. The zopiclone–ethanol combination has failed to produce an additive impairment in various psychomotor tests (Seppälä *et al.*, 1982b; Kuitunen *et al.*, 1990b). Although the present and presumably new Ω-agonists can differ from traditional BZDs (see Burt and Kamatchi, 1991), which could lead to different drug–drug interactions, all those results should be documented in rigorous cross-over studies, with at least two dose levels.

Pharmacokinetic Interactions

Many researchers interested in pharmacokinetics have tried to rationalize the altered central effects of psychotropic drugs as resulting from pharmaco-kinetic alterations produced by other concomitant drugs which are known to modify the kinetics of BZDs (Abernethy *et al.*, 1984). However, unequivocal proof has been reached only exceptionally. The clearest proof of an important pharmacokinetic mechanism is the erythromycin-induced inhibition of mid-azolam metabolism mediated via cytochrome P450 IIIA. One week treatment with erythromycin doubled the plasma concentrations of midazolam and po-tentiated midazolam (15 mg) effects on digit symbol substitution and saccadic eye movements (Aranko *et al.*, 1991). A comparable interaction of trolean-domycin and triazolam (Warot *et al.*, 1987) is also convincing. A minor yet statistically significant enhancement of triazolam responses by erythromycin (750 mg) given 1 hour before midazolam has been shown in our laboratory (Vanakoski and Mattila, unpublished). Concerning diazepam, inhibition or induction of its metabolism, thus resulting in important alterations in its phar-macodynamics, remains speculative thus far because diazepam has an almost equally active metabolite (nordiazepam) and because records of performance have often been inadequate. Induced glucuronide conjugation of diazepam and nordiazepam after their induced hydroxylation might reduce their com-bined effect if measured adequately.

Summary

Psychotropic drugs are commonly used with ethyl alcohol or/and with other drugs, thus resulting in numerous interactions. Their consequences vary from lethal toxicity to behavioural impairment, depending on the effects of the drugs concerned, the doses of drugs and alcohol given and their route of administra-tion. Pharmacokinetic interactions refer to altered tissue concentrations of alco-hol or drugs or both, indirectly evaluated by measuring their concentrations in the plasma. Pharmacodynamic interactions refer to the combined actions which primarily take place at the tissue (receptor?) level, without or with an important pharmacokinetic component of interaction. Human psychomotor performance and its impairment by psychotropic drugs and their combinations have impor-tant implications for driving fitness and capability in occupational tasks. Ethics and methodological problems restrict the full analysis of drug–alcohol and drug–drug interactions of psychotropic drugs in man.

Considerable intersubject and intrasubject variation in responses to single drugs and their combinations in performance tests result from several factors, such as the drugs concerned (pharmacokinetics and pharmacodynamics), per-formance tests (reliability; sensitivity), the trial design (placebo and random-ization; single doses versus maintenance; parallel groups versus cross-over study; environment; statistics) and the individual characteristics of the test subjects (age and disease; the amount of practice; personality and 'accident proneness'). All these factors should be optimally balanced in the study design to allow drawing relevant conclusions from the reliable results. Pertinent implications of the results to real life still necessitate a moderate to good validity of the tests used. Although this kind of ideal investigation is uncommon, even less glorious studies may give valuable information provided that they are honest and adequately controlled. The number of healthy volunteers should not be doubled or tripled too easily to meet with the rules of statistics if the required statements are too accurate and mainly for promotional needs.

Alcohol increases, mainly in the additive manner, the psychomotor and cognitive effects of hypnotics, benzodiazepines and sedative antidepressants, and probably of neuroleptics, though there are few reports of them. Although alcohol retards the metabolism of several psychotropic drugs and modifies the protein binding of some drugs, their combined effect may occur at the receptor level in most cases. Newer benzodiazepines and Ω-agonists may differ from old benzodiazepines in their interactions, partly for pharmacokinetic reasons. There are no definite alcohol antagonists for human use.

The combined effects of sedative psychotropic drugs on performance are little investigated, although the symptomatic use of benzodiazepines in combination with other drugs is common. Diazepam increases the decremental effects on performance of anti-epileptics (?), neuroleptics and sedative antidepressants, while stimulating antidepressants (nomifensine, bupropion, etc.) can counteract benzodiazepine effects as methylxanthines and amphetamines do. Novel serotoninergic antidepressants (fluoxetine, etc.) and anxiolytics (buspirone, etc.) are interesting in the sense that they do not add to the decremental effects of alcohol on performance, yet buspirone is subjectively sedative. It does not add much to the diazepam-induced impairment of performance.

References

Abernethy, D.R., Greenblatt, D.J., Ochs, H.R., and Shader, R.I. (1984). Benzodiazepine drug–drug interactions commonly occurring in clinical practice. *Curr. Med. Res. Opin.*, **8** (Suppl. 4), 80–93.

Allen, D., and Lader, M. (1989). Interactions of alcohol with amitriptyline, fluoxetine and placebo in normal subjects. *Int. Clin. Psychopharmacol.*, **4** (Suppl. 1), 7–14.

Aranko, K., Mattila, M.J., and Seppälä, T. (1983). Development of tolerance and cross-tolerance to the psychomotor actions of lorazepam in man. *Br. J. Clin. Pharmacol.*, **15**, 545–52.

Aranko, K., Mattila, M.J., Nuutinen, A., and Pellinen, J. (1985a). Benzodiazepines, but not antidepressants or neuroleptics, induce dose-dependent development of tolerance in psychiatric patients. *Acta Psychiatr. Scand.*, **72**, 434–46.

Aranko, K., Seppälä, T., Pellinen, J., and Mattila, M.J. (1985b). Interaction of diazepam or lorazepam with alcohol: Psychomotor effects and bioassayed serum levels after single and repeated doses. *Eur. J. Clin. Pharmacol.*, **28**, 559–65.

Aranko, K., Olkkola, K.T., Hiller, A., and Saarnivaara, L. (1991). Clinically important interaction between erythromycin and midazolam. *Br. J. Clin. Pharmacol.*, **33**, 217P–218P.

Attwood, D.A., Williams, R.D., McBurney, L.J., and Frecker, R.C. (1981). Cannabis, alcohol and driving: Effects on selected closed-course task. In: Goldberg, L. (ed.), *Alcohol, Drugs and Traffic Safety,* Vol. III—T80, Stockholm, Almqvist & Wicksell, pp. 938–53.

Berlin, I., Cournot, A., Zimmer, R., Pedarriosse, A.M, Manfredi, R., Molinier, P., and Puech, A.J. (1990). Evaluation and comparison of the interaction between alcohol and moclobemide or clomipramine in health subjects. *Psychopharmacology,* **100**, 40–45.

Bond, A., and Lader, M. (1974). The use of analogue scales in rating subjective feelings. *Br. J. Med. Psychol.,* **47**, 211–18.

Borland, R.G., and Nicholson, A.N. (1984). Visual motor co-ordination and dynamic visual activity. *Br. J. Clin. Pharmacol.,* **18**, 69S–72S.

Broadbent, D.E. (1984). Performance and its measurement. *Br. J. Clin. Pharmacol.,* **18**, 5S–9S.

Brogden, R.N., and Goa, K.L. (1988). Flumazenil: A preliminary review of its benzodiazepine antagonist properties, intrinsic activity and therapeutic use. *Drugs,* **35**, 448–67.

Bührer, M., Maitre, P.O., Crevoisier, C., and Stanski, D.R. (1990). Electroencephalographic effects of benzodiazepines. II. Pharmacodynamic modeling of the electroencephalographic effects of midazolam and diazepam. *Clin. Pharmacol. Ther.,* **48**, 555–67.

Burt, D.R., and Kamatchi, G.L. (1991). $GABA_A$ receptor subtypes: From pharmacology to molecular biology. *FASEB J.,* **5**, 2916–23.

Castleden, C.M., and George, C.F. (1979). Increased sensitivity to benzodiazepines in the elderly. In: Crooks, J., and Stevenson, I.H. (eds), *Drugs and the Elderly: Perspectives in Geriatric Clinical Pharmacology,* London: Macmillan, pp. 169–78.

Ciraulo, D.A., and Barnhill, J. (1986). Pharmacokinetic mechanisms of ethanol–psychotropic drug interactions. *Nat. Inst. Drug. Abuse Res. Monogr.,* **68**, 73–8.

Classen, W., and Laux, G. (1990). Psychometric alterations in treatment with the MAO-A-inhibitor moclobemide. *J. Neural Transm.,* **32** (Suppl.), 185–188.

Cohen, A.F., Posner, J., Ashby, L., Smith, R., and Peck, A.W. (1984). A comparison of methods assessing the sedative effects of diphenhydramine on skills related to car driving. *Eur. J. Clin. Pharmacol.,* **27**, 477–82.

Curry, S.H. (1977). Homergic interactions, isobols and drug concentrations in blood. In: Grahame-Smith, D.G. (ed.), *Drug Interactions,* Macmillan: London, pp. 87–99.

Dingemanse, J., Danhof, M., and Breimer, D.D. (1988). Pharmacokinetic–pharmacodynamic modeling of CNS drug effects: An overview. *Pharmacol. Ther.,* **38**, 1–58.

Dorian, P., Sellers, E.M., Reed, K.L., Warsh, J.J., Hamilton, C., Kaplan, H.L., and Fan, T. (1983). Amitriptyline and ethanol: Pharmacokinetic and pharmacodynamic interaction. *Eur. J. Clin. Pharmacol.,* **25**, 325–31.

Dorian, P., Sellers, E.M., Kaplan, H.L., Hamilton, C., Greenblatt, D.J., and Abernethy, D. (1985). Triazolam and ethanol interaction: Kinetic and dynamic consequences. *Clin. Pharmacol. Ther.,* **37**, 558–62.

Eison, A.S., and Temple, J.L., Jr (1986). Buspirone: A review of its pharmacology and current perspectives on its mechanism of action. *Am. J. Med.,* **80** (Suppl. 3b), 1–9.

Ellinwood, E.H., Jr, and Nikaido, A.M. (1987). Perceptual–neuromotor pharmacodynamics of psychotropic drugs. In: Melzer, H.Y. (ed.), *Psychopharmacology: The Third Generation of Progress,* New York: Raven Press, pp. 1457–66.

Fagan, D., Tiplady, B., and Scott, B.D. (1987). Effects of ethanol on psychomotor performance. *Br. J. Anaesth.,* **59**, 961–5.

Fagan, D., Lamont, M., Jostell, K.-G., Tiplady, B., and Scott, D.B. (1990). A study of the psychometric effects of chlormethiazole in healthy young and elderly subjects. *Age Ageing,* **19**, 395–402.

Ferrara, S.D., and Giorgetti, R. (eds.) (1992). Methodology in man–machine interaction and epidemiology on drugs and traffic safety. Experiences and guidelines from an international Workshop, Padova: Addiction Research Foundation of Italy (ARFI).

File, S., and Lister, R. (1983). Does tolerance to lorazepam develop with once weekly dosing? *Br. J. Clin. Pharmacol.*, **16**, 645–50.

Greenblatt, D.J., Ehrenberg, B.L., Gunderman, J., Lockniskar, A., Savone, J.M., Harmatz, J.S., and Shader, R.I. (1989). Pharmacokinetic and electroencephalographic study of intravenous diazepam, midazolam and placebo. *Clin. Pharmacol. Ther.*, **45**, 356–65.

Grübel-Mathyl, U. (1986). Effects of neuroleptics on aspects relevant to driving fitness (preliminary evaluation). In O'Hanlon, J.F., and deGier, J.J. (eds.), *Drugs and Driving*, London: Taylor and Francis, pp. 241–247.

Häkkinen, S. (1976). Traffic accidents and psychomotor test performance: A follow-up study. *Mod. Probl. Pharmacopsychiatry*, **11**, 51–6.

Haynes, W.G., and Webb, D.J. (1991). Ethics of volunteer research: The role of new EC guidelines. *Br. J. Clin. Pharmcol.*, **32**, 671–6.

Hindmarch, I. (1980). Psychomotor function and psychoactive drugs. *Br. J. Clin. Pharmacol.*, **10**, 189–209.

Hindmarch, I., and Gudgeon, A.C. (1982). Loprazolam (HR 158) and flurazepam with ethanol compared or tests of psychomotor ability. *Eur. J. Clin. Pharmacol.*, **23**, 509–12.

Hindmarch, I., and Subhan, Z. (1986). The effects of antidepressants taken with and without alcohol on information processing, psychomotor performance and car handling ability. In: O'Hanlon, J.F., and deGier, J.J. (eds), *Drugs and Driving*, London: Taylor & Francis, pp. 231–40.

Hindmarch, I., Kerr, J.S., and Sherwood, N. (1991). The effects of alcohol and other drugs on psychomotor performance and cognitive function. *Alcohol and Alcoholism*, **26**, 71–9.

Irving, A. (1988). A proposed investigation into drug impairment testing methodology. *Int. Clin. Psychopharmacol.*, **3** (Suppl. 1), 99–109.

Keats, A.S. (1985). The effects of drugs on respiration in man. *Ann. Rev. Pharmacol. Toxicol.*, **25**, 41–65.

Klebel, E. (1981). Problems and opportunities of experimental design in psychopharmacological research. In: Goldberg, L. (ed.), *Alcohol, Drugs and Traffic Safety*, Vol. III—T80, Stockholm: Almqvist & Wicksell, pp. 895–908.

Koelega, H.S. (1989). Benzodiazepines and vigilance performance: A review. *Psychopharmacology*, **98**, 146–56.

Kuitunen, T., Mattila, M.J., Seppälä, T., Aranko, K., and Mattila, M.E. (1990a). Actions of zopiclone and carbamazepine, alone and in combination, on human skilled performance in laboratory and clinical tests. *Br. J. Clin. Pharmacol.*, **30**, 453–461.

Kuitunen, T., Mattila, M.J., and Seppälä, T. (1990b). Actions and interactions of hypnotics on human performance: single doses of zopiclone, triazolam and alcohol. *Int. J. Psychopharmacol.*, **5** (Suppl. 2), 115–130.

Laisi, U., Linnoila, M., Seppälä, T., Himberg, J.-J., and Mattila, M.J. (1979). Pharmacokinetic and pharmacodynamic interactions of diazepam with different interactions of diazepam with different alcoholic beverages. *Eur. J. Clin. Pharmacol.*, **16**, 263–70.

Langer, Z., and Arbilla, S. (1988). Imidazopyridines as a tool for the characterization of benzodiazepine receptors: a proposal for a pharmacological classification as omega receptor subtypes. *Pharmacol. Biochem. Behav.*, **29**, 76–766.

Larkin, J.G., McKee, P.J.W., and Brodie, M.J. (1992). Rapid tolerance to acute psychomotor impairment with carbamazepine in epileptic patients. *Br. J. Clin. Pharmacol.*, **33**, 111–114.

Levander, S., Hägemark, Ö. and Ståhle, M. (1985). Peripheral antihistamine and central sedative effects of three H_1-receptor antagonists. *Eur. J. Clin. Pharmacol.,* **28**, 523–9.

Linnoila, M. (1983). Benzodiazepines and performance. In: Costa, E. (ed.), *The Benzodiazepines: From Molecular Biology to Clinical Practice*, New York: Raven Press, pp. 267–78.

Linnoila, M., and Häkkinen, S. (1974). Effects of diazepam or codeine, alone or in combination with alcohol on simulated driving. *Clin. Pharmacol. Ther.,* **15**, 368–73.

Linnoila, M., and Mattila, M.J. (1973). Drug interactions on psychomotor skills related to driving. *Eur. J. Clin. Pharmacol.,* **5**, 186–94.

Linnoila, M., and Mattila, M.J. (1981). How to antagonize ethanol-induced inebriation. *Pharmacol. Ther.,* **15**, 99–109.

Linnoila, M., Guthrie, S., and Lister, R. (1986). Mechanisms of drug-induced impairment of driving. In: O'Hanlon, J.F., and deGier, J.J. (eds), *Drugs and Driving*, London: Taylor & Francis, pp. 29–49.

Linnoila, M., Stapleton, J.M., Lister, R., Moss, H., Lane, E., Granger, A., Greenblatt, D.J., and Eckardt, M.J. (1990a). Effects of adinazolam and diazepam, alone and in combination with ethanol, on psychomotor and cognitive performance and on autonomic nervous system reactivity in healthy volunteers. *Eur. J. Clin. Pharmacol.,* **38**, 371–7.

Linnoila, M., Stapleton, J.M., Lister, R., Moss, H., Lane, E., Granger, A., and Eckardt, M.J. (1990b). Effects of single doses of alprazolam and diazepam, alone and in combination with ethanol, on psychomotor and cognitive performance and on autonomic nervous systems reactivity in healthy volunteers. *Eur. J. Clin. Pharmacol.,* **39**, 21–8.

Marangos, P., Paul, A., Goodwin, F., Syapin, P., and Skolnick, P. (1979). Purinergic inhibition of diazepam binding to rat brain. *Life Sci.,* **24**, 851–8.

Mattila, M.J. (1984). Interactions of benzodiazepines on psychomotor skills. *Br. J. Clin. Pharmacol.,* **18**, 21S–26S.

Mattila, M.J. (1990). Alcohol and drug interactions. *Ann. Med.,* **22**, 363–9.

Mattila, M.J., and Nuotto, E. (1983). Caffeine and theophylline counteract diazepam effects in man. *Med. Biol.,* **61**, 337–43.

Mattila, M., Seppälä, T., and Mattila, M.J. (1986a). Combined effects of busiprone and diazepam on objective and subjective tests of performance in healthy volunteers. *Clin. Pharmacol. Ther.,* **40**, 620–6.

Mattila, M.J., Mattila, M., and Konno, K. (1986b). Acute and subacute actions and interactions with diazepam of temelastine (SK&F 93944) and diphenhydramine on human performance. *Eur. J. Clin. Pharmacol.,* **31**, 291–8.

Mattila, M.J., Mattila, M., Konno, K., and Saarialho-Kere, U. (1988a). Actions and interactions with ethanol or diazepam of remoxipride on psychomotor skills and mood in healthy volunteers. *J. Psychopharmacol.,* **2**, 138–49.

Mattila, M.J., Mattila, M., and Saarialho-Kere, U. (1988b). Acute effects of sertraline, amitriptyline, and placebo on the psychomotor performance of healthy subjects over 50 years of age. *J. Clin. Psychiatry,* **49** (Suppl.), 52–8.

Mattila, M.J., Mattila, M., and Aranko, K. (1988c). Objective and subjective assessments of the effects of flupentixol and benzodiazepines on human psychomotor performance. *Psychopharmacology,* **95**, 323–8.

Mattila, M., Seppälä, T., and Mattila, M.J. (1988d). Anxiogenic effects of yohimbine in healthy subjects: Comparison with caffeine and antagonism by clonidine and diazepam. *Int. Clin. Psychopharmacol.,* **3**, 215–29.

Mattila, M.E., Mattila, M.J., Vrijmoed-de Vries, M.C., and Kuitunen, T. (1989). Actions and interactions of psychotropic drugs on human performance and mood:

Single doses of ORG 3770, amitriptyline, and diazepam. *Pharmacol. Toxicol.*, **65**, 81–8.

Mattila, M.J., Mattila, M.E., Olkkola, K.T., and Scheinin, H. (1991). Effect of dexmedetomidine and midazolam on human performance and mood. *Eur. J. Clin. Pharmacol.*, **41**, 217–23.

Mattila, M.E., Mattila, M.J., and Nuotto, E. (1992). Caffeine moderately antagonizes the effects of triazolam and zopiclone on the psychomotor effects of healthy subjects. *Pharmacol. Toxicol.*, **70**, 286–289.

McManus, I.C., Ankier, S.I., Norfolk, J., Phillips, M., and Priest, R.G. (1983). Effects on psychological performance of the benzodiazepine loprazolam, alone and with alcohol. *Br. J. Clin. Pharmac.*, **16**, 291–300.

Moscowitz, H. (1981). Alcohol–drug interactions. In: Goldberg, L. (ed.), *Alcohol, Drugs and Traffic Safety*, Vol. III—T80, Stockholm: Almqvist & Wicksell, pp. 881–94.

Moscowitz, H. (1984). Attention tasks as skilled performance measures of drug effect. *Br. J. Clin. Pharmacol.*, **18**, 51S–61S.

Moser, E., Hüther, K.J., Koch-Weser, J., and Lundt, P.V. (1978). Effects of terfenadine and diphenhydramine alone or in combination with diazepam or alcohol on psychomotor performance and subjective feelings. *Eur. J. Clin. Pharmacol.*, **14**, 417–23.

Neuvonen, P.J., Pentikäinen, P.J., Jostell, K.-G., and Syvälahti, E. (1981). Effect of ethanol on the pharmacokinetics of chlormethiazole in humans. *Int. J. Clin. Pharmacol. Ther. Toxicol.*, **19**, 552–560.

Nicholson, A.N. (1988). The significance of impaired performance. *Int. Clin. Psychopharmacol.*, **3** (Suppl. 1), 117–27.

Nicholson, A.N., and Ward, J. (eds) (1984). Psychotropic drugs and performance. *Br. J. Clin. Pharmacol.*, **18** (Suppl. 1), 15–139S.

Nicholson, A.N., Pascoe, P.A., Turner, C., Ganellin, C.R., Greengrass, P.M., Casy, A.F., and Mercer, A.D. (1991). Sedation and histamine H_1-receptor antagonism: Studies in man with the enantiomers of chlorpheniramine and dimethindene. *Br. J. Pharmac.*, **104**, 270–6.

Niemand, D., Martinell, S., Arvidsson, S., Svedmyr, N., and Ekström-Jodal, B. (1984). Aminophylline inhibition of diazepam sedation: Is adenosine blockade of GABA receptors the mechanism? *Lancet*, **i**, 463–4.

Nuotto, E., and Mattila, M.J. (1990). Actions and interactions of alcohol in performance tests. In: Ollat, H., and Parvez, H. (eds), *Progress in Alcohol Research, Vol. 2, Alcohol and Behaviour: Basic and Clinical Aspects*, Utrecht: VSP, pp. 117–29.

Ochs, H.R., Miller, L.G., Greenblatt, D.J., and Shader, R.I. (1987). Actual versus reported benzodiazepine usage by medical outpatients. *Eur. J. Clin. Pharmacol.*, **32**, 383–8.

O'Hanlon, J.F. (1984). Driving performance under the influence of drugs: Rationale for, and application of, a new test. *Br. J. Clin. Pharmacol.*, **18**, 121S–129S.

O'Hanlon, J.F., and deGier, J.J. (eds) (1986). *Drugs and Driving*, London: Taylor and Francis.

Palva, E.S., Linnoila, M., Saario, I., and Mattila, M.J. (1979). Acute and subacute effects of diazepam on psychomotor skills: Interaction with alcohol. *Acta Pharmacol. Toxicol.*, **45**, 257–64.

Palva, E.S., Linnoila, M., Routledge, P., and Seppälä, T. (1982). Actions and interactions of diazepam and alcohol on psychomotor skills in young and middle-aged subjects. *Acta Pharmacol. Toxicol.*, **50**, 257–64.

Parrott, A.C. (1991). Performance tests in human psychopharmacology (1): Test reliability and standardization. *Hum. Psychopharmacol.*, **6**, 1–9.

Parrott, A.C., Hindmarch, I., and Stonier, P.D. (1982). Nomifensine, clobazam and Hoe 8476: Effects on aspects of psychomotor performance and cognitive ability. *Eur. J. Clin. Pharmacol.*, **23**, 309–13.

Patat, A., Klein, M.J., Hucher, M., and Granier, J. (1988). Acute effects of amitriptyline on human performance and interactions with diazepam. *Eur. J. Clin. Pharmacol.*, **35**, 585–592.

Peck, A.W., and Hamilton, M. (1983). Psychopharmacology of bupropion in normal volunteers. *J. Clin. Psychiatry*, **44**, 202–5.

Perez-Reyes, M., Hicks, R.E., Bumberry, J., Jeffcoat, A.R., and Cook, C.E. (1988). Interaction between marijuana and ethanol: effects on psychomotor performance. *Alcoholism*, **12**, 268–276.

Pieters, M.S.M., Jennekens-Schinkel, A., Schoemaker, H.C., and Cohen, A.F. (1992). Self-selection for personality variables among healthy volunteers. *Br. J. Clin. Pharmacol.*, **33**, 101–106.

Rohrbaugh, J., Stapleton, J.M., Parasuraman, R., Frohwein, H., Eckardt, M.J., and Linnoila, M. (1987). Alcohol intoxication in humans: Effect on vigilance performance. In: Lindros, K.O., Ylikahri, R., and Kiianmaa, K. (eds), *Advances in Biomedical Alcohol Research. Supplement 1 to Alcohol and Alcoholism*, Oxford: Pergamon Press, pp. 97–102.

Saarialho-Kere, U. (1988). Studies on the psychopharmacology of analgesic drug combinations in man. Doctoral thesis, University of Helsinki.

Saarialho-Kere, U., Julkunen, H., Mattila, M.J., and Seppälä, T. (1988). Psychomotor performance of patients with rheumatoid arthritis: Cross-over comparison of dextropropoxyphene plus amitriptyline, indomethacin, and placebo. *Pharmacol. Toxicol.*, **63**, 286–92.

Saario, I., Linnoila, M., and Mattila, M.J. (1976). Modification by diazepam or thioridazine of the psychomotor skills related to driving: A subacute trial in neurotic outpatients. *Br. J. Clin. Pharmacol.*, **3**, 165–71.

Saletu, B., Darragh, A., Salmon, P., and Coen, R. (1989). EEF brain mapping in evaluating the time-course of the central action of DUP 996: a new acetylcholine releaser. *Br. J. Clin. Pharmacol.*, **28**, 1–16.

Samson, H.H., and Harris, R.A. (1992). Neurobiology of alcohol abuse. *Trends Pharmacol. Sci.*, **13**, 206–211.

Sanders, A.F. (1986). Drugs, driving and the measurement of human performance. In: O'Hanlon, J.F, and deGier, J.J. (eds), *Drugs and Driving*, London: Taylor & Francis, pp. 1–16.

Sanders, A.F., and Wauschkuhn, C.H. (1988). Drugs and information processing in skilled performance. *Psychopharmacology Series*, **6**, 23–47.

Schmidt, G., and Bösche, J. (1981). Effects of high levels of diazepam and alcohol in practice. In: Goldberg, L. (ed.), *Alcohol, Drugs and Driving*, Vol. III—T80, Stockholm: Almquist & Wicksell, pp. 984–95.

Sellers, E.M., and Busto, U. (1982). Benzodiazepines and ethanol: Assessment of the effects and consequences of psychotropic drug interactions. *J. Clin. Psychopharmacol.*, **4**, 249–62.

Sellers, E.M., and Holloway, M.R. (1978). Drug kinetics and alcohol ingestion. *Clin. Pharmacokin.*, **3**, 440–52.

Sellers, E.M., Carr, G., Bernstein, J.G., Sellers, S., and Koch-Weser, J. (1972). Interaction of chloral hydrate and ethanol in man. II. Haemodynamics and performance. *Clin. Pharmacol. Ther.*, **13**, 209–15.

Sellers, E.M., Naranjo, C.A., Giles, H.G., Frecker, R.C., and Beeching, M. (1980). Intravenous diazepam and oral ethanol interaction. *Clin. Pharmacol. Ther.*, **28**, 638–45.

Seppälä, T., and Linnoila, M. (1983). Effects of zimeldine and other antidepressants on skilled performance: a comprehensive review. *Acta Psychiatr. Scand.*, **68** (Suppl. 308), 515–522.

Seppälä, T., Linnoila, M., and Mattila, M.J. (1978). Psychomotor skills in depressed out-patients treated with *l*-tryptophan, doxepin, or chlorimipramine. *Ann. Clin. Res.,* **10**, 214–21.

Seppälä, T., Linnoila, M., and Mattila, M.J. (1979). Drugs, alcohol and driving. *Drugs,* **17**, 389–400.

Seppälä, T., Aranko, K., Mattila, M.J., and Shotriya, R.C. (1982a). Effects of alcohol on buspirone and lorazepam actions. *Clin. Pharmacol. Ther.,* **32**, 201–7.

Seppälä, T., Dreyfus, J.F., Saario, I., and Nuotto, E. (1982b). Zopiclone and flunitrazepam in healthy subjects: Hypnotic activity, residual effects on performance and combined effects with alcohol. *Drugs Exp. Clin. Res.,* **8**, 35–47.

Seppälä, T., Mattila, M.J., Palva, E.S., and Aranko, K. (1986). Combined effects of anxiolytics and alcohol on psychomotor performance in young and middle-aged subjects. In: O'Hanlon, J.F., and deGier, J.J. (eds), *Drugs and Driving,* London: Taylor & Francis, pp. 179–189.

Shaw, L. and Sichel, H. (1971). *Accident Proneness,* Oxford: Pergamon Press.

Silverstone, T. (1988). The influence of psychiatric disease and its treatment on driving performance. *Int. Clin. Psychopharmacol.,* **3** (Suppl. 1), 59–66.

Starmer, G.A. (1986). A review of the effects of analgesics on driving performance. In: O'Hanlon, J.F., and deGier, J.J. (eds), *Drugs and Driving,* London: Taylor & Francis, pp. 251–69.

Starmer, G.A., and Bird, K.D. (1984). Investigating drug–ethanol interactions. *Br. J. Clin. Pharmacol.,* **18**, 27S–35S.

Strömberg, C. (1988). Psychomotor performance and sedation: Human and animal experiments with atypical antidepressants and ethanol. Doctoral thesis, University of Helsinki.

Strömberg, C., and Mattila, M.J. (1987). Acute comparison of clovoxamine, alone and in combination with ethanol, on human psychomotor performance. *Pharmacol. Toxicol.,* **60**, 374–9.

Strömberg, C., Suokas, A., and Seppälä, T. (1988). Interaction of alcohol with maprotiline or nomifensine: Echocardiographic and psychometric effects. *Eur. J. Clin. Pharmacol.,* **35**, 593–9.

Strömberg, C., Suokas, A., Seppälä, T., and Kupari, M. (1991). Echocardiographic and psychometric effects of amitriptyline or imipramine plus alcohol. *Eur. J. Clin. Pharmacol.,* **40**, 349–54.

Subhan, Z., and Hindmarch, I. (1983). The effects of midazolam in conjunction with alcohol on iconic memory and free recall. *Neuropsychobiology,* **9**, 230–234.

Trimble, M.R. (1987). Anticonvulsant drugs and cognitive function: A review of the literature. *Epilepsia,* **28** (Suppl. 3), S37–S45.

Volkerts, E.R., Brookhuis, K.A., and O'Hanlon, J.F. (1987). The effects of treatment with buspirone, diazepam and lorazepam on driving performance in real traffic. In: *Alcohol, Drugs, and Traffic Safety—T86, Excerpta Medica Int. Congr. Ser.,* **721**, 217–21.

Warot, D., Bergougnan, L., Lamiable, D., Berlin, I., Bensimon, G., Danjou, P., and Puech, A.J. (1987). Troleandomycin–triazolam interaction in healthy volunteers: Pharmacokinetic and psychometric evaluation. *Eur. J. Clin. Pharmacol.,* **32**, 389–93.

Yocca, F.D. (1990). Neurochemistry and neurophysiology of buspirone and gepirone: Interactions at presynaptic and postsynaptic 5-HT_{1A} receptors. *J. Clin. Psychopharmacol.,* **10**, 6S–12S.

11

Measures of Neuroleptic Effects on Cognition and Psychomotor Performance in Healthy Volunteers

David J. King

The Queen's University of Belfast, Northern Ireland

Introduction and Rationale

Accurate measurement of the cognitive and psychomotor effects of neuroleptics is important for a number of reasons: to describe different adverse effect and safety profiles; to relate pharmacodynamic effects to pharmacokinetic parameters; and as a means of exploring the basis of their antipsychotic action at a neuro- and psychophysiological level. Recent reviews have all focused on studies in schizophrenic patients. Medalia *et al.* (1988) reviewed the literature according to the effects on different types of neuropsychological tests; Spohn and Strauss (1989) concentrated on the importance of study design; and Cassens *et al.* (1990) contrasted the effects of single and chronic dosing schedules. I have previously compared the findings in schizophrenia with those in healthy volunteers (King, 1990). It is clear from this that variables due to the clinical state of patients greatly confound the interpretation of drug effects especially on neuropsychological tests and, although a body of sound knowledge of the effects in volunteers should form the basis for studies in schizophrenia, such has not been the case.

Methodological Issues

In reviewing this literature one is struck by the great variety of tests and methodologies used and, not surprisingly, little consistency in the reported findings. Generally speaking the clinical studies have been sophisticated in the

Human Psychopharmacology, Vol. 4. Edited by I. Hindmarch and P. D. Stonier
© 1993 John Wiley & Sons Ltd

neuropsychological tests of information processing but naive in pharmacological method and vice versa with the volunteer studies. Recurring
problems, which have not always been recognized, are: the effects of practice
and fatigue; variation in motivation, cooperation or attention; both inter- and
intra-individual variation; differences in sensitivity between tests of similar
functions; and lack of selectivity of tests said to measure a particular function.
Further problems arise in trial design, e.g. many early studies may have
missed peak drug effects because of testing at only one or two time points. It
has also not always been appreciated that sedation or extrapyramidal symptoms (EPS) may, in themselves, be a sufficient explanation for the observed
effects on information processing or memory.

Studies with Phenothiazines

Kornetsky *et al.* (1957) were the first to study the effects of chloropromazine
(CPZ) in comparison with secobarbital, meperidine and LSD, in ten normal
volunteers. They reported that CPZ (200 mg) and secobarbital (200 mg)
caused similar impairments in motor (pursuit-rotor) and psychomotor (digit
symbol substitution (DSST) and symbol-copying) tasks. In subsequent studies
(Mirsky and Kornetsky, 1964) they demonstrated that, whereas secobarbital
caused more cognitive effects than CPZ (using the DSST), CPZ had greater
effects than secobarbital on sustained attention (using the continuous performance test (CPT) of Rosvold *et al.*, 1956). They also showed that it was the
paced component of the CPT which was important in detecting the effect of
CPZ (Kornetsky and Ozrack, 1964). It was therefore proposed that CPZ
acted preferentially on that portion of the ascending reticular activating system responsible for *tonic* (sustained) cortical arousal as opposed to *phasic*
(brief) cortical arousal. However, subsequent studies with the CPT produced
inconsistent results (Medalia *et al.*, 1988) and it now seems clear that a general
decrease in brain-stem arousal does not account for the beneficial effect of
neuroleptics (Janke and Debus, 1972; Hartley, 1983).

In another series of studies, using a similar set of psychomotor tests and a
wide range of subjective ratings, Di Mascio *et al.* (1963a, 1963b) compared the
effects of four doses of CPZ (25, 50, 100 and 200 mg), promethazine (25, 50,
100, 200 mg), perphenazine (2, 4, 8 and 16 mg) and trifluoperazine (2, 4, 8 and
16 mg) in 36 student volunteers. The aliphatic phenothiazines invariably impaired psychomotor performance and speed (but not accuracy) of cognitive
functions, while the piperazines, even at the highest dose, either had no effect
or actually improved performance (e.g. on tapping speed, pursuit-rotor time,
symbol copying and serial addition). Others, however, reported a depressant
effect of piperazine phenothiazines (Idestrom, 1960; Nakra *et al.*, 1975).

Subsequent studies, using much lower doses, have usually confirmed impairments with phenothiazine derivatives in general, in a variety of tests.

Besser and Duncan (1967) found a peak effect of CPZ (50 mg) at 4 hours and persistence for 8 hours, on auditory flutter fusion and visual critical flicker fusion threshold (CFFT). Both CPZ and thioridazine in doses of 1.0 mg/kg impaired tracking, pursuit-rotor and simulated driving tests (Milner and Landauer, 1971). Stone *et al.* (1969), however, thought they had observed a beneficial effect of CPZ (50 mg) on short-term memory. Nevertheless, the test was administered to 40 volunteers in a single group only 45 minutes after drug ingestion and, since the effects of pentobarbital (100 mg), scopolamine (0.6 mg) and placebo were indistinguishable, the findings with chlorpromazine were probably spurious. Meyer *et al.* (1983) reported some paradoxical effects, with thioridazine 1.0 mg/kg producing greater impairments than 1.5 mg/kg on some tests. However, there were only four volunteers, the tests are poorly described, the times of dosing and testing are not given and inappropriate statistics were used. Inconsistent findings with thioridazine (50 mg) were reported in an eight-volunteer study by Szabadi *et al.* (1980). In that study, although digit cancellation and motor coordination were impaired, DSST and symbol copying appeared to have been improved by thioridazine. Nevertheless, in a subsequent study, using essentially similar methodology, the same group reported highly consistent impairments with thioridazine (50 mg) on digit cancellation, DSST, symbol copying, CFFT, finger tapping and motor coordination (Theofilopoulos *et al.*, 1984).

In view of Kornetsky and Orzack's (1964) findings with the CPT measure of sustained attention one might expect that vigilance tests would produce the most consistent findings. Typically, however, these tests last for an hour or more and the results are not easily related to drug effects, especially after single doses. Much of this work has been reviewed by Hartley (1983). Loeb *et al.* (1965), using a 1 hour auditory vigilance task, first showed that amphetamine prevented a decline in performance over time and that CPZ (50 mg) impaired the effective sensitivity of detections (d') over time, but the actual number of detections, false responses and the response latency were similar to placebo. Visual vigilance tasks, however, may be more sensitive to drug effects than auditory vigilance tasks. Hartley *et al.* (1977) showed that both CPZ (25 mg and 75 mg) and noise separately impaired performance on a 1 hour visual vigilance task, but there was no impairment when CPZ and noise were applied together. It would appear that noise causes supra-optimal and CPZ suboptimal arousal and that these actions cancel each other out when noise and CPZ are applied simultaneously. Hartley (1983) also repeated the observation first made by Kornetsky and Orzack (1964) that CPZ impaired tests of attention which were paced but not those which were unpaced.

Does tolerance occur with repeated dosing in volunteers? Liljequist *et al.* (1975, 1978) were unable to detect any effect of CPZ 20 mg t.i.d. or thioridazine 10 mg t.i.d. for 2 weeks on memory, learning or psychomotor performance in 20 volunteers. Neither were any psychomotor effects detected by Saario (1976) after thioridazine 10 mg t.i.d. for 1 week followed by 20 mg t.i.d. for a second week in 20 volunteers. Nevertheless, since no impairments with single dosing at these levels was described, tolerance could not be assumed to have occurred. However, Isah *et al.* (1991) have recently shown typical psychomotor impairments (on choice reaction time, CFFT and letter cancellation) with single doses of prochlorperazine (PCZ) (12.5 mg i.v. or 50 mg orally) in volunteers, but neither subjective nor psychometric changes after 25 mg b.d. for 14 days. During chronic dosing the steady state levels of PCZ in the plasma were similar to those after a single 50 mg dose, and there was accumulation of the *N*-desmethyl metabolite (which was undetectable after single dosing). Thus tolerance to the psychomotor effects of phenothiazines does also seem to occur in volunteers as had earlier been observed in patients (Kornetsky *et al.*, 1959; Cassens *et al.*, 1990).

Thus, given a properly designed trial with 8–12 subjects, conventional psychomotor tests, such as the CPT, DSST, choice reaction time, CFFT, letter cancellation and finger tapping, will usually detect phenothiazines in single doses equivalent to 50 mg CPZ from about 2 to 8 hours (with peak effects at 4 hours) post-dosing. These are, however, really rather non-specific tests and the effects are probably secondary to sedation (as indicated by concomitant visual analogue ratings) and to which tolerance occurs with repeat dosing.

Studies with Haloperidol (HPL)

Clearly studies with non-sedative neuroleptics would be of greater value in identifying a relevant neuro- or psychophysiological basis for an antipsychotic action. However, although human volunteer studies with HPL have been reported for 24 years, there is still anxiety about the ability of volunteers to tolerate adequate doses to produce objective measures without akathisia and dysphoria. In some of these studies excessively high doses have been used, e.g. 5 mg i.v. (Belmaker and Wald, 1977), and 0.5 mg/kg orally or 0.125 mg/kg i.v. (Magliozzi *et al.*, 1985), but others have had problems with 2 mg i.m. (depression lasting 16 hours in one subject; Pfeiffer *et al.*, 1968), or even 5 mg orally (akathisia up to 5 days and dysphoria for up to 6 weeks; Anderson *et al.*, 1981). Magliozzi *et al.* (1989) reported akathisia in 5 of 12 subjects given 4 mg HPL, but in only 2 of 9 given 10 mg. Four of the latter group, however, had drowsiness which may have masked akathisia. In our own experience also, about a third of volunteers develop akathisia after 5 mg HPL orally. Incidentally, Isah *et al.* (1991) also found akathisia in 3 of 7 subjects after single doses of prochlorperazine (12.5 mg i.v. or 50 mg orally), and 4 of 10 were unable to tolerate repeat dosing with 25 mg b.d.

Thus many human volunteer studies have attempted to detect HPL effects with 1 or 2 mg doses. The studies reporting objective psychomotor test results are summarized in Table 1. The use of very low doses seems to have given misleading results, with the suggestion of improvement in cognition in some tests. Thus James and James (1973) reported DSST performance improved with HPL compared with chlordiazepoxide, but inspection of their data suggests that HPL was indistinguishable from placebo. Similarly, Parrott and Hindmarch (1975) reported impairment of CFFT but improved CRT latency with HPL, but again the latter effect was not statistically significant nor different from placebo. In our own recent study (King and Henry, 1992) similar changes in total CRT 3 hours after HPL (1 mg) (in males but not in females)

Table 1. Psychomotor studies with haloperidol in human volunteers

Study	Dose (mg)	n	Reported effect
1. Janke and Debus (1972)	1, 2	13	↑Tapping speed (low 'workload') (1–1.5 h) ↓Tapping speed (high 'workload') No change in word fluency
2. James and James (1973)	0.3 t.i.d. × 24 h	138	↑DSST*
3. Parrott and Hindmarch (1975)	1	6	↓CFFT; ↑CRT (latency) (2 h)*
4. Saletu et al. (1983a, 1983b)	2	10	↑Simple and complex RT (4 h) ↓LC and CFFT (6 h)
5. Saarrialho-Kere (1988)	0.5 b.d × 48 h	12	No effect on CFFT, CRT, Maddox wing or tracking
6. Frey et al. (1989)	0.75 i.v.	6	No effect on CFFT
7. McClelland et al. (1987)	3	12	↓RIPT (4 h)
8. McClelland et al. (1990)	3	12	↓RIPT (4 h–48 h) ↓FFT (6 h)
9. Magliozzi et al. (1989)	4 10	12 9	Dose-dependent ↓DSST (4–6 h) No change in FCT
10. Mungas et al. (1990)	4 10	14 10	No effect on verbal or spatial learning or memory
11. King and Henry (1992)	1	20	↑CRT (3 h) (males only) ↑Visual RT (4.5 h) (males and females)

*Not statistically significantly different from placebo.
↑: improvement; ↓: impairment of function.

Abbreviations: CFFT, critical flicker fusion threshold; CRT, choice reaction time; FCT, flexibility of closure test; FFT, 2 flash fusion threshold; LC, letter cancellation; RIPT, rapid information-processing task; RT, reaction time.

and a decreased (improved) visual reaction time at 4.5 hours were the only statistically significant results with HPL. However, there were no similar trends at other time points and, since a dose-dependent effect could not be demonstrated, these isolated findings may have been spurious.

Inspection of Table 1 shows a great variety of improvements and impairments. Apparent improvements are seen with 1 mg shortly after dosing. The most reliable results seem to be found using at least 2 mg, with 12 or more volunteers and testing from 4 hours post-dosing onward. It is also of interest that in three studies reporting variable or no effects of HPL, elevations in plasma prolactin were found nevertheless (Saletu *et al.*, 1983a, 1983b; Saarialho-Kere, 1988; Frey *et al.*, 1989).

Studies with Atypical Neuroleptics

The development of new antipsychotics with little or no tendency to cause EPS should make human volunteer studies more valuable and easier to interpret. Clozapine (50 mg) has been shown to cause impairments in a range of conventional psychomotor tests as well as EEG changes after 2 and 4 hours (Saletu *et al.*, 1987) but the highly sedative nature of this compound makes these results difficult to interpret.

Sulpiride, either in single doses of 100 mg (Bartfai and Wiesel, 1986) or chronic low doses of 50 mg t.i.d. for 2 weeks (Liljequist *et al.*, 1975), has not been shown to cause any psychomotor or cognitive impairment in conventional tests. Similarly, von Aschoff *et al.* (1974), using electro-oculogram nystagmography, found that sulpiride (300 mg daily for 1 week) was devoid of any effect on the velocity or latency of saccadic eye movements and, in fact, saccadic accuracy was slightly improved. McClelland *et al.* (1990), however, reported that 400 mg of sulpiride caused delayed impairments on a rapid information-processing task (RIPT) at 24 hours. Remoxipride, in single doses of 30 and 60 mg, caused impairments in CFFT, CRT latency and continuous attention between 4 and 6 hours (Fagan *et al.*, 1988). Performance on DSST and a tracking test were also impaired by 100 mg doses of remoxipride between 4.5 and 6 hours (Mattila *et al.*, 1988). Further studies with these two drugs, which are also relatively non-sedative, particularly using more specific tests of central nervous system (CNS) function, are awaited with interest.

The Search for New Test Strategies

None of the tests so far developed has been shown to be selective for a particular psychomotor of cognitive function, nor have they distinguished between the effects of neuroleptics and other drugs with central depressant properties such as the benzodiazepines. Such a test would be a real advance and should throw some light on how the neuroleptics, which have generally negative effects in volunteers, are associated with such beneficial neuropsychological effects in schizophrenic patients.

Rapid Information-processing Task (RIPT)

This test has been developed from the work of Posner and Keele (1967) and, although similar to the CPT of Rosvold *et al.* (1956), requires a higher level of performance sustained over 400 seconds (McClelland *et al.*, 1990). Five different letters, in both lower and upper cases, are presented singly on a visual display unit (VDU) in pseudo-random order, at a rate of one per second. The subject has to indicate consecutive presentations of the same letter, irrespective of case. It appears to be a very sensitive test, and McClelland *et al.* (1990) have used it successfully to detect chlorpromazine (50 mg), haloperidol (3 mg) and sulpiride (400 mg). Nevertheless, it appears to be an non-specific test since highly significant impairments in all six measured variables were produced by lorazepam (2.5 mg) (Leigh *et al.*, 1991).

Continuous Attention Test (CAT)

This is another computerized test of sustained attention, developed by Tiplady (1988). It is a non-verbal task. The subject is shown a series of different patterns of shaded squares in a 3×3 design over a period of 8 minutes and has to indicate when two identical patterns occur consecutively. This test has been shown to be sensitive to remoxipride (30 and 60 mg) (Fagan *et al.*, 1988), but its relative specificity for neuroleptics compared to benzodiazepines has yet to be determined.

Perceptual Maze Test (PMT)

Elithorn *et al.* (1982) developed a computerized neuropsychological test system which included a series of perceptual mazes of progressive difficulty depending on the subject's performance (Smith *et al.*, 1978). This is a visuospatial and cognitive task requiring planning and sustained attention for 20–30 minutes. It has been shown to be associated with increased metabolic activity in the left frontal area and both occipital poles, in positron emission tomographic studies (Nybäck *et al.*, 1985). It did not, however, detect HPL (1 mg) at 4.5 hours in our hands (King and Henry, 1992). This may partly have been because of the inherent interest of the puzzles, but also because the level of difficulty was such that there was a marked learning effect during the practice sessions, after which a plateau of performance was reached. This test also failed to detect amitriptyline (50 mg) (King and Devaney, 1988) or diazepam (10 mg) (King *et al.*, 1991a).

Eye Movements

The use of measures of smooth pursuit and saccadic eye movements in psycho-pharmacology has been extensively reviewed in an earlier volume in this series (Bittencourt and Tedeschi, 1991). Glue (1991) has also described how saccadic eye movements can also be used to measure changes in benzodiazepine receptor sensitivity either following pharmacological challenge or in anxiety disorders.

Saccadic eye movements are the fastest movements in the body, with angular velocities of up to 600° per second. They are regulated by a pulse generator in the paramedian pontine reticular formation (Fuchs and Kaneko, 1981) and are very sensitive to central depressant drug effects (Griffiths *et al.*, 1984). Impairments in peak saccadic velocity appear to be a non-specific measure, closely linked to the level of sedation since they can be observed after alcohol (Griffiths *et al.*, 1984), temazepam (Bittencourt *et al.*, 1981; King and Bell, 1988), chlorpromazine (King *et al.*, 1990) and promethazine (King *et al.*, 1991b). However, a direct link with sedation has been disputed by Glue (1991) on the grounds that: (1) with incremental doses of midazolam significant changes in saccade parameters occur prior to changes in self-rated sedation; (2) there are no close correlations between clonidine-induced sedation and reductions in saccade parameters; and (3) thyrotrophin-releasing hormone (TRH) has been shown to reverse lorazepam-induced sedation but not the associated slowing of saccades. Thus in certain circumstances the link with sedation is not invariable. Nevertheless, the value of measures of saccadic eye movements in studies of neuroleptics is as a relatively pure test of brain-stem arousal in the detection of non-specific sedative properties.

The role of dopamine in the control of saccades is unclear. Saccadic latencies are abnormally slow in Parkinson's disease and improve following dopamine (Hotson *et al.*, 1986) but, while we found that chlorpromazine (50 and 100 mg) reduced peak saccadic velocity (King *et al.*, 1990), haloperidol (1.5 and 5 mg) did not (King and Bell, 1990).

The findings of our studies in this area have been summarized in Table 2.

Table 2. Drug effects on peak saccadic velocity and conventional psychomotor tests (% change from placebo)

	VARS (alert)	CFFT	PSV	CPT	DSST	CRT
Tempazepam (20 mg)	−25**	−8**	−25**	n.s.	−15**	11**
Lorazepam (2.5 mg)	−59**	−10**	−24**	40**	−25**	28**
Promethazine (50 mg)	−45**	−17**	−18**	10*	−17*	11*
Chlorpromazine (100 mg)	−70*	−9**	−24**	n.s.	−8**	6*
Haloperidol (5 mg)	n.s.	n.s.	n.s.	−1**	−3*	n.s.

n.s., non-significant; *$p < 0.05$; **$p < 0.01$.

CFFT, critical flicker fusion threshold; CPT, continuous performance test; CRT, choice reaction time; DSST, digit symbol substitution test; PSV, peak saccadic velocity; VARS, visual analogue rating scale.

Percentage changes are given to allow comparisons between three different studies and are the percentage differences from placebo at the time of peak effect. The table also shows the corresponding results for conventional psychomotor tests and subjective ratings of sedation. It is clear that:

(1) HPL differed from all the other drugs in only having effects on the CPT and DSST.
(2) None of the tests distinguished neuroleptics from benzodiazepines or promethazine.
(3) Peak saccadic velocity was the most sensitive and reliable of the objective tests.
(4) Impaired brain-stem arousal, as originally posited by Mirsky and Kornetsky (1964), does *not*, in fact, account for the antipsychotic action of neuroleptic drugs.

Smooth pursuit eye movements, on the other hand, which are frequently impaired in both schizophrenic patients and their relatives (Holzman, 1985), have not been used as extensively in psychopharmacology. This is because it seemed that they were less sensitive to drug effects, probably because the methodology for measuring the accuracy of tracking and the identification of saccadic intrusions was somewhat cruder and less objective. The first studies failed to detect either CPZ (up to 1.334 mg/kg) or diazepam (up to 0.284 mg/kg) in volunteers (Holzman *et al.*, 1975). Studies in patients taking drugs chronically revealed effects of lithium (Holzman *et al.*, 1991) but not of neuroleptics (Levy *et al.*, 1984). More recent work with more refined methods of measurement, however, has shown that these movements are as sensitive to benzodiazepines as saccadic eye movements, in volunteers (Bittencourt *et al.*, 1983). We are currently investigating the effect of neuroleptics on smooth pursuit eye movements. Since they involve more attentional processing (Shagass *et al.*, 1976) and centres outside the brain stem, including the frontal eye fields (Levin, 1984; Holzman, 1985; Carpenter, 1988), we predict that they will be sensitive to both sedative and non-sedative neuroleptics.

'Frontal Lobe' Tests

Many workers have used tests thought to be relatively specific for frontal lobe functions both in the investigation of the neuropsychological deficits in schizophrenia and to investigate neuroleptic effects. These include a range of tests of planning, card sorting, Stroop colour–word interference, verbal fluency, visual search and attentional control. The hazards of inferring that any of these tests are, in fact, selective for frontal lobe function have been discussed by Shallice *et al.* (1991). Impairments on such tests, therefore, may help to define the processes on which neuroleptics exert their effects, but not necessarily the brain regions involved.

One interesting example of these tests is the Posner covert orientation of attention test used by Clark *et al.* (1989) in studies of droperidol and clonidine. In this task responses are measured to targets 25° lateral to the left or right while the eyes remain fixed to a central point. The targets are preceded by either neutral, valid (true) or invalid (false) cues, and the 'benefits' of valid cueing, or the 'costs' of invalid cueing, can be measured. Although droperidol and clonidine were found to increase overall response times, both drugs reduced the cost of invalid cueing, implying improved attentional processing by facilitating the shifting of attention. These effects were contrasted with those of amphetamine, which enhances attention during vigilance tasks but impairs the disengagement of attention. These data imply, however, that either dopamine antagonism or decreased adrenergic transmission would improve attentional mechanisms, but only the former has been found to be effective in schizophrenia. Furthermore, other tests of attentional shifting, using card-sorting and word fluency tests, found *impairments* after HPL (in patients with spasmodic torticollis) (Berger *et al.*, 1989).

It is important to recognize, however, that impairments of lower levels of function (such as motor speed or alertness) may have non-specific effects on such tests. Indeed, the simpler tests are often *more* sensitive to drug effects than complex ones. For instance, Herbert *et al.* (1983) detected both oxazepam (30 mg) and zetidoline (10 and 20 mg) with a choice serial reaction time test which lasted 10 minutes, but Baddeley logical reasoning for 5 minutes was only sensitive to the higher dose of zetidoline, and a 5-minute visual search test was not affected by either drug. Thus the duration of a test rather than its inferred 'cognitive load' may be more important for its sensitivity to drug effects. This may also partly account for the success of the RIPT, which lasts between 6 and 7 minutes, in detecting neuroleptics (see above). Indeed, if cognitive load is interesting, rather than monotonous, the test may be quite insensitive to drug effects. Thus Magliozzi *et al.* (1989) found the DSST was impaired by both 4 and 10 mg HPL, whereas a more complex, and presumably more interesting, 'flexibility of closure test' (where complex geometric figures had to be reproduced) was not. Szabadi *et al.* (1980) also found mere digit cancellation to be more sensitive to thioridazine than the DSST. Both interest and duration of a test would therefore seem to be important by affecting motivation: a test should be both long and monotonous to be sensitive to drug effects. Thus the RIPT, digit cancellation and DSST seem to be better than most of the interesting 'frontal lobe' tests in detecting neuroleptic drugs.

Conclusions

What lessons can be learned from this review about the measurement of neuroleptic drug effects on cognitive and psychomotor function in normal volunteers?

(1)   The same principles that apply to psychopharmacological testing in general are all important. Thus the effects of practice and motivation (interest versus monotony), the duration of the test and study design will all affect the apparent sensitivity of the test.

(2)   Sedation may have non-specific effects on any test, and the test battery must include simple measures of sedation, and both a placebo and a benzodiazepine should be included as negative and positive controls, respectively.

(3)   The paced versus the unpaced nature of the test *may* be particularly relevant for neuroleptic effects, as has frequently been suggested (Kornetsky and Orzack, 1964; Hartley, 1983; Broadbent, 1984), but as yet no test has been found which reliably distinguishes neuroleptics from benzodiazepines.

(4)   Neuroleptics impair all functions tested in human volunteers. Earlier studies suggesting improvement in some cognitive functions with low doses of non-sedative neuroleptics were misleading.

(5)   Tolerance to the effects of repeated doses on cognitive and psychomotor function occurs in human volunteers as in patients.

(6)   The problem of how drugs, which impair attention in normals, are effective in improving attention in schizophrenic patients remains. Whether this is because (a) an overall decrease in attention in schizophrenia helps to restore a 'filter' mechanism and improve selectivity of attention (McClelland *et al.*, 1990), (b) improved shifting of attention occurs in spite of an overall slowing of response (Clark *et al.*, 1989), (c) inhibition of subcortical mesolimbic hyperactivity improves cortical function and attention indirectly, by reducing interference from these lower structures (King, 1990), or (d) some other mechanism; remains to be resolved.

Acknowledgements

I am indebted to Dr M. F. Mannion for his help with Table 2 and Mrs Mavis Scullion for her patience and expertise in the preparation of the manuscript.

References

Anderson, B.G., Reker, D., and Cooper, T.B. (1981). Prolonged adverse effects of haloperidol in normal subjects. *N. Eng. J. Med.*, **305**, 643–4.

Bartfai, A., and Wiesel, F.A. (1986). Effect of sulpiride on vigilance in healthy subjects. *Int. J. Psychophysiol.*, **4**, 1–5.

Belmaker, R.H., and Wald, D. (1977). Haloperidol in normals. *Br. J. Psychiatry*, **131**, 222–3.

Berger, H.J.C., van Hoof, J.J.M., van Spaendonck, K.P.M., Horstink, M.W.I., van den Bercken, J.H.L., Jaspers, R., and Cools, A.R. (1989). Haloperidol and cognitive shifting. *Neuropsychologia*, **27**, 629–39.

Besser, G.M., and Duncan, C. (1967). The time course of action of single doses of diazepam, chlorpromazine and some barbiturates as measured by auditory flutter fusion and visual flicker fusion thresholds in man. *Br. J. Pharmacol. Chemother.,* **30**, 341–8.

Bittencourt, P.R.M., and Tedeschi, G. (1990). The oculomotor system: Multiple pharmacodynamic models. In: Hindmarch, I., and Stonier, P.D. (eds), *Human Psychopharmacology, Measures and Methods,* Vol. 3, Chichester: Wiley, pp. 39–60.

Bittencourt, P.R.M., Wade, P., Smith, A.T., and Richens, A. (1981). The relationship between peak velocity of saccadic eye movements and serum benzodiazepine concentration. *Br. J. Clin. Pharmacol.,* **12**, 523–33.

Bittencourt, P.R.M., Wade, P., Smith, A.T., and Richens, A. (1983). Benzodiazepines impair smooth pursuit eye movements. *Br. J. Clin. Pharmacol.,* **15**, 259–62.

Broadbent, D.E. (1984). Performance and its measurement. *Br. J. Clin. Pharmacol.,* **18** (Suppl. 1), 5S–9S.

Carpenter, R.H.S. (1988). *Movements of the Eyes* (2nd edn), London: Pion, Ch. 9, pp. 210–92.

Cassens, G., Inglis, A.K., Appelbaum, P.S., and Gutheil, T.G. (1990). Neuroleptics: Effects on neuropsychological function in chronic schizophrenic patients. *Schizophr. Bull.,* **16**, 477–99.

Clark, C.R., Geffen, G.M., and Geffen, L.B. (1989). Catecholamines and the covert orientation of attention in humans. *Neuropsychologia,* **27**, 131–9.

DiMascio, A., Havens, L.L., and Klerman, G.L. (1963a). The psychopharmacology of phenothiazine compounds: A comparative study of the effects of chlorpromazine, promethazine, trifluoperazine and perphenazine in normal males. I: Introduction, aims and methods. *J. Nerv. Ment. Dis.,* **136**, 15–28.

DiMascio, A., Havens, L.L., and Klerman, G.L. (1963b). The psychopharmacology of phenothiazine compounds: A comparative study of the effects of chlorpromazine, promethazine, trifluoperazine, and perphenazine in normal males: II: Results and discussion. *J. Nerv. Ment. Dis.,* **136**, 168–86.

Elithorn, A., Mornington, S., and Stavrou, A. (1982). Automated psychological testing: Some principles and practice. *Int. J. Man–Machine Studies,* **17**, 246–63.

Fagan, D., Scott, D.B., and Mitchell, M. (1988). The psychomotor effects of remoxipride in healthy volunteers. *Neurosc. Lett. Suppl.,* **32**, S45.

Frey, S., Bente, G., Fuchs, A., Preiswerk, G., Glatt, A., and Imhof, P. (1989). Spontaneous motor activity in healthy volunteers after single doses of haloperidol. *Int. Clin. Psychopharmacol.,* **4**, 39–53.

Fuchs, A.F., and Kaneko, C.R.S. (1981). A brain stem generator for saccadic eye movements. *Trends Neurosci.,* November, 283–6.

Glue, P. (1991). The pharmacology of saccadic eye movements. *J. Psychopharmacol.,* **5**, 377–87.

Griffiths, A.N., Marshall, R.W., and Richens, A. (1984). Saccadic eye movement analysis as a measure of drug effects on human psychomotor performance. *Br. J. Clin. Pharmacol.,* **18**, 73S–82S.

Hartley, L.R. (1983). Arousal, temporal and spatial uncertainty and drug effects. *Prog. Neuro-psychopharmacol. Biol. Psychiatry,* **7**, 29–37.

Hartley, L., Couper-Smartt, J., and Henry, T. (1977). Behavioural antagonism between chlorpromazine and noise in man. *Psychopharmacology,* **55**, 97–102.

Herbert, M., Standen, P.J., Short, A.H., and Birmingham, A.T. (1983). A comparison of some psychological and physiological effects exerted by zetidoline (DL308) and by oxazepam. *Psychopharmacology,* **81**, 335–9.

Holzman, P.S. (1985). Eye movement dysfunctions and psychosis. *Int. Rev. Neurobiol.*, **27**, 179–205.

Holzman, P.S., Levy, D.L., Uhlenhuth, E.H., Proctor, L.R., and Freedman, D.X. (1975). Smooth-pursuit eye movements, and diazepam, CPZ and secobarbital. *Psychopharmacologia*, **44**, 111–15.

Holzman, P.S., O'Brian, C., and Waternaux, C. (1991). Effects of lithium treatment on eye movements. *Biol. Psychiatry*, **29**, 1001–15.

Hotson, J.R., Langston, E.B., and Langston, J.W. (1986). Saccade responses to dopamine in human MPTP-induced parkinsonism. *Ann. Neurol.*, **20**, 456–63.

Idestrom, C.M. (1960). Experimental psychologic methods applied in psychopharmacology. *Acta Psychiatr. Neurol. Scand.*, **35**, 302–13.

Isah, A.O., Rawlins, M.D., and Bateman, D.N. (1991). Clinical pharmacology of prochlorperazine in healthy young males. *Br. J. Clin. Pharmacol.*, **32**, 677–84.

James, B., and James, N. McI. (1973). Low dosage haloperidol and induced anxiety in normal volunteers. *NZ Med. J.*, **78**, 210–12.

Janke, W., and Debus, G. (1972). Double-blind psychometric evaluation of pimozide and haloperidol versus placebo in emotionally labile volunteers under two different work load conditions. *Pharmakopsychiatry*, **1**, 34–51.

King, D.J. (1990). The effect of neuroleptics on cognitive and psychomotor function. *Br. J. Psychiatry*, **157**, 799–811.

King, D.J., and Bell, P. (1988). The effect of temazepam on psychomotor performance and saccadic eye movements. *J. Psychopharmacol.*, **2**, 135 (Abstract).

King, D.J., and Bell, P. (1990). Differential effects of temazepam and haloperidol on saccadic eye movements and psychomotor performance. *Br. J. Clin. Pharmacol.*, **29**, 590P.

King, D.J., and Devaney, N. (1988). Clinical pharmacology of sibutramine hydrochloride (BTS 54524), a new antidepressant, in healthy volunteers. *Br. J. Clin. Pharmacol.*, **26**, 607–11.

King, D.J., and Henry, G. (1992). The effect of neuroleptics on cognitive and psychomotor function: a preliminary study in healthy volunteers. *Br. J. Psychiatry*, **160**, 647–53.

King, D.J., Bell, P., Best, S.J., and Mannion, M. (1990). A comparison of the effects of chlorpromazine and temazepam on saccadic eye movements and psychomotor performance. *Br. J. Clin. Pharmacol.*, **30**, 309P–310P.

King, D.J., Bell, P., Bratty, J.R., and McEntegart, D.J. (1991a). A preliminary study of the effects of flosequinan on psychomotor function in healthy volunteers. *Int. Clin. Psychopharmacol.*, **6**, 155–68.

King, D.J., Best, S.J., Montgomery, R.C., and Mannion, M.F. (1991b). A comparison of the effects of promethazine and lorazepam on saccadic eye movements and psychomotor performance. *Br. J. Clin. Pharmacol.*, **31**, 239P.

Kornetsky, C., and Orzack, M.H. (1964). A research note on some of the critical factors on the dissimilar effects of chlorpromazine and secobarbital on the digit symbol substitution and continuous performance tests. *Psychopharmacologia*, **6**, 79–86.

Kornetsky, C., Humphries, O., and Evarts, E.V. (1957). Comparison of psychological effects of certain centrally acting drugs in man. *AMA Arch. Neurol. Psychiatry*, **77**, 318–24.

Kornetsky, C., Pettit, M., Wynne, R., and Evarts, E.V.A. (1959). A comparison of the psychological effects of acute and chronic administration of chlorpromazine and secobarbital (quinalbarbitone) in schizophrenic patients. *J. Med. Sci.*, **105**, 190–8.

Leigh, T.J., Link, C.G.G., and Fell, G.L. (1991). Effects of granisetron and lorazepam, alone and in combination, on psychometric performance. *Br. J. Clin. Pharamcol.,* **31,** 333–6.

Levin, S. (1984). Frontal lobe dysfunctions in schizophrenia. I. Eye movement impairments. *J. Psychiatr. Res.,* **18,** 27–55.

Levy, D.L., Lipton, R.B., Yasillo, N.J., Peterson, J., Pandey, G., and Davis, J.M. (1984). Psychotropic drug effects on smooth pursuit eye movements: A summary of recent findings. In: Gale, A.G., and Johnson, F. (eds), *Theoretical and Applied Aspects of Eye Movement Research,* Amsterdam: Elsevier, pp. 497–505.

Liljequist, R., Linnoila, M., Mattila, M.J., Saario, I., and Seppala, T. (1975). Effect of two weeks' treatment with thioridazine, chlorpromazine, sulpiride, and bromazepam, alone or in combination with alcohol, on learning and memory in man. *Psychopharmacologia,* **44,** 205–8.

Liljequist, R., Linnoila, M., and Mattila, M.J. (1978). Effect of diazepam and chlorpromazine on memory functions in man. *Eur. J. Clin. Pharmacol.,* **13,** 339–43.

Loeb, M., Hawkes, J., Evans, P., and Alluisi, E.A. (1965). Influence of *d*-amphetamine, benactyzine and chlorpromazine on performance in an auditory vigilance task. *Psychonomic Sci.,* **3,** 29–30.

McClelland, G.R., Cooper, S.M., and Raptopoulos, P. (1987). Paroxetine and haloperidol: Effects on psychomotor performance. *Br. J. Clin. Pharmacol.,* **24,** 268P–269P.

McClelland, G.R., Cooper, S.M., and Pilgrim, A.J. (1990). A comparison of the central nervous system effects of haloperidol, chlorpromazine and sulpiride in normal volunteers. *Br. J. Clin. Pharmacol.,* **30,** 795–803.

Magliozzi, J.R., Gillespie, H., Lombrozo, L., and Hollister, L.E. (1985). Mood alteration following oral and intravenous haloperidol and relationship to drug concentration in normal subjects. *J. Clin. Pharmacol.,* **25,** 285–90.

Magliozzi, J.R., Mungas, D., Laubly, J.N., and Blunden, D. (1989). Effect of haloperidol on a symbol digit substitution task in normal adult males. *Neuropsychopharamcology,* **2,** 29–37.

Mattila, M.J., Mattila, M.E., Konno, K., and Saarialho-Kere, U. (1988). Objective and subjective effects of remoxipride, alone and in combination with ethanol or diazepam, on performance in healthy subjects. *J. Psychopharmacol.,* **2,** 138–49.

Medalia, A., Gold, J., and Merriam, A. (1988). The effect of neuroleptics on neuropsychological test results of schizophrenics. *Arch. Clin. Neuropsychol.* **3,** 249–71.

Meyer, F.P., Neubüser, G., Weimeister, O., and Walther, H. (1983). Influence of thioridazine on human cognitive, psychomotor, and reaction performance as well as subjective feelings. *Int. J. Clin. Pharmacol. Ther. Toxicol.,* **21,** 192–6.

Milner, G., and Landauer, A.A. (1971). Alcohol, thioridazine and chlorpromazine effects on skills related to driving behaviour. *Br. J. Psychiatry,* **118,** 351–2.

Mirsky, A.F., and Kornetsky, C. (1964). On the dissimilar effects of drugs on the digit symbol substitution and continuous performance tests: A review and preliminary integration of behavioral and physiological evidence. *Psychopharmacologia,* **5,** 161–77.

Mungas, D., Magliozzi, J.R., Laubly, J.N., and Blunden, D. (1990). Effects of haloperidol on recall and information processing in verbal and spatial learning. *Prog. Neuro-Psychopharmacol Biol. Psychiatry,* **14,** 181–93.

Nakra, B.R.S., Bond, A.J., and Lader, M.H. (1975). Comparative psychotropic effects of metoclopramide and prochlorperazine in normal subjects. *J. Clin. Pharmacol.,* May/June, 449–454.

Nybäck, H., Blomqvist, G., Greitz, T., Levander, S., Nyman, H., Sedvall, G., Sjögren, I., Stone-Elander, S., and Widén, L. (1985). Brain metabolism and neuropsychological test performance in healthy volunteers and patients with Alzheimer's dementia. *IVth World Congress of Biological Psychiatry*, Philadelphia, Abstract No. 419.6.

Parrott, A.C., and Hindmarch, I. (1975). Haloperidol and chlorpromazine: Comparative effects upon arousal and performance. *IRCS Med. Sci.*, **3**, 562.

Pfeiffer, C.C., Goldstein, L., and Murphree, H.B. (1968). Effects of parenteral administration of haloperidol and chlorpromazine in man. I. Normal subjects: Quantitative EEG and subjective response. *J. Clin. Pharmacol.*, **8**, 79–88.

Posner, N.I., and Keele, S.W. (1967). Decay of visual information from a single letter. *Science*, **158**, 137–9.

Rosvold, H.E., Mirsky, A.F., Sarason, I., Bransome, E.D., and Beck, L.H. (1956). A continuous performance test of brain damage. *J. Consul. Psychol.*, **20**, 343–50.

Saarialho-Kere, U. (1988). Psychomotor, respiratory and neuroendocrinological effects of nalbuphine and haloperidol, alone and in combination, in healthy subjects. *Br. J. Clin. Pharmacol.*, **26**, 79–87.

Saario, I. (1976). Psychomotor skills during subacute treatment with thioridazine and bromazepam, and their combined effects with alcohol. *Ann. Clin. Res.*, **8**, 117–23.

Saletu, B., Grünberger, J., Linzmayer, L., and Dubini, A. (1983a). Determination of pharmacodynamics of the new neuroleptic zetidoline by neuroendocrinologic, pharmaco-EEG, and psychometric studies. Part I. *Int. J. Clin. Pharmacol. Ther. Toxicol.*, **21**, 489–95.

Saletu, B., Grünberger, J., Linzmayer, L., and Dubini, A. (1983b). Determination of pharmacodynamics of the new neuroleptic zetidoline by neuroendocrinologic, pharmaco-EEG, and psychometric studies. Part II. *Int. J. Clin. Pharmacol. Ther. Toxicol.*, **21**, 544–51.

Saletu, B., Grünberger, J., Linzmayer, L., and Anderer, P. (1987). Comparative placebo-controlled pharmacodynamic studies with zotepine and clozapine utilizing pharmaco-EEG and psychometry. *Pharmacopsychiatry*, **20**, 12–27.

Shagass, C., Roemer, R.A., and Amadeo, M. (1976). Eye-tracking performance and engagement of attention. *Arch. Gen. Psychiatry*, **33**, 121–5.

Shallice, T., Burgess, P.W., and Frith, C.D. (1991). Can the neuropsychological case-study approach be applied to schizophrenia? *Psychol. Med.*, **21**, 661–73.

Smith, J., Jones, D., and Elithorn, A. (1978). *The Perceptual Maze Test*, London: Medical Research Council.

Spohn, H.E., and Strauss, M.E. (1989). Relation of neuroleptic and anticholinergic medication to cognitive functions in schizophrenia. *J. Abnorm. Psychol.*, **98**, 367–80.

Stone, G.C., Callaway, E., Jones, R.T., and Gentry, T. (1969). Chlorpromazine slows decay of visual short-term memory. *Psychonomic Sci.*, **16**, 229–30.

Szabadi, E., Bradshaw, C.M., and Gaszner, P. (1980). The comparison of the effects of DL-308, a potential new neuroleptic agent, and thioridazine on some psychological and physiological functions in healthy volunteers. *Psychopharmacology*, **68**, 125–34.

Theofilopoulos, N., Szabadi, E., and Bradshaw, C.M. (1984). Comparison of the effects of ranitidine, cimetidine and thioridazine on psychomotor functions in healthy volunteers. *Br. J. Clin. Pharmacol.*, **18**, 135–44.

Tiplady, B. (1988). A continuous attention test for the assessment of the acute behavioural effects of drugs. *Psychopharmacol. Bull.*, **24**, 213–16.

von Aschoff, J.C., Becker, W., and Weinert, D. (1974). Computer-nystagmographie als neue Bestimmungsmethode von Vigilanz und Reaktionsverhalten unter Psychopharmaka. *Arzneim-Forsch. (Drug Res.)*, **24**, 1085–7.

12

Assessment of Anticonvulsant Drugs in Patients with Bipolar Affective Illness

Robert M. Post, Terence A. Ketter, Kirk Denicoff, Gabriele S. Leverich and Kirstin Mikalauskas

National Institute of Mental Health, Bethesda, Maryland, USA

Introduction

Assessment strategies in bipolar illness are complicated by the highly varied time domains with which the clinician and investigator must deal. That is, one is concerned about acute antimanic and antidepressant responsivity over a time frame of days to weeks on the one hand, and longer-term prevention of episodes over a period of years to decades on the other. In addition, there is increasing recognition of new syndromes such as recurrent brief depression and recurrent brief mania where severe symptomatology may emerge episodically over a period of several days and rapidly return to baseline. Moreover, there is increasing recognition of ultradian fluctuations occurring within manic and depressive episodes. Thus, the methods one utilizes in the acute and long-term assessment of bipolar affective disorder must be either varied enough or flexible enough to capture these differential time domains and provide an accurate assessment of response to pharmacological interventions.

Initial Diagnostic Assessment

In the initial evaluation of a patient, particularly for entry into a clinical trial, a formal diagnostic assessment should be utilized. This might include the schedule for affective disorders and schizophrenia (SADS) (Endicott and Spitzer, 1978), the diagnostic interview schedule (DIS) (Robins *et al.*, 1981), the structured clinical interview for the DSM-III-R (SCID) (Spitzer *et al.*, 1988), or

Human Psychopharmacology, Vol. 4. Edited by I. Hindmarch and P. D. Stonier
© 1993 John Wiley & Sons Ltd

similar techniques, in order to apply the ICD9 diagnostic criteria. The similarities and differences among these techniques and their assets and liabilities are reviewed by Altshuler *et al.* (1991).

Once the diagnosis for bipolar affective illness is arrived at, we highly recommend systematic retrospective and prospective life charting of the course of illness, for both the clinician and clinical research investigator (Squillace *et al.*, 1984; Roy-Byrne *et al.*, 1985; Post *et al.*, 1988; Leverich *et al.*, 1990; Leverich and Post, 1992). The prior course of illness can, in fact, help in making a more accurate diagnosis. The verification of discrete episodes of mood elevation or depression in the context of 'well intervals' with good interim functioning provides the hallmark of the bipolar diagnosis and course of illness. For patients entering acute and long-term prophylactic clinical trials, it additionally provides a critical stratification technique for the number of prior affective episodes, which appears to be an increasingly important variable in outcome studies, at least with long-term prophylaxis with lithium carbonate. For example, Gelenberg *et al.* (1989) reported that lithium was largely ineffective in patients with more than three prior episodes. Similarly, O'Connell *et al.* (1991) reported that lithium (supplemented with a variety of other modalities) was effective in a subgroup of patients with relatively fewer prior episodes (3.5), while it yielded fair or poor responses in those with 5.3 and 7.7 prior episodes, respectively. Thus, accurate assessment of number of prior episodes may be a critical variable in assignment of patients to randomized clinical trials as well as in the assessment of alternative strategies in the clinical treatment of individual patients.

Moreover, we would recommend the use of life-charting techniques in bipolar illness for a variety of other reasons (Table 1). When utilized with the patient, it enhances the process of medicalization of the illness, the sense of patient participation in the assessment and treatment of his own illness, and thus enhances the therapeutic alliance and, ultimately, compliance with clinical pharmacotherapeutics. The patient and physician can 'at a glance' ascertain the prior course of illness which appears to be the best, if not infallible predictor of subsequent illness, and thus might help to guide pharmacotherapeutics. Since life charting also involves systematic assessment of the efficacy of prior pharmacological intervention, this also represents an invaluable guide to future treatment, particularly in the context of switching treating physicians or institutions where records are often not easily transferred with the patient or busy clinicians have limited time to integrate voluminous medical records. We advise that the patient be in possession of his prior life chart and assist in the prospective following of his illness, much the way a diabetic continues to monitor his blood or urine glucose levels in relationship to self-administered insulin in order to maximize and optimize treatment.

Table 1. Benefits of life charting

Document prior course	*Patient as active partner*
Partial response	*Increase compliance*
Psychosocial precipitants	*Directs future clinical trials*
Seasonal variation	*and need for combinations*
Tolerance patterns	*Target psychotherapy*
Cycle acceleration	*Develop early-warning system*
TCA, MAOI	

In addition to these assets, life charting also assists the patient and therapist in assessing whether episodes are associated with psychosocial stressors, anniversary reactions, seasonal variations, or other important potential zeitgebers (including endocrine determinants such as menarche, childbirth and menopause, in addition to exogenously administered hormones) as well as presentations secondary to medical illnesses and/or complicating drug and alcohol abuse. In many patients, a transition occurs from episodes that were initially associated with or precipitated by psychosocial stressors to episodes that occur more spontaneously and autonomously (Post, 1992). Thus, life charting may assist in the identification of initially precipitated episodes that then begin to emerge spontaneously, and the clinician may then be in a position to alter psycho- and pharmacotherapeutic approaches accordingly. Elsewhere, we have discussed the possibility that more psychodynamic interventions may be helpful with an illness that is closely associated with psychosocial stressors, but once the illness has begun to occur autonomously and spontaneously, more behavioural, cognitive, interpersonal and focused therapies may be of importance (Post, 1992). In this fashion, we suggest that the life-charting process may assist in the long-term longitudinal evaluation of both psychosocial and pharmacotherapeutic interventions, particularly over long-term time domains.

A life chart can be readily and rapidly constructed on the basis of a short telephone consultation or an extremely detailed life chart constructed with extensive and ongoing consultation with patient, family, previous physicians and utilization of previous hospital records. The method for developing a life chart has been discussed in detail elsewhere and will be only briefly reviewed here (Squillace *et al.*, 1984; Roy-Byrne *et al.*, 1985; Post *et al.*, 1988; Leverich *et al.*, 1990; Leverich and Post, 1992). As illustrated in Figure 1, course of illness is charted at three levels of severity of manic and depressive episodes, with treatments further coded above these episodes, and important life events and psychosocial stresses intercalated below the mood and behaviour baseline. The assessment of manic and depressive episodes is linked to severity of

214

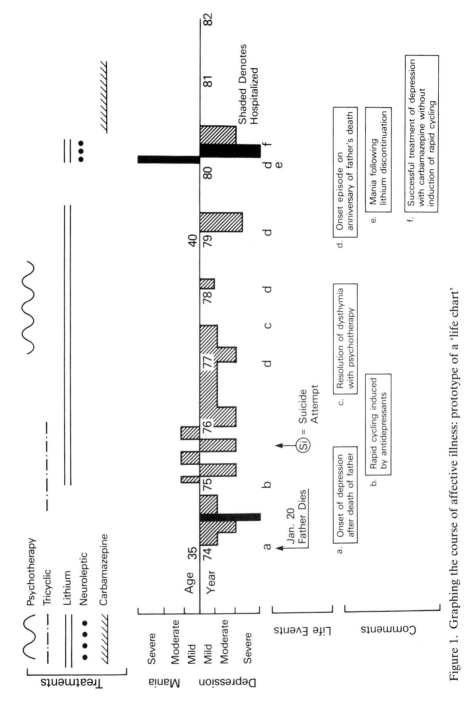

Figure 1. Graphing the course of affective illness: prototype of a 'life chart'

functional incapacitation, assisting in the retrospective categorization of the severity of episodes, at least in a global fashion. For example, mild depressive episodes are those where the patient's mood is distinctly different from normal but not associated with functional incapacitation in their usual social or occupational role. In a moderate depression, the patient has substantial difficulty in these usual roles but remains able to function. The severe category is when the patient is unable to function or is hospitalized—hospitalization is additionally indicated by a dark shading of the episode. In order to be conservative regarding episode counts, we have arbitrarily chosen to consider only moderate or severe depressive episodes as distinct and separate occurrences. In contrast, we have used any level of manic behaviour in the episode count, as bipolar patients tend to deny hypomanic symptoms in the first place and often underestimate their occurrence; often information from family members and others is required in order to chart hypomanic episodes accurately. When episodes have clearly occurred at some time in the past but the timing or duration cannot be precisely described, we have included these episodes in the life chart, but denote them with a broken line.

Treatments, including medications and psychotherapy, can be charted above the mood line in order better to elucidate acute and long-term responsiveness in relationship to single or multiple therapies and their dose adjustments. Psychosocial stressors and other important life events are charted below the mood line. Further examples of life charts and their elucidation of various phenomena in the assessment of the long-term course of affective illness and its response to pharmacotherapy are illustrated in a variety of figures in the section on long-term prophylaxis.

Assessment of Acute Antidepressant Response

Altshuler *et al.* (1991) have outlined a variety of observer and self-rated scales for the assessment of acute antidepressant response. The standard in the field has been the Hamilton Depression Rating Scale (Hamilton, 1960), which is particulary useful for assessment of behavioural and somatic features of depression. The scale was originally developed to be used as an index of severity in individuals already diagnosed as suffering from depression and is often used for severity of entry criteria to studies, with a minimum cut-off of 17 or 20 being utilized. The original scale involved 21 items, 17 of which were scored; 9 of the items are scored on a 5-point scale 0–4, and 8 on a 3-point scale 0–2, all reflecting the presence or absence of symptoms. The four unscored symptoms (diurnal variation, paranoia, obsessions–compulsions, and depersonalization) were not considered related to the severity of depression. Over the past several years, the scale has been modified to include additional items. A 24-item scale including three cognitive items—helplessness, hopelessness and worthlessness—has been developed but most raters still score

only the original 17 items (Hedlund and Vieweg, 1979). Rosenthal and Heffeman (1986) have adopted the scale and supplemented items to include more
atypical depressive symptoms such as those occurring in bipolar patients and
in those with seasonal affective disorders (SADs). These items include hypersomnia and hyperphagia and carbohydrate craving.

Because of the emphasis of the Hamilton Scale on vegetative symptoms
such as weight, appetite and sleep, it is not sensitive to changes on a daily
basis. Moreover, there is no self-rating scale that closely approximates the
observer-rated items. This difficulty is obviated with the Carroll rating scale
and with the recently developed Inventory for Depressive Symptomatology
developed by Rush and associates (1986). The utility of concurrently used
observer and subjective ratings of depression is emphasized for both the
clinician and the investigator. Many investigators have noted the marked
differences in temporal dimensions of clinical response, as well as marked
associations in subjective versus objective measures of clinical response
(Altshuler *et al.*, 1991; Murphy *et al.*, 1982). Particularly in bipolar patients,
nurses and physicians often notice considerable improvement before the
patient is able to observe these changes in mood, energy, appetite and sleep.
Subtle gradations in symptomatology may be missed altogether by the bipolar patient who may have a disorder of affective assessment as well as
affective expression (Rubinow and Post, 1992) (see Figure 3 in Altshuler *et
al.*, 1991).

The study of Cowdry and Gardner (1988) also emphasizes the qualitative
aspects of differential subjective and objective responses. In their double-
blind study of patients with borderline personality disorder, they demonstrated that the anticonvulsant carbamazepine had a marked effect on dyscontrol acts, with decreases in self-mutilatory and aggressive behaviour as
assessed by the physician. Physicians rated this improvement as a marked part
of the clinical response compared with placebo and markedly in contrast to
the anticonvulsant alprazolam (Xanax), which was associated with disinhibition and an increase in dyscontrol acts. However, in contrast to this notable
rating of clinical improvement in the objective dyscontrol domain, the patients subjectively did not feel a marked antidepressant response from this
agent and, in fact, rated the monoamine oxidase inhibitor tranylcypromine
(Parnate) as more efficacious on mood response. Thus, these data emphasize
not only the importance of dual collection of subjective and objective ratings,
but also of the assessment of a variety of sign and symptom domains with
appropriate rating scales in order to 'capture' different components of clinical
response that may be selectively associated with different pharmacological
manipulations.

We have recently become impressed with patients' reports of marked and
discrete mood fluctuations occurring with extreme rapidity, in a manner of
minutes to hours (Kramlinger and Post, 1988, 1993; George *et al.*, 1993).

Thus, utilizing subjective ratings in order to capture this phenomenon more systematically may be of critical importance in assessing the impact of psychopharmacological agents on what we have called ultra-ultra-rapid cycling or ultradian cycling, where discrete mood shifts occur at a rate faster than once every 24 hours. This kind of phenomenon emphasizes the importance of adapting the frequency of self- and observer-rated observations to the appropriate time domain. It had previously been considered that patients with 48-hour cycling represented the maximum frequency of oscillation in classical bipolar illness (Bunney and Hartmann, 1965; Gelenberg *et al.*, 1978). This underestimation of the frequency of cycling possible in a bipolar patient may have been due in part to utilization of measures no more frequent than once or twice every 24 hours, such as in the Bunney–Hamburg Rating Scale.

The importance of frequency of ratings and observations in different time domains is illustrated in Figure 2, where life charting can be presented in a rapid-cycling bipolar patient over a period of years (in the top line), over a period of days (utilizing systematic nursing assessments on a once or twice-daily basis), as well as in a matter of hours on the lower line (representing ultra-ultra-rapid or ultradian fluctuations in mood). In this latter instance, self-ratings every 2 hours were used to assess these ultradian fluctuations. Moreover, in this and other instances, we were able to verify these ultradian shifts in patients utilizing concurrent 2-hour nursing ratings as well (Kramlinger and Post, 1992). However, in most instances this frequency of nursing observation is impractical, and for patients and investigators who wish to track the faster frequencies we would suggest the use of visual analogue self-ratings once appropriate verification of scale utilization has been achieved in comparison with physician or nurse observations. It is perhaps worthy of note, even in a preliminary fashion, that we have observed that patients with these ultra-ultra-rapid or ultradian fluctuations in mood appear to require combination therapy in order to demonstrate complete clinical response. This often involves lithium in conjunction with carbamazepine (Kramlinger and Post, 1989a, 1989b), or lithium plus valproate (Calabrese and Delucchi, 1989). Clearly, much further work is required in order to elucidate whether ultradian patterns are associated with specific profiles of clinical response. Nonetheless, for this purpose, we wish to emphasize the importance of the systematization of these clinical observations so that appropriate associations to ultimate psychopharmacological response can, in fact, be ascertained.

As noted above, if one wishes to assess pharmacological response over rapid time domains, one may require different ratings from those typically utilized in once-weekly or once-monthly Hamilton Depression Ratings. For this purpose, we have found the Bunney–Hamburg Scale of considerable utility (Bunney and Hamburg, 1963). We have trained nursing staff to make

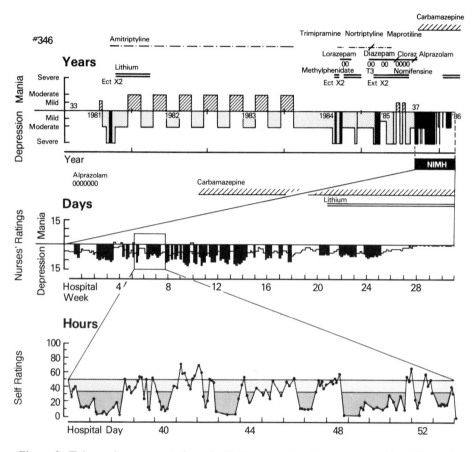

Figure 2. Telescopic representation of affective episodes: focus on monthly, daily and hourly durations

global judgements of depression, mania, anxiety, anger, psychosis and functional incapacity on the basis of twice-daily consensus of all nurses involved in each daily nursing shift (Post *et al.*, 1986b, 1987b). These kinds of data provide the ability to differentiate time courses of clinical antidepressant effects of different modalities. For example, as illustrated in Figure 3a, the response to sleep deprivation often occurs literally overnight and then is transient with relapse following the next day's sleep (Post *et al.*, 1987c). In contrast, response to electroconvulsive therapy (even though it is rapid in onset) often is associated with considerable lag to achievement of maximum degree of therapeutic response, in our series requiring approximately 2 weeks. In contrast, typical antidepressants appear to demonstrate their response (in responders) over even longer time domains, requiring up to 3 weeks in order to show maximum degree of clinical efficacy. We have observed this pattern with both the anti-convulsant carbamazepine as well as with lithium. This appears to be typical of traditional antidepressant modalities and helps explain the controversial nature of the time course of clinical antidepressant response, which is often described as occurring with a considerable lag. While some responsive patients may begin to demonstrate improvement in the first several weeks (Figure 3a and b), on the average, however, the time frame to maximum degree of antidepressant response appears to be considerably delayed, often requiring 3–4 weeks of treatment. Thus, in the current psychopharmacological era, where rapidity of onset of the antidepressant response is highly sought after by clinicians and the pharmaceutical industry alike, it is important to utilize instruments that can adequately assess this degree of rapidity of response. Daily observer- and self-ratings may be required in order to differentiate these time domains and, ultimately, relate differences in onset to different molecular actions of the antidepressant modalities (Post *et al.*, 1987c). In particular, Baxter *et al.* (1986) and Grube and Hartwich (1990) have demonstrated that acute antidepressant response to sleep deprivation can be achieved in one night and perhaps extended by concurrent lithium treatment. This provides a potential rationale for combining the acute treatment response to sleep deprivation with a longer-acting psychopharmacological agent. Daily ratings may be required in order to capture and verify this phenomenon.

In addition, we have observed that response to sleep deprivation can occur either in the early morning hours or in the late afternoon and show relapses (or not) after an afternoon nap or the full night's recovery sleep. In order to capture this phenomenon, obviously more frequent ratings are required, and we have utilized 2-hour self- and nurse-ratings for this purpose (Roy-Byrne *et al.*, 1984; Gerner *et al.*, 1979; Gill *et al.*, 1992). Gill *et al.* have, in addition, noted that the duration of antidepressant response to sleep deprivation may vary as a function of duration of depressive episodes, with minimal responses occurring early in an episode in bipolar patients, but more sustained and complete responses occurring in mid and late phases of depressive episodes, respectively. These data also emphasize the importance of frequent monitoring not only in order to assess the amplitude and duration of an acute response such as to that of sleep deprivation, but also to assess the dynamic phenomenological and neurobiological changes occurring within depressive episodes.

This caveat is also emphasized in the studies of Delgado and associates (1988, 1990, 1991), who studied acute perturbations in mood following acute depletion of plasma tryptophan. In patients who showed good clinical responses to antidepressant modalities, acute depletion of plasma tryptophan (associated with decreased brain serotoninergic function) was associated with acute exacerbations of mood. These severe depressive exacerbations were transient, however, and most of the patients returned to baseline with

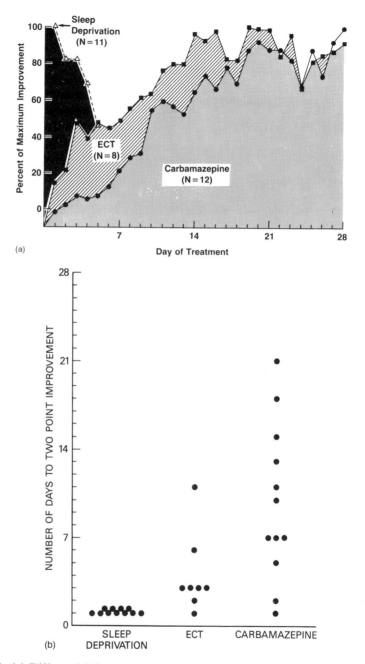

(a)

(b)

Figure 3. (a) Differential time course of therapeutic response in depression. (b) Differential onset of improvement in depression after sleep deprivation, ECT and carbamazepine

trytophan repletion by 12–24 hours later. These investigators have gone on to demonstrate that tryptophan depletion reverses the effects of serotoninergically active antidepressants but not those associated with primary effects on noradrenergic metabolism, such as that achieved with desipramine. This elegant series of studies documents the need for frequent ratings, in this case twice-daily, in order to document profound but transient changes in mood associated with psychopharmacological manipulations crucial for dissecting mechanistic bases of antidepressant actions.

Acute Antimanic Effects

As illustrated in Figure 4, the anticonvulsant carbamazepine can exert acute antimanic effects of time course similar to that achieved by the antipsychotic neuroleptics (thioridazine and chlorpromazine). In these instances, drugs were initiated on a double-blind basis, often in the context of a patient's emergent deterioration in an acute manic episode, often requiring seclusion. Within several days of institution of treatment with carbamazepine or

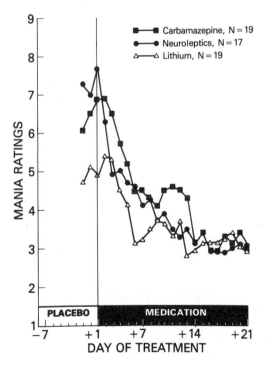

Figure 4. Time course of antimanic effects of carbamazepine compared to lithium and neuroleptics

neuroleptics, substantial improvement was observed, with highly significant effects occurring within the first week of treatment. These observations, paralleled by a variety of other investigators, have been documented utilizing blind global mania ratings on the Bunney–Hamburg Mania Scale (Post *et al.*, 1987b). The Beigel–Murphy Mania Scale (Beigel *et al.*, 1971), which divides symptoms into both frequency and intensity, is highly effective but also cumbersome and time consuming and has not been systematically utilized by many groups and has even been abandoned by the Murphy group itself. In contrast, the Young Mania Rating Scale (MRS) is easy to administer, sensitive to severity of manic symptoms, and has been found to reflect significant treatment differences (Young *et al.*, 1978). The Bech–Rafaelson Mania Rating Scale (BRMS) (Bech *et al.*, 1978) has also been reported to have adequate inter-observer reliability.

Recently, it has been documented that patients with dysphoric manias show inadequate responses acutely or in the long term to lithium carbonate (Post *et al.*, 1989; Prien *et al.*, 1988; Himmelhoch and Garfinkel, 1986; Secunda *et al.*, 1987). At the same time, it is apparent that some patients with dysphoric mania respond to the anticonvulsants carbamazepine (Post *et al.*, 1987b, 1989) or valproate (McElroy *et al.*, 1988, 1990; Calabrese and Delucchi, 1989, 1990; Freeman *et al.*, 1992). Thus, ratings of concurrent anxiety and depressive symptomatology in the context of the full-blown manic episode (Figure 5) become important in the assessment of ultimate relationship to pharmacological response, as well as potential elucidation of neurobiological substrates (Post *et al.*, 1989). In this latter instance, degree of dysphoric mania has been associated with increase in CSF noradrenaline (norepinephrine), a finding that has, in part, been replicated using markers of urinary noradrenergic function by Swann and associates (1991). These latter investigators also documented that patients with dysphoric mania showed increased incidence of cortisol hypersecretion, similar to that observed in patients with primary depressive disorders. Taken together, these observations highlight the importance of the assessment of combined symptomatology utilizing discrete rating assessments in order to characterize the continuum of dysphoria occurring in the manic syndrome or to devise subgroups, where appropriate, in order to assess psychopharmacological response and pathophysiological mechanisms.

Psychosensory Symptoms: Relationship to Anticonvulsant Response in Affective Illness?

One of the issues arising in the assessment of anticonvulsants in psychiatric patients is whether response is dependent on covert electrophysiological paroxysms (seizures) in what otherwise appear to be patients with primary affective disorders. A variety of approaches have been addressed to this issue, as discussed in detail elsewhere (Post, 1986; Post *et al.*, 1986a, 1991a, 1991c). One

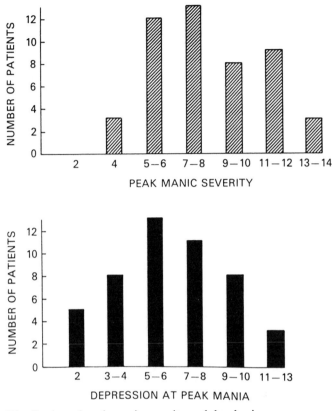

Figure 5. Distribution of peak manic severity and dysphoria

approach to this problem has been to ask patients with primary affective disorder whether they experience paroxysmal psychosensory and psychomotor phenomena typical of patients with complex partial seizures of the temporal lobe (psychomotor epilepsy) (Table 2). Silberman and associates (1985) developed a scale in order to systematically assess these transient distortions of sensation, experience and motor phenomena (Silberman–Post Psychosensory Rating Scale (SPPRS)). They found that patients with primary affective disorders did show a high incidence of these signs and symptoms, particularly in concurrence with their manic and depressive episodes and not in the well interval, but the occurrence of these phenomena was not selectively linked to those patients who responded to anticonvulsants. In fact, those with greater numbers of psychosensory symptoms appeared to show better responses to lithium carbonate. Figure 6 illustrates the lack of association of acute antidepressant or acute antimanic response and the number of psychosensory symptoms experienced (Ketter, Bierer and Post, unpublished observations). However, Hayes and Goldsmith (1991) have reported that patients who

Table 2. Transient sensory, cognitive and affective phenomena in affective illness. Frequency of symptoms in affectives, epileptics and controls

	Affective	Epileptic	Controls
	(%, $n = 44$)	(%, $n = 37$)	(%, $n = 30$)
Affectives > controls			
Speeded thoughts	68**	19	7
Slowed thoughts	50**	8	3
Sudden, intense, unexplained fear	25#	14	7
Sudden, intense, unexplained depression	23*	8	3
Formed visual hallucinations	20*	14	3
Sudden, intense, unexplained pleasurable sensations	16*	8	3
Autoscopic states	14*	5	0
Sudden, intense, unexplained sexual sensation	14*	5	0
Altered sound quality	11*	8	0
Affectives and epileptics > controls			
Illusions of significance	66**	27*	0
Jumbled thoughts	36**	65**	0
Altered sound intensity	27**	27**	0
Altered odour intensity	27**	11#	0
Formed auditory hallucinations	25*	16#	0
Altered colour intensity	20**	22**	0
Olfactory hallucinations	18*	22**	3
Derealization	18#	16*	3
Metamorphopsia	16#	19#	3
Altered distance	16*	14#	0
Epigastric hallucinations	11#	57**	0
Amnestic episodes	11#	73**	0
Epileptics > controls			
Motor automatisms	2	81**	0
Speech arrest	0	70**	0
Vestibular hallucinations	9	35**	3
Gustatory hallucinations	9	27**	3
Time disorientation	9	38**	0
Body part dissociations	7	19*	0
Tactile distortions	7	14*	0
Altered body size	9	11#	0
Perception of surroundings as bizarre			
Unformed auditory hallucinations	5	11#	0
No group differences			
Déjà vu	73	54	63
Altered light intensity	23	24	10
Unformed visual hallucinations	18	22	10
Altered odour quality	16	14	7
Depersonalization	14	19	10

Sudden, intense, unexplained rage	11	14	3
Sudden, intense, unexplained dysphoria (other than rage or depression)	9	8	3
Slowed time perception	7	5	0
Jamais vu	5	5	3
Speeded time perception	5	5	3

#Different from controls $p < 1$.
*Different from controls $p < 0.05$.
**Different from controls $p < 0.01$.

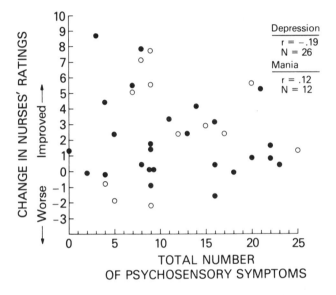

Figure 6. Psychosensory symptoms do not predict antidepressant (●) or antimanic (○) response to carbamazepine

respond to anticonvulsants (as opposed to lithium) in long-term prophylaxis appear to have greater numbers of self-assessed psychosensory symptoms.

Thus, it remains an open issue as to whether the occurrence of psychosensory symptoms relates selectively to disturbances of the temporal lobe and whether the occurrence of these phenomena is associated with differential response to the anticonvulsant agents versus the non-anticonvulsant mood stabilizer lithium in patients with primary affective disorder. In our patients with primary affective disorder, we have not found an increased incidence of abnormal or even borderline abnormal electroencephalograms (EEGs) and have so far not found evidence of 'hot spots' on positron emission tomography (PET) scans utilizing 17-fluorodeoxyglucose, which might be expected to occur during acute seizure activity. Rather, evidence of hypometabolism has been observed in either frontal areas (Baxter *et al.*, 1989) or temporal areas

(Post *et al.*, 1987a) in affectively ill patients, which is more consistent with the interictal hypometabolism observed in patients with complex partial seizures (Engel *et al.*, 1982; Theodore *et al.*, 1987). Indeed, patients with depressive symptoms secondary to epilepsy (Bromfield *et al.*, 1990, 1992), Parkinson's disease (Mayberg *et al.*, 1990a) or Huntington's disease (Mayberg *et al.*, 1990b) may also have decreased inferior frontal lobe metabolism compared to euthymic controls with the same neurological disorder. The relationship of psychosensory symptoms to regional alterations in EEG, cerebral glucose metabolism and blood flow achieved with discrete activation of temporal lobe structures with the local anaesthetic procaine (Kellner *et al.*, 1987; Ketter *et al.*, 1992, unpublished observations; Ryback and Gardner, 1991) remains to be further investigated.

However, we wish to note that the life chart process can be modified in order to deal with the relationship between seizures and bipolar affective disorder when the two do occur concomitantly. Thus, we suggest the utility of life-charting techniques in patients with primary seizure disorders who may have concurrent mood disturbances, which does appear to occur in a high proportion of patients (Altshuler, 1991; Robertson and Trimble, 1983). Another use of life charting is illustrated in Figure 7 in relationship to a differential diagnosis and sequential evolution of signs and symptoms associated with both an ictal and an affective process (Post *et al.*, 1991b). In this instance, seizure-like episodes occurred at an approximate rate of four times per year in 1979, with progressive acceleration in their frequency until they were occurring at an approximate frequency of once per month in 1987, and then at even faster frequencies in 1989. Four years following their onset, a full-blown affective psychosis occurred, with recurrence and cyclicity developing in 1987–1989. The life charting of this complicated case history demonstrates an acceleration in both the frequency of seizures and in affective episodes with their associated marked effect on social and occupational functioning. These affective episodes were inadequately responsive to lithium and neuroleptics, but both seizures and affective illness responded dramatically to institution of the anticonvulsant carbamazepine, as illustrated in 1989–1990. Thus, life charting may be important in sequencing the onset of two different medical phenomena and in the ultimate establishment of the primary or secondary nature of the affective disorder. Moreover, this kind of representation would be helpful in the elucidation of phenomena such as forced normalization which can be associated with psychosis exacerbation in the successfully treated seizure patient (Wolf, 1991; Landolt, 1953, 1958; Wolf and Trimble, 1985; Vaillancourt, 1988; Pakalnis *et al.*, 1987).

These very condensed and preliminary observations highlight the multiple associations of seizures and psychosis which can be either direct or inverse; the suggestion of an inverse relationship led to the initial utilization of electroconvulsive therapy for the treatment of psychosis and, in particular,

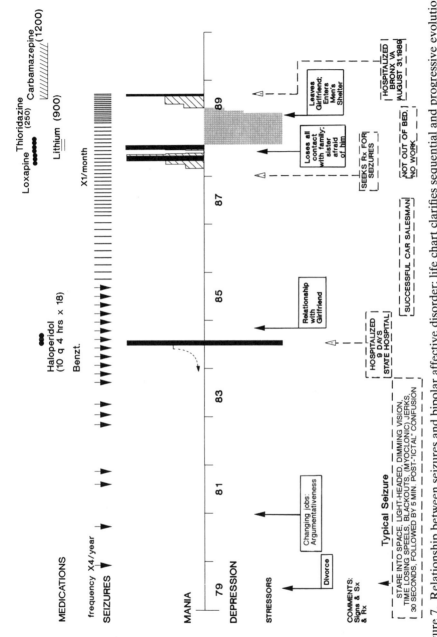

Figure 7. Relationship between seizures and bipolar affective disorder: life chart clarifies sequential and progressive evolution

depressive disorders. Recently, Hauser and associates (1989) and Ketter and associates (1992a) have observed marked exacerbation in affective symptomatology in patients undergoing anticonvulsant withdrawal; these observations can be captured both with life-chart methodology and with systematic assessment of psychiatric symptoms on Hamilton Depression, Young Mania, Zung Anxiety and Brief Psychiatric Rating Scales, as well as the mini-mental status or other quick bedside assessments for confusional elements and cognitive impairment in the context of seizure-induced exacerbation of behavioural and affective symptoms.

Long-term Assessment of Prophylactic Efficacy of the Anticonvulsants in the Affective Disorders

Greenhouse *et al.* (1991), Frank and Associates (1991), Kraemer *et al.* (1987), Gelenberg *et al.* (1992), Prien *et al.* (1991), Kraemer and Pruyn (1990) and Kraemer and Telch (1992) have emphasized methodological problems in the assessment, randomization and maintenance of patients in long-term prophylactic studies. Greenhouse *et al.* (1991) emphasize that following the achievement of acute responses through different pharmacological manipulations, a re-randomization to prophylaxis introduces a variety of methodological confounds that may not be easily mitigated by statistical analysis. Rather, they suggest several solutions to this problem, including continuing the patients into the prophylactic phase following acute stabilization with the same agent. In this fashion, various carry-over effects and other methodological problems related to the re-randomization may be obviated. Relatively few long-term systematic double-blind, controlled clinical trials utilizing the anticonvulsants in psychiatric patients have been conducted despite recent wide use of these agents. Prien and Gelenberg (1989) have highlighted a variety of methodological concerns involved in the prophylactic studies of carbamazepine versus lithium. They cite difficulties with small number of subjects, heterogeneous groups, adjunctive antidepressant and other medicines, and high drop-out rates, typified in the study of Placidi *et al.* (1986) and also clearly evident in the more recent study of Small *et al.* (1991).

Prien and Gelenberg (1989) do indicate that mirror image designs and systematic clinical trials in an on–off–on fashion can help in the assessment of the long-term efficacy of anticonvulsants such as carbamazepine, however. One such patient is illustrated in Figure 8, where repeated institution of treatment with carbamazepine was associated with marked improvement in mood, behaviour, and psychosis and amount of time in seclusion, and repeated placebo substitution was associated with deterioration in these indices. Moreover, as discussed in detail in the manuscript (Post *et al.*, 1984), this patient also demonstrates selective response among the anticonvulsant agents. This patient responded well to the anticonvulsant carbamazepine but not to phenytoin or valproate. We have observed other instances where patients have responded to valproate and not carbamazepine (see Figure 4 in Post *et al.*, 1984) and to combination therapy with valproate and carbamazepine (Ketter *et al.*, 1992b) and not monotherapy with either agent. Thus, the anticonvulsants cannot be considered as a unitary class in terms of psychotropic response, just as there appears to be selective response among the anticonvulsant agents within the epilepsies.

Figure 9 illustrates another pattern of response to the psychotropic effects of the anticonvulsants during long-term prophylaxis. This is an extension of the same patient graphed in Figure 2, with an emphasis on prospective follow-up using life-chart methodology. As illustrated in the middle portion of Figure 2, the patient showed an inadequate response to carbamazepine alone, but with lithium augmentation (when lithium had previously been ineffective with other agents) the patient showed a complete remission of symptoms. As illustrated in Figure 9, this essentially complete remission was sustained for approximately 3 years, punctuated by only minor and transient periods of depression. However, in 1989, episodes of depression began to emerge with increasing severity and duration, in spite of attempts at adjunctive treatment. Thus, this patient illustrates the phenomenon of the development of apparent tolerance to the psychotropic effects of the anticonvulsant carbamazepine. We have observed this pattern in approximately one-half the patients showing an initial good response to carbamazepine when followed for a period of 2–10 years (Post *et al.*, 1990).

Figure 10 illustrates an illness index in the two groups of patients, who appear to show either a sustained response (top) over periods as long as 10 years or some degree of escape from initial good response in the second or third year of treatment (Figure 10, bottom), i.e. a tolerance pattern as typified by the patient in Figure 9. The illness index is constructed using life-chart methodology and combines duration of time ill with the severity assessment, utilizing 0.25 for mild, 0.50 for moderate and 1.0 for severe. Thus, a score of 20 would represent 20 weeks of complete incapacitation or 40 weeks of moderately severe illness. When viewed in this fashion, it is apparent that a subgroup of patients do appear to demonstrate a pattern of emergence of tolerance to the psychotropic effects of carbamazepine when used either alone or in combination with lithium, while another group appears to show sustained and stable long-term prophylaxis. These data are presented in order to re-emphasize the utility of the life-chart approach for systematic prospective documentation of the degree and pattern of response of patients in long-term clinical trials.

This prospective life charting can be accomplished on the basis of weekly to monthly telephone interviews with the patient (Leverich *et al.*, 1990) or with more systematic utilization of patient's self-assessments of their mood fluctuations on a 100 mm line scale ranging from 0 (worst they have ever felt) to 50

230

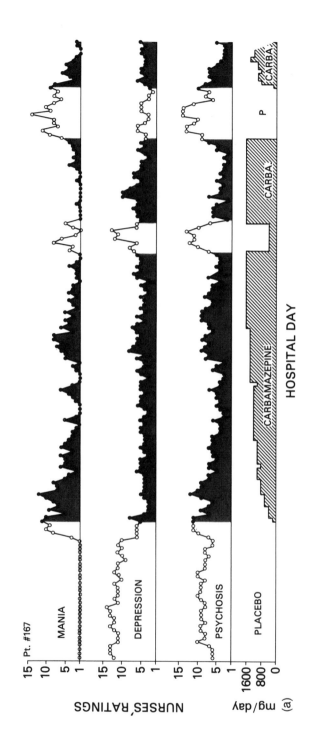

(euthymic or normal usual self) to 100 (most high ever). The clinician can then utilize these self-assessments in order to establish the degree of functional incapacitation accompanying the appropriate mood fluctuations and derive a systematic life chart (Denicoff *et al.*, 1992, unpublished observations). In this fashion, both numbers of episodes and severity can be assessed for pharmacological trials (Post *et al.*, 1990).

In addition, one can then utilize a variety of measures of loss of prophylactic efficacy in assessment of any drug response. These might include time to first mild, moderate or severe episode as well as time to the need for first medication supplementation or hospitalization. Thus, the prospective life charting for assessment of pharmacological response in prophylactic trials provides for flexibility in endpoint measures in the assessment of drug efficacy. In our study of the long-term effects of carbamazepine, we observed that the patients who showed the more rapid deterioration in the 4 years prior to starting the clinical trial with carbamazepine were the ones who showed the pattern of escape from carbamazepine prophylaxis or tolerance. This analysis emphasizes the utility of the life-chart approach in combining retrospective data with prospective data on clinical outcome.

While tolerance to the antinociceptive effects of carbamazepine has been well recognized in the neurological literature (Pazzaglia and Post, 1992), there is considerable controversy as to whether tolerance does or does not develop to the anticonvulsant effects of carbamazepine. Perhaps this is, in part, a function of how systematically a record of seizure occurrence is assessed in

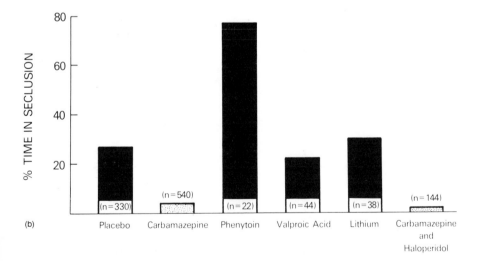

Figure 8. (a) (opposite) Antimanic effect of carbamazepine in a lithium-resistant manic-depressive patient. (b) (above) Carbamazepine decreases time required in seclusion in a manic-depressive patient

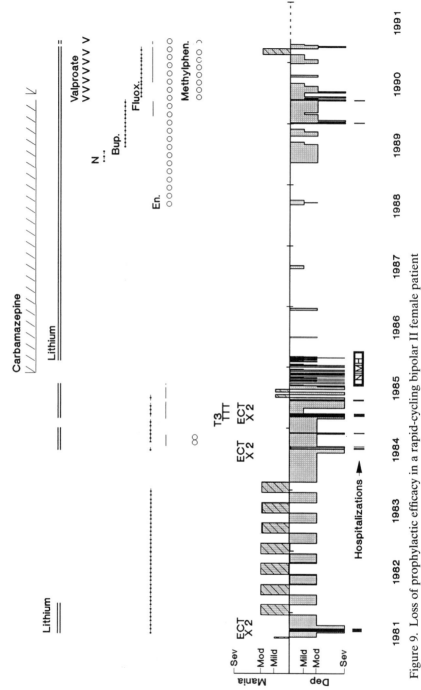

Figure 9. Loss of prophylactic efficacy in a rapid-cycling bipolar II female patient

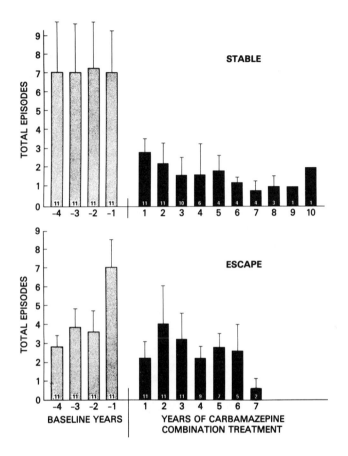

Figure 10. Persistence of carbamazepine prophylaxis: (episodes per year)

long-term clinical trials, as well as the duration of clinical trials. In the initial studies of lithium efficacy, complete responses were observed over relatively short periods of time. However, with longer time frames of observation, there appears to be a subgroup of patients who also demonstrate loss of prophylactic efficacy to lithium carbonate (Maj *et al.*, 1989). We would wonder whether the same phenomenon would not occur in the assessment of the anticonvulsant effects of carbamazepine in epileptic patients, in that some patients achieve refractoriness, not via the route of initial non-responsiveness, but due to the fact that they develop loss of efficacy or tolerance. The clinician and investigator are faced with clinical decisions as to how best to treat this patient subsequently in the face of this loss of efficacy. Systematic pharmacological

234

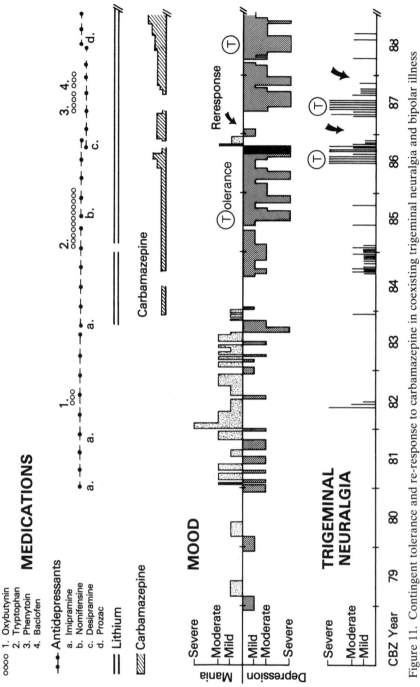

Figure 11. Contingent tolerance and re-response to carbamazepine in coexisting trigeminal neuralgia and bipolar illness

trials have not been conducted in order to ascertain the best treatment procedure. Nonetheless, preclinical data suggest the possibility that tolerance development to carbamazepine may be of the conditioned or contingent variety and, following a period of drug discontinuation, the patient may re-respond to the same agent (Pazzaglia and Post, 1992). Such a patient showing an apparent re-response is illustrated in Figure 11, based on retrospective assessment of mood and pain symptoms in a patient with concurrent bipolar illness and trigeminal neuralgia. In this instance, periods of drug discontinuation once the patient became refractory appeared to be associated with renewed response, at least for a short period of time. Again, these data illustrate the utility of retrospective and prospective life charting in the long-term assessment of drug efficacy and patterns of response, including loss of efficacy over time, and in elucidating potential strategies that require more systematic assessment in controlled clinical trials.

In contrast to the utility of a period of drug discontinuation in a patient who has lost responsiveness, we would emphasize that the opposite can occur in a patient who is discontinued in the face of successful long-term prophylaxis. As illustrated in Figure 12, a patient with an excellent acute response to lithium continued well for 1½ years until she discontinued lithium in 1980. This was associated with a rapid relapse into a manic and depressive episode and, with the reinstitution of lithium, the patient remained well for the next 6½ years. In this instance, it was suggested that she no longer needed lithium treatment and she tapered her dose. This was followed by the rapid re-emergence of symptoms and, despite reinstitution of lithium at previously effective doses (and then at higher and even toxic dose with adjunctive supplementation with the anticonvulsant carbamazepine), the patient showed no evidence of response. We have observed this phenomenon in a small series of patients and have noted that other investigators have observed the same phenomenon as well, which we have labelled discontinuation-induced refractoriness (Post, 1990; Post *et al.*, 1992). Thus, it would appear that termination of successful treatment may, in some instances, lead to the development of refractoriness. This appears to contrast with discontinuation of an agent that has already lost effectiveness (Figure 11), which may be associated with a re-response. We present these case vignettes in order to re-emphasize the utility of the life-charting perspective in elucidating these differential patterns, in order both to warn clinicians about the potential liabilities of drug discontinuation, and to raise issues for further pharmacological trials as to new treatment interventions that might be helpful in these instances of loss of treatment response.

The potential clinical impact of systematic prospective life charting of the course of illness is further illustrated in Figure 13. In this instance, the patient was clearly a well-documented non-responder to lithium as revealed by life charting. He experienced repeated hospitalizations despite adequate lithium

236

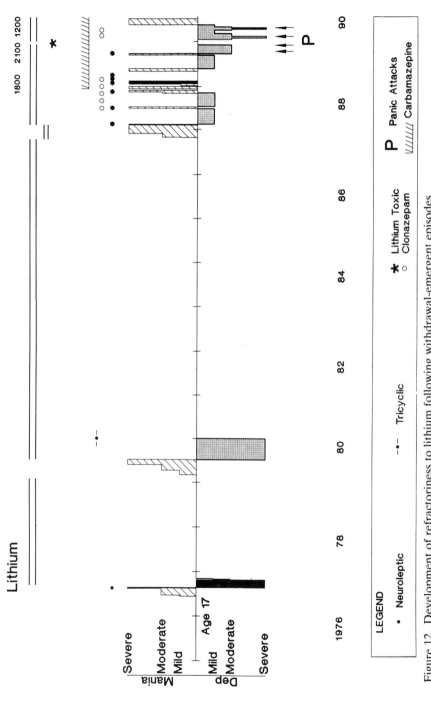

Figure 12. Development of refractoriness to lithium following withdrawal-emergent episodes

237

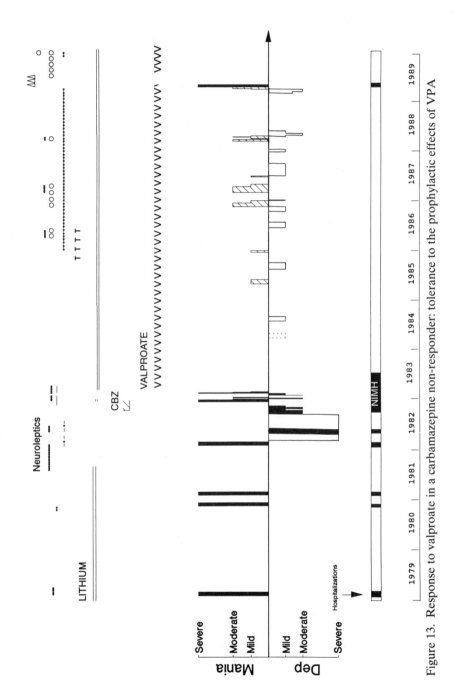

Figure 13. Response to valproate in a carbamazepine non-responder: tolerance to the prophylactic effects of VPA

levels. It is noteworthy that the patient also suffered from extremely dysphoric mania, with high levels of depression, anxiety, and even panic attacks occurring in the course of his manic episodes. Upon the emergence of a manic episode in the context of his National Institute of Mental Health (NIMH) hospitalization, the patient was treated with carbamazepine and then lithium adjunctively. He did not respond adequately to this combination so valproate supplementation was substituted, which achieved a remarkable antimanic effect. The patient showed a sustained long-term prophylactic response to valproate and lithium, whereas lithium alone or adjunctively with other agents had previously been ineffective. This patient again illustrates the principle that non-response to one anticonvulsant agent does not predetermine response or non-response to another with a potentially different mechanism of action (Post *et al.*, 1984; Post, 1990). The point to be emphasized in this patient's life chart, however, is that when he subsequently developed a breakthrough episode in 1989 and required a brief rehospitalization in another institution, the prescribed discharge regimen was lithium and the anticonvulsant valproate was discontinued. Upon mailing a copy of this patient's life chart to the new treating physician, the wisdom of this return to a previously ineffective treatment was reassessed and adjunctive valproate was re-administered, with resumption of a good response.

We believe this case, illustrated in Figure 13, dramatically demonstrates the clinical as well as research utility of systematic assessment of retrospective and prospective course of illness in arriving at appropriate decisions for successful pharmacotherapy. Bipolar illness is virtually always recurrent and an illness that deserves systematic, long-term assessment, potentially for the duration of the patient's lifetime. More systematic and precise methodologies need to be developed than those currently routinely employed in order to assess the outcome in bipolar illness and its response to treatment more effectively and uniformly.

Recently, we have been impressed with the degree of morbidity that occurs in patients who are even classed as good responders in most conventional psychopharmacological studies. The prospective life-chart methodology reveals that many patients have long periods of sustained mild or moderate episode and symptom occurrence despite otherwise achieving a good response measured by the criterion of lack of a full-blown relapse requiring hospitalization (Denicoff *et al.*, unpublished, 1992). As the psychopharmacology of affective disorders becomes increasingly complex and sophisticated, we urge that the assessment tools keep pace with this process so that drug therapies can be optimized and maximally titrated against side-effects profiles.

We are currently engaged in the computerization of life-chart methodology which would facilitate the process of conversion to quantitative data sets readily subject to data and statistical analysis (Leverich and Post, 1993). Moreover, utilizing this technology, one is able to define phases of patients' illness according to the pattern of recurrence. George *et al.* (1993) have emphasized the utility of modelling the course of affective illness with mathematical equations derived from chaos theory. These models suggest that variations in a single parameter could account for the progression of affective illness from isolated intermittent episodes to more continuous cycling and, finally, to ultra-ultra-rapid cycling with its apparently chaotic oscillations.

Conclusions

In this chapter we hope to have illustrated a variety of techniques for the acute and long-term assessment of manic and depressive episodes in patients with bipolar illness, and their potential response to anticonvulsant and other psychotropic modalities. We have emphasized the critical importance of the time domains of clinical response and the frequency and intensity of clinical observations necessary for appropriate assessment of pharmacological response, both acutely and prophylactically.

The recurrent nature of the affective disorders presents unique problems and opportunities in the treatment and assessment of the disorder. Life-charting methodologies need to be updated and improved so that adequate representation of the course of affective disorders can be systematically gleaned within and across clinical and research investigations. This is all the more critical in light of the dearth of studies on long-term prophylaxis in the bipolar disorders. The life-chart methodology and its improved derivatives offer the clinician the ability to become a clinical investigator in the exploration of clinical pharmacological responsivity in each individual patient, using that patient as their own control. These techniques can further be utilized in the assessment of the impact and efficacy of psychological as well as pharmacological interventions in bipolar patients.

In this fashion, it is hoped that uncontrolled observations well documented with appropriate rating systems can provide the groundwork for more controlled, randomized series in larger patient populations. These, in turn, might provide the groundwork for the most highly controlled randomized, double-blind clinical designs with the newly introduced anticonvulsants (Post, 1990), as well as with a series of new treatment options which should be forthcoming based on the rapid advances in the basic and clinical neurosciences. Systematic assessment of the life course of bipolar illness should enable each patient not only to achieve a more optimal treatment outcome but, in this fashion, contribute to the accumulation of knowledge for the better treatment of this potentially lethal and disabling medical disorder.

R. M. Post et al.

References

Altshuler, L.L. (1991). Depression and epilepsy. In: Theodore, W.H., and Devinsky, O. (eds), *Epilepsy and Behavior*, New York: Wiley–Liss, pp. 47–65.

Altshuler, L.L., Post, R.M., and Fedio, P. (1991). Assessment of affective variables in clinical trials. In: Mohr, E., and Brouwers, P. (eds), *Handbook of Clinical Trials*, Amsterdam: Swets & Zeitlinger, pp. 141–64.

Baxter, L.R., Jr, Liston, E.H., Schwartz, J.M., Altshuler, L.L., Wilkins, J.N., Richeimer, S., and Guze, B.H. (1986). Prolongation of the antidepressant response to partial sleep deprivation by lithium. *Psychiatry Res., 19*, 17–23.

Baxter, L.R., Jr, Schwartz, J.M., Phelps, M.E., Mazziotta, J.C., Guze, B.H., Selin, C.E., Gerner, R.H., and Sumida, R.M. (1989). Reduction of prefrontal cortex glucose metabolism common to three types of depression. *Arch. Gen. Psychiatry, 46*, 243–50.

Bech, P., Rafaelsen, O.J., Kramp, P., and Bolwig, T.G. (1978). The mania rating scale: Scale construction and inter-observer agreement. *Neuropharmacology, 17*, 430–1.

Beigel, A., Murphy, D., and Bunney, W. (1971). The manic state rating scale: Scale construct, reliability, and validity. *Arch. Gen. Psychiatry, 25*, 256–62.

Bromfield, E.B., Altshuler, L., Leiderman, D.B., Balish, M., Ketter, T.A., Devinsky, O., Post, R.M., and Theodore, W.H. (1990). Cerebral metabolism and depression in patients with complex partial seizures. *Epilepsia, 31*, 625–6.

Bromfield, E.B., Altshuler, L., Leiderman, D.B., Balish, M., Ketter, T.A., Devinsky, O., Post, R.M., and Theodore, W.H. (1992). Cerebral metabolism and depression in patients with complex partial seizures. *Arch. Neurol., 49*, 617–623.

Bunney, W.E., Jr, and Hamburg, D.A. (1963). Methods for reliable longitudinal observation of behavior. *Arch. Gen. Psychiatry, 9*, 280–94.

Bunney, W.E., Jr, and Hartmann, E.L. (1965). Study of a patient with 48-hour manic-depressive cycles. Part I. *Arch. Gen. Psychiatry, 12*, 611–18.

Calabrese, J.R., and Delucchi, G.A. (1989). Phenomenology of rapid cycling manic depression and its treatment with valproate. *J. Clin. Psychiatry, 50*, 30–4.

Calabrese, J.R., and Delucchi, G.A. (1990). Spectrum of efficacy of valproate in 55 patients with rapid-cycling bipolar disorder. *Am. J. Psychiatry, 147*, 431–4.

Cowdry, R.W., and Gardner, D.L. (1988). Pharmacotherapy of borderline personality disorder. *Arch. Gen. Psychiatry, 111*, 111–19.

Delgado, P. (1991). Serotonin depletion studies in affective disorders. Presentation, *Yale Symposium on Neurobiology of Affective Disorders*.

Delgado, P.L., Goodman, W.K., Price, L.H., Landis, H., and Aghajanian, G.K. (1988). Behavioral effects of acute tryptophan-depletion in depressed and obsessive compulsive disorder (OCD) patients. *ACNP Abstracts*, 184.

Delgado, P.L., Charney, D.S., Price, L.H., Aghajanian, G.K., Landis, H., and Heninger, G.R. (1990). Serotonin function and the mechanism of antidepressant action: Reversal of antidepressant-induced remission by rapid depletion of plasma tryptophan. *Arch. Gen. Psychiatry, 47*, 411–18.

Endicott, J., and Spitzer, R.L. (1978). A diagnostic interview: The schedule for affective disorders and schizophrenia. *Arch. Gen. Psychiatry, 35*, 837–44.

Engel, J., Jr, Kuhl, D.E., and Phelps, M.E. (1982). Patterns of human local cerebral glucose metabolism during epileptic seizures. *Science, 218*, 64–6.

Frank, E., Prien, R.J., Jarrett, R.B., Keller, M.B., Kupfer, D.J., Lavori, P.W., Rush, A.J., and Weissman, M.M. (1991). Conceptualization and rationale for consensus definitions of terms in major depressive disorder: Remission, recovery, relapse, and recurrence. *Arch. Gen. Psychiatry, 48*, 851–5.

Freeman, T.W., Clothier, J.L., Pazzaglia, P., Lesem, M.D., and Swann, A.C. (1992). A double-blind comparison of valproate and lithium in the treatment of acute mania. *Am. J. Psychiatry,* **149**, 108–11.

Gelenberg, A.J., Klerman, G.L., Hartmann, E.L., and Salt, P. (1978). Recurrent unipolar depressions with a 48-hour cycle: Report of a case. *Br. J. Psychiatry,* **133**, 123–9.

Gelenberg, A.J., Kane, J.M., Keller, M.B., Lavori, P., Rosenbaum, J.F., Cole, K., and Lavelle, J. (1989). Comparison of standard and low serum levels of lithium for maintenance treatment of bipolar disorder. *N. Engl. J. Med.,* **321**, 1489–93.

Gelenberg, A.J., Prien, R.F., Keller, M.B., Frank, E., and Post, R.M. (1992). Bipolar disorder. In: Robinson, D., and Prien, R. (eds), *Clinical Evaluation of Psychotropic Drugs: Principles and Guidance,* New York: Raven Press, in press.

George, M.S., Jones, M., Post, R.M., Putnam, F., Mikalauskas, K., and Leverich, G. (1993). The longitudinal course of affective illness: mathematical models involving chaos theory. *J. Psychiatr. Res.,* submitted.

Gerner, R.H., Post, R.M., and Gillin, J.C. (1979). Biological and behavioral effects of one night's sleep deprivation in depressed patients and normals. *J. Psychiatr. Res.,* **15**, 21–40.

Gill, D.S., Ketter, T.A., and Post, R.M. (1993). Increasing antidepressant response to sleep deprivation as a function of time into depressive episode in bipolar patients. *Acta Psychiatr. Scand.,* in press.

Greenhouse, J.B., Stangl, D., Kupfer, D.J., and Prien, R.F. (1991): Methodologic issues in maintenance therapy clinical trials. *Arch. Gen. Psychiatry,* **48**, 313–18.

Grube, M., and Hartwich, P. (1990). Maintenance of antidepressant effect of sleep deprivation with the help of lithium. *Eur. Arch. Psychiatry Neurol. Sci.,* **240**, 60–1.

Hamilton, M. (1960). A rating scale for depression. *J. Neurol. Neurosurg. Psychiatry,* **12**, 56–62.

Hauser, P., Devinsky, O., De Bellis, M., Theodore, W.H., and Post, R.M. (1989). Benzodiazepine withdrawal delirium with catatonic features: Occurrence in patients with partial seizure disorders. *Arch. Neurol.,* **46**, 696–9.

Hayes, S.G., and Goldsmith, B.K. (1991). Psychosensory symptomatology in anticonvulsant-responsive psychiatric illness. *Ann. Clin. Psychiatry,* **3**, 27–35.

Hedlund, J., and Vieweg, B. (1979). The Hamilton Rating Scale for Depression: A comprehensive review. *J. Operational Psychiatry,* **10**, 149–62.

Himmelhoch, J.M., and Garfinkel, M.E. (1986). Sources of lithium resistance in mixed mania. *Psychopharmacol. Bull.,* **22**, 613–20.

Kellner, C.H., Post, R.M., Putnam, F., Cowdry, R.W., Gardner, D., Kling, M.A., Minichiello, M.D., Trettau, J.R., and Coppola, R. (1987). Intravenous procaine as a probe of limbic system activity in psychiatric patients and normal controls. *Biol. Psychiatry,* **22**, 1107–26.

Ketter, T.A., Malow, B.A., White, S.R., Post, R.M., and Theodore, W.H. (1992a). Anticonvulsant withdrawal-emergent psychopathology. *Am. Acad. Neurol.,* Abstract.

Ketter, T.A., Pazzaglia, P.J., and Post, R.M. (1992b). Synergy of carbamazepine and valproic acid in affective illness: Case report and review of literature. *J. Clin. Psychopharmacol.,* **12**, 276–281.

Kraemer, H.C., Pruyn, J.P. (1990). The evaluation of different approaches to randomized clinical trials: Report on the 1987 MacArthur Foundation Network I Methodology Workshop. *Arch. Gen. Psychiatry,* **47**, 1163–9.

Kraemer, H.C., and Telch, C.R. (1992). Selection and utilization of outcome measures in psychiatric clinical trials: Report on the 1988 MacArthur Foundation Network I Methodology Institute. *Neuropsychopharmacology,* **7**, 85–94.

Kraemer, H.C., Pruyn, J.P., Gibbons, R.D., Greenhouse, J.B., Grochocinski, V.J., Waternaux, C., and Kupfer, D.J. (1987). Methodology in psychiatric research: Report on the 1986 MacArthur Foundation Network I Methodology Institute. *Arch. Gen. Psychiatry,* **44**, 1100–6.

Kramlinger, K.G., and Post, R.M. (1988). Ultra-rapid cycling bipolar affective disorder. Presented at the Annual Meeting of the Psychiatric Research Society, Park City, Utah, March 10–12.

Kramlinger, K.G., Post, R.M. (1989a). The addition of lithium carbonate to carbamazepine: Antidepressant efficacy in treatment-resistant depression. *Arch. Gen. Psychiatry,* **46**, 794–800.

Kramlinger, K.G., and Post, R.M. (1989b) Adding lithium carbonate to carbamazepine: Antimanic efficacy in treatment-resistant mania. *Acta Psychiatr. Scand.,* **79**, 378–85.

Kramlinger, K.G., and Post, R.M. (1993). Ultra-rapid and ultradian cycling in bipolar affective illness. *Arch. Gen. Psychiatry,* in press.

Landolt, H. (1953). Some clinical electroencephalographical correlations in epileptic psychoses (twilight states). *Electroencephalogr. Clin. Neurophysiol.,* **5**, 121.

Landolt, H. (1958). Serial EEG investigation during psychotic episodes in epileptic patients and during schizophrenic attacks. In: de Mass, L. (eds), *Lectures on Epilepsy,* Amsterdam: Elsevier, pp. 91–133.

Leverich, G.S., and Post, R.M. (1992). The National Institute of Mental Health Life Charting Method and Manual. Unpublished monograph.

Leverich, G.S., Post, R.M., and Rosoff, A.S. (1990). Factors associated with relapse during maintenance treatment of affective disorders. *Int. Clin. Psychopharmacol.,* **5**, 135–56.

Maj, M., Pirozzi, R., and Kemali, D. (1989). Long-term outcome of lithium prophylaxis in patients initially classified as complete responders. *Psychopharmacology (Berlin),* **98**, 535–8.

Mayberg, H.S., Starkstein, S.E., Peyser, C.E., Folstein, S.E., Dannals, R.F., Folstein, M.F., and Wagner, H.N., Jr (1990a). Cerebral glucose utilization in Huntington's disease: Inferior frontal hypometabolism identifies patients with major depression. *Soc. Neurosci. Abstracts,* **16**, 139.

Mayberg, H.S., Starkstein, S.E., Sadzot, B., Preziosi, T., Andrezejewski, P.L., Dannals, R.F., Wagner, H.N., Jr, and Robinson, R.G. (1990b). Selective hypometabolism in the inferior frontal lobe in depressed patients with Parkinson's disease. *Ann. Neurol.,* **28**, 57–64.

McElroy, S.L., Keck, P.E., Jr, Pope, H.G., Jr, and Hudson, J.I. (1988). Valproate in the treatment of rapid-cycling bipolar disorder. *J. Clin. Psychopharmacol.,* **8**, 275–9.

McElroy, S.L., Pope, H.G., Jr, Keck, P.E., Jr and Hudson, J.I. (1990). A placebo-controlled study of valproate in mania. *Abstracts of the 143rd Annual Meeting of the American Psychiatric Association,* p. 167, Abs. #NR312.

Murphy, D.L., Pickar, D., and Alterman, I.S. (1982). Methods for the quantitative assessment of depressive and manic behavior. In: Burdock, E.I., Sudilovsky, A., and Gershon, S. (eds), *The Behavior of Psychiatric Patients: Quantitative Techniques for Evaluation,* New York: Marcel Dekker, pp. 355–92.

O'Connell, R.A., Mayo, J.A., Flatow, L., Cuthbertson, B., and O'Brien, B.E. (1991). Outcome of bipolar disorder on long-term treatment with lithium. *Br. J. Psychiatry,* **159**, 123–9.

Pakalnis, A., Drake, M.E., Kuruvilla, J., and Kellum, J.B. (1987). Forced normalization: Acute psychosis after seizure control in seven patients. *Arch. Neurol.,* **44**, 289–92.

Pazzaglia, P.J., and Post, R.M. (1992). Contingent tolerance and re-response to carbamazepine: A case study in a patient with trigeminal neuralgia and bipolar disorder. *J. Neuropsychiatry Clin. Neurosci.*, **41**, 76–81.

Placidi, G.F., Lenzi, A., Lazzerini, F., Cassano, G.B., and Akiskal, H.S. (1986). The comparative efficacy and safety of carbamazepine versus lithium: A randomized, double-blind 3-year trial in 83 patients. *J. Clin. Psychiatry*, **47**, 490–4.

Post, R.M. (1986). Does limbic system dysfunction play a role in affective illness? In: Doane, B.K., and Livingston, K.E. (eds), *The Limbic System: Functional Organization and Clinical Disorders*, New York: Raven Press, pp. 229–49.

Post, R.M. (1990). Prophylaxis of bipolar affective disorders. *Int. Rev. Psychiatry*, **2**, 277–320.

Post, R.M. (1992). The transduction of psychosocial stress into the neurobiology of recurrent affective disorder. *Am. J. Psychiatry*, **149**, 999–1010.

Post, R.M., Berrettini, W.H., Uhde, T.W., and Kellner, C.H. (1984). Selective response to the anticonvulsant carbamazepine in manic-depressive illness: A case study. *J. Clin. Psychopharamcol.*, **4**, 178–85.

Post, R.M., Uhde, T.W., Joffe, R.T., and Bierer, L. (1986a). Psychiatric manifestations and implications of seizure disorders. In: Extein, I., and Gold, M. (eds), *Medical Mimics of Psychiatric Disorders*, Washington, DC: American Psychiatric Association Press, pp. 35–91.

Post, R.M., Uhde, T.W., Roy-Byrne, P.P., and Joffe, R.T. (1986b). Antidepressant effects of carbamazepine. *Am. J. Psychiatry*, **143**, 29–34.

Post, R.M., Delisi, L.E., Holcomb, H.H., Uhde, T.W., Cohen, R., and Buchsbaum, M.S. (1987a). Glucose utilization in the temporal cortex of affectively ill patients: Positron emission tomography. *Biol. Psychiatry*, **22**, 46–54.

Post, R.M., Uhde, T.W., Roy-Byrne, P.P., and Joffe, R.T. (1987b). Correlates of antimanic response to carbamazepine. *Psychiatry Res.*, **21**, 71–83.

Post, R.M., Uhde, T.W., Rubinow, D.R., and Huggins, T. (1987c). Differential time course of antidepressant effects following sleep deprivation, ECT, and carbamazepine: Clinical and theoretical implications. *Psychiatry Res.*, **22**, 11–19.

Post, R.M., Roy-Byrne, P.P., and Uhde, T.W. (1988). Graphic representation of the life course of illness in patients with affective disorder. *Am. J. Psychiatry*, **145**, 844–8.

Post, R.M., Rubinow, D.R., Uhde, T.W., Roy-Byrne, P.P., Linnoila, M., Rosoff, A., and Cowdry, R.W. (1989). Dysphoric mania: Clinical and biological correlates. *Arch. Gen. Psychiatry*, **46**, 353–8.

Post, R.M., Leverich, G.S., Rosoff, A.S. and Altshuler, L.L. (1990). Carbamazepine prophylaxis in refractory affective disorders: a focus on long-term followup. *J. Clin. Psychopharmacol.*, **10**, 318–27.

Post, R.M., Altshuler, L.L., Ketter, T.A., Denicoff, K., and Weiss, S.R.B. (1991a) . Antiepileptic drugs in affective illness: Clinical and theoretical implications. In: Smith, D.B., Treiman, D.M., and Trimble, M.R. (eds), *Advances in Neurology, Vol. 55, Neurobehavioral Problems in Epilepsy*, New York: Raven Press, pp. 239–77.

Post, R.M., Kahn, R.S., and Findling, R.N. (1991b). Interfaces between seizures and affective disorders: Evolution and longitudinal course. *Mt Sinai J. Med.*, **58**, 310–323.

Post, R.M., Weiss, S.R.B., Clark, M., Nakajima, T., and Ketter, T.A. (1991c). Seizures as an evolving process: Implications for neuropsychiatric illness. In: Theodore, W.H., and Devinsky, O. (eds), *Epilepsy and Behavior*, New York: Wiley–Liss, pp. 361–87.

Post, R.M., Leverich, G.S., Altshuler, L.L., and Mikalauskas, K. (1992). Lithium discontinuation-induced refractoriness: Preliminary observations. *Am. J. Psychiatry*, **149**, 1727–1729.

Prien, R.F., and Gelenberg, A.J. (1989). Alternatives to lithium for preventive treatment of bipolar disorder. *Am. J. Psychiatry,* **146**, 840–8.

Prien, R.F., Himmelhoch, J.M., and Kupfer, D.J. (1988). Treatment of mixed mania. *J. Affective Disord.,* **15**, 9–15.

Prien, R.F., Carpenter, L.L., and Kupfer, D.J. (1991). The definition and operational criteria for treatment outcome of major depressive disorder: A review of the current research literature. *Arch. Gen. Psychiatry,* **48**, 796–800.

Robertson, M.M., and Trimble, M.R. (1983). Depressive illness in patients with epilepsy: A review. *Epilepsia,* **24**, S109–S116.

Robins, L.N., Helzer, J.E., Croughan, J., and Ratcliff, K.S. (1981). National Institute of Mental Health Diagnostic Interview Schedule: Its history, characteristics, and validity. *Arch. Gen. Psychiatry,* **38**, 381–9.

Rosenthal, N.E., and Heffeman, M.M. (1986). Bulimia, carbohydrate craving and depression: A central connection? In: Wurtman, R.J., and Wurtman, J.J. (eds), *Nutrition and the Brain,* Vol. 6, New York: Raven Press, pp. 139–66.

Roy-Byrne, P.P., Uhde, T.W., and Post, R.M. (1984). Antidepressant effects of one night's sleep deprivation: Clinical and theoretical implications. In: Post, R.M., and Ballenger, J.C. (eds), *Neurobiology of Mood Disorders,* Baltimore: Williams & Wilkins, pp. 817–35.

Roy-Byrne, P.P., Post, R.M., Uhde, T.W., Porcu, T., and Davis, D.D. (1985). The longitudinal course of recurrent affective illness: Life chart data from research patients at NIMH. *Acta Psychiatr. Scand. Suppl.,* **71**, 5–34.

Rubinow, D.R., and Post, R.M. (1992). Impaired recognition of affect in facial expression in depressed patients. *Biol. Psychiatry,* **31**, 947–953.

Rush, A.J., Giles, D.E., Schlesser, M.A., Fulton, C.L., Weissenburger, J., and Burns, C.A. (1986). The inventory for depressive symptomatology (IDS): Preliminary findings. *Psychiatry Res.,* **18**, 65–87.

Ryback, R.S., and Gardner, E.A. (1991). Limbic system dysrhythmia: A diagnostic electroencephalogram procedure utilizing procaine activation. *J. Neuropsychiatry Clin. Neurosci.,* **3**, 321–9.

Secunda, S.K., Swann, A., Katz, M.M., Koslow, S.H., Croughan, J., and Chang, S. (1987). Diagnosis and treatment of mixed mania. *Am. J. Psychiatry,* **144**, 96–8.

Silberman, E.K., Post, R.M., Nurnberger, J., Theodore, W., and Boulenger, J.-P. (1985). Transient sensory, cognitive, and affective phenomena in affective illness: A comparison with complex partial epilepsy. *Br. J. Psychiatry,* **146**, 81–9.

Small, J.G., Klapper, M.H., Milstein, V., Kellams, J.J., Miller, M.J., Marhenke, J.D., and Small, I.F. (1991). Carbamazepine compared with lithium in the treatment of mania. *Arch. Gen. Psychiatry,* **48**, 915–21.

Spitzer, R.L., Williams, J.B.W., Gibbon, M. and First, M.B. (1988). *Structural Clinical Interview for DSM-III-R,* New York: NY State Psychiatric Institute.

Squillace, K., Post, R.M., Savard, R., and Erwin, M. (1984). Life charting of the longitudinal course of recurrent affective illness. In: Post, R.M., and Ballenger, J.C. (eds), *Neurobiology of Mood Disorders,* Baltimore: Williams & Wilkins, pp. 38–59.

Swann, A.C., Secunda, S.K., Katz, M.M., Maas, J.W., and Croughan, J. (1991). Syndromal specificity of mixed manic states. *Abstracts, ACNP NA,* 122.

Theodore, W.H., Fishbein, D., Deitz, M., and Baldwin, P. (1987). Complex partial seizures: Cerebellar metabolism. *Epilepsia,* **28**, 319–23.

Vaillancourt, P.D. (1988). Forced normalization [letter]. *Arch. Neurol.,* **45**, 138.

Wolf, P. (1991). Acute behavioral symptomatology at disappearance of epileptiform EEG abnormality: Paradoxical or 'forced' normalization. In: Smith, D.B., Treiman,

D.M., and Trimble, M.R. (eds), *Advances in Neurology, Vol. 55, Neurobehavioral Problems in Epilepsy,* New York: Raven Press, pp. 127–42.

Wolf, P. and Trimble, M.R. (1985). Biological antagonism and epileptic psychosis. *Br. J. Psychiatry,* **146**, 272–6.

Young, R.C., Biggs, J.T., Ziegler, V.E., and Meyer, D.A. (1978). A rating scale for mania: Reliability, validity and sensitivity. *Br. J. Psychiatry,* **133**, 429–35.

Index

Index compiled by Liza Weinkove